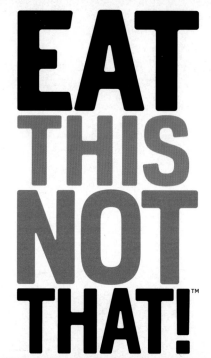

EAT THIS NOT THAT!™

SUPERMARKET SURVIVAL GUIDE

The No-Diet Weight Loss Solution

BY DAVID ZINCZENKO
WITH MATT GOULDING

RODALE

P9-DNP-373

PRAISE FOR *EAT THIS, NOT THAT!* AND *EAT THIS, NOT THAT! FOR KIDS!*

"*EAT THIS, NOT THAT!* is gonna freak the weight right off of you."
—Ellen DeGeneres

"Food marketers have packed our foods with hundreds of
hidden calories. *EAT THIS, NOT THAT!* helps you find out where they are,
and carve a path to a healthier, leaner, happier you."
—Mehmet Oz, MD, vice chair of surgery at Columbia University and
author of *You: On a Diet*

"It will change the length of your child's life.
This is a book you guys need to absolutely check out!"
—Rachel Ray

"Once you open it, just try to put it down."
— *The Washington Post*

"The sheer volume of products evaluated (a dozen
or more per categories) makes [the supermarket] section
perhaps the most valuable to harried parents.
And the compact size of the book means it's perfect
for tucking into a purse or grocery tote."
— *Chicago Tribune*

"There's a forehead-slapper on practically every one of the 300 pages."
— *Rocky Mountain News*

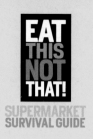

DEDICATION

For the men and women working in America's fields, farms, and supermarkets. Because of your hard work, we have the choices that can keep us lean, healthy, and happy.

Mention of specific companies, organizations, or authorities in this book does not imply endorsement by the author or publisher, nor does mention of specific companies, organizations, or authorities imply that they endorse this book, its author, or the publisher.

Internet addresses and telephone numbers given in this book were accurate at the time it went to press.

The brand-name products mentioned in this book are trademarks or registered trademarks of their respective companies. This book is intended as a reference volume only, not as a medical manual. The information given here is designed to help you make informed decisions about your health.

It is not intended as a substitute for any treatment that may have been prescribed by your doctor. If you suspect that you have a medical problem, we urge you to seek competent medical help.

Eat This, Not That! is a registered trademark of Rodale Inc.
© 2009 by Rodale Inc.

All rights reserved. No part of this publication may be reproduced or transmitted in any form or by any means, electronic or mechanical, including photocopying, recording, or any other information storage and retrieval system, without the written permission of the publisher.

Rodale books may be purchased for business or promotional use or for special sales. For information, please write to: Special Markets Department, Rodale Inc., 733 Third Avenue, New York, NY 10017

Printed in the United States of America

Rodale Inc. makes every effort to use acid-free ♾, recycled paper ♻.

Book design by George Karabotsos

All interior photos by Mitch Mandel and Thomas MacDonald/Rodale Images, with the exception of the following: page 46: © Christina Peters/StockFood (broccolini), Steven Mark Needham/FoodPix/Jupiter Images (corn), © iStockphoto (carrots, pluot, and tomato), © Lew Robertson/StockFood (cauliflower); pages 58–59: © iStockphoto; cover photos and pages 60–61, 73, 75, 77, 79, 81, 83: © Jeff Harris; recipe photos on pages 289–298: © Yunhee Kim; recipe photos on pages 300 and 303: © Tim Turner

Library of Congress Cataloging-in-Publication Data

Zinczenko, David.
    Eat this, not that, supermarket survival guide : the no-diet weight loss solution / David Zinczenko with Matt Goulding.
        p. cm.
    Includes index.
    ISBN-13 978–1–60529–838–2 paperback
    ISBN-10 1–60529–838–7 paperback
    1. Nutrition—Popular works.   2. Weight loss—Popular works.   3. Consumer education—Popular works.
  I. Goulding, Matt. II. Title.
  RA784.Z562 2008
  613.2′5—dc22   2008047534

Distributed to the trade by Macmillan

14 16 18 20 19 17 15 13 paperback

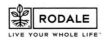

RODALE
LIVE YOUR WHOLE LIFE™

We inspire and enable people to improve their lives and the world around them

For more of our products visit **rodalestore.com** or call 800-848-4735

ACKNOWLEDGMENTS

This book is the product of thousands of hours spent in the market aisles, hundreds of conversations with industry experts, and the collective smarts, dedication, and raw talent of dozens of individuals. Our undying thanks to all of you who have inspired this project in any way. In particular:

Steve Murphy, who captains the ship called Rodale Inc. with grace, courage, and remarkable vision. Thanks for continuing to make this the best publishing company on the planet.

The Rodale family, whose dedication to improving the lives and well-being of their readers is apparent in every book and magazine they put their name on.

George Karabotsos, whose vision has once again turned a jumble of words and numbers into something that's impossible to put down.

Stephen Perrine, with whom we've conferred over many a fast-food lunch and who never met an exclamation mark he didn't like.

Clint Carter, whose supermarket savvy is apparent in every chapter.

The entire *Men's Health* editorial staff: A smarter, more inspiring group of writers, editors, researchers, designers, and photo directors does not exist, in the magazine world or beyond.

To the Rodale book team: Chris Krogermeier, Nancy Bailey, Erana Bumbardatore, Sara Cox, Jackie Dornblaser, Susan Eugster, Jennifer Giandomenico, Tara Long, Tom MacDonald, Mitch Mandel, Sonya Maynard, Melissa Reiss, Jean Rogers, Emma Sanders, Steve Schirra, Troy Schnyder, Marc Sirinsky, Sara Vignieri, and Nikki Weber. Your extraordinary sacrifices of time and sanity brought another project to reality in record time.

The doctors, researchers, and nutritionists whose expertise helped inform this book: David Katz, MD; Matthew Kadey, RD; and Mary Story, PhD, RD, among others.

Special thanks to: Adam Campbell, John Dixon, Riva Fischel, Sophie Fitzgerald, Carolyn Kylstra, Anna Maltby, Vikki Nestico, Robb Rice, and Michelle Stark.

And to the people who matter most to us in this world: Sorry for all the talk about calorie counts.

—Dave and Matt

The Choice Is Yours

It can be a place of wonder and excitement, of bright shiny colors, delectable scents, and enticingly sweet delights. It's a place packed with temptations and miracles, where the great bounty of American prosperity becomes unmistakable and where every hunger and thirst can be satiated in myriad ways.

But it can also be a place of great danger, where marketing ploys, and outright lies can rob you of your fitness, your health, your vitality—and in the end, even your life.

I'm talking, of course, about the American supermarket.

When Roald Dahl wrote *Charlie and the Chocolate Factory* nearly half a century ago, he demonstrated how a crafty food marketer could wow us with wonder and treats, at the same time putting us in grave danger with his reckless disregard for our health. And while there isn't anything on the supermarket shelves that will turn your child into an enormous blueberry à la Violet Beauregarde (at least, not yet), there are plenty of foods for sale— plenty—that will blow up your waistline and batter your bathroom scale.

Many of these caloric offenders are obvious—you'll never beat the rap in food court by claiming you didn't know the double-cheese-and-pepperoni calzones were a health hazard—but a lot of the worst offenders are double agents. They pose as healthy choices, often labeled with such comforting words as "fortified," "lite," "all-natural," and even "multigrain," but you'd be surprised to discover how often these words mean nothing. Indeed, food packaging can be so deceptive that you often have no way of knowing which foods will lead you to a lifetime of leanness and which will undermine every effort you make to control your body—and your life.

Until now.

If you want to eat great food and still stay slim, pack in the most nutrition for your food dollar, learn the simple secret swaps that will protect your body without penalizing your taste buds, and avoid the fat bombs and caloric catastrophes that await you on your next shopping trip, you've come to the right place. Because eating healthier, smarter, and better doesn't have to mean sacrifice, self-denial, and hunger pangs. Nor does it require hours sweating away in the gym or pounding the roadways.

It simply means knowing a handful of rules—and knowing when to Eat This, Not That.

WHY YOUR WEIGHT IS NOT YOUR FAULT

Ever go to a parent-teacher night at an elementary school and try to squeeze into your fourth grader's desk chair? Embarrassing, right? Our adult bodies are simply wider, heavier, and differently proportioned than our children's are.

Well, if we could build a time machine and travel back—not to Cro-Magnon days but to our grandparents' day—we'd find much the same thing. Our chairs would be smaller. So would our clothing. And guess what else would be smaller?

Our meals and snacks.

Consider, for example, the humble bag of potato chips, washed down with a Coke. Since the days when Fonzie was ruling the drive-ins and diners of America, the average salty snack portion has increased by 93 calories, and soft drink portions have increased by 49 calories, according to the Nation-wide Food Consumption Survey and the Continuing Survey of Food Intakes, which together create a sample of more than 63,000 people. So if you were to indulge in a bag of chips and a soda once a day, you'd be eating 142 more calories every day than Fonzie did. And that's just in one snack! (No wonder it was so easy for the Fonz to be cool.) It takes 3,500 calories to create a pound of fat on your body. By eating the same snack every day that people from our grandparents' era did, we automatically ingest enough calories to add a pound of flab to our frames every 25 days—or 14 pounds of fat a year!

But it's not just our snack foods that are loaded with more calories. The supersizing of the American diet has affected all of our foods, and nowhere is that more apparent than at the supermarket. For example, in 1971 the average American male consumed 2,450 calories a day; the average woman, 1,542. But by the year 2000, American men were averaging 2,618 daily calories (up 7 percent), while women were eating 1,877 calories (a whopping 22 percent increase, or 335 more calories every day!).

As a result, since the 1970s the obesity rate in this country has doubled, with two-thirds of our population now overweight. The health condition most directly tied to obesity—diabetes—now eats up one in every five dollars Americans spend on health care, and a recent study at Harvard found that obesity may soon surpass tobacco as the number one cause of cancer deaths. And the future looks even more bleak for our children: No matter what your weight may have been growing up, because of the way we're packaging and selling foods at restaurants and supermarkets, your child faces four times the risk of obesity as you did.

WHO BLEW UP THE FOOD?

A lot of people want to blame the obesity epidemic on too much TV, too little exercise, and too much gluttony. But that's blaming the victim, in my opinion. Why should guys give up Sunday afternoons with pizza and John Madden—and why should women give up Sunday nights with a bowl of ice cream and *Brothers & Sisters* on the tube? Indulgences like that make life worth living. And really— did they not have cheeseburgers and fries (and television) back in the 1970s?

Indeed, I'd argue that Americans are working harder than ever to keep themselves in shape. Every year, we spend an estimated $542 million on health and fitness books, $18.5 billion on health club memberships, and $5.2 billion on diet foods and weight loss programs. And that's not to mention the popularity of weight loss challenge programs like *The Biggest Loser* and fitness magazines like *Bicycling, Runner's World, Women's Health,* and *Men's Health.* When all is said and done, we'll have spent close to $60 billion this year on trying to keep the pounds off.

But unless you understand how food marketers have altered the reality of our weekly trip to the supermarket, it's impossible to truly see where the battle lines fall in the fight against fat. See, the food industry spends $30 billion a year on advertising—nearly half of it pitching convenience foods, candy, soda, and desserts. And while they're busy using dancing leprechauns and talking teddy bears to sell you on how the new shrink-wrapped food of the month is going to make you the most popular mom or dad on the block, they're obscuring the real story. And the real story is this: The food we consume today is simply different from the food that Americans ate 20 or 30 years ago. And the reasons are as simple as they are sneaky.

❋ **We've added extra calories to traditional foods.** In the early 1970s, food manufacturers, looking for a cheaper ingredient to replace sugar, came up with a substance called high-fructose corn syrup. This new invention made perfect sense: Corn was cheap and adundant—thanks to heavy government subsidies—and Americans had an ever-escalating desire for sweet foods. Today, HFCS is in an unbelievable array of foods—everything from breakfast cereals to bread, from ketchup to pasta sauce, from juice boxes to iced tea. While most current research concludes that the body metabolizes HFCS in the same way it does ordinary sugar, this synthetic sweetener has a few sneaky "advantages" over table sugar: 1) It's cheaper to produce, 2) it has a longer shelf life, and 3) its liquid form makes it easy to incorporate into the types of products that never received the sugar treatments before (read: whole wheat bread). So Grandma's pasta sauce now comes in a jar, and it's loaded with stuff just perfect for adding meat to your bones—and flab on your belly.

❋ **We've been trained to supersize it.** It seems like Economics 101: If you can get a lot more food for just a few cents more, then it makes all the sense in the world to upgrade to the "value meal." And since this trick has worked so well for fast-food marketers, your average product in the supermarket has become Hulkified as well. The problem is the way we look at food—we should be looking at cutting down on our calories, not adding to them.

❋ **We've laced our food with time bombs.** A generation ago, it was hard for food manufacturers to create baked goods that would last on store shelves. Most baked goods require oils, and oil leaks at room temperature. But since the 1960s, manufac-turers have been baking with—and restaurateurs have been frying with—something called trans fat. Trans fat is cheap and effective: It makes potato chips crispier and cookies tastier, and it lets fry-cooks make pound after pound of fries without smoking up their kitchens. The downside: Trans fat increases your bad cholesterol, lowers your good cholesterol, and greatly increases your risk of heart disease.

✱ **Our fruits and vegetables aren't as healthy as they once were.**
Researchers in a study in the *Journal of the American College of Nutrition* tested 43 different garden crops for nutritional content and discovered that 6 out of 13 nutrients showed major declines between 1950 and 1999: protein, calcium, phosphorus, iron, riboflavin, and ascorbic acid (vitamin C). Researchers say the declines are probably due to farmers' efforts to achieve higher yields and plants that grow faster and can be picked earlier. As a result, the plants aren't able to make or take in nutrients at the same rate.

✱ **Even the animals we eat are different today.** Here's a terrifying statistic: The average piece of chicken has 266 percent more fat than it did in 1971, while its protein content has dropped by a third, according to researchers at the Institute of Brain Chemistry and Human Nutrition at the London Metropolitan University. Because we no longer eat chickens that roam the farm eating bugs and grasses—today they're kept in cages and fed antibiotic-laced soy and corn and other unnatural foods—today's chicken is actually higher in fat than it is in protein. (If that is what modern food management is doing to chickens, imagine what it's doing to us!)

✱ **We're drinking more calories than ever.** A study from the University of North Carolina found that we consume 450 calories a day from beverages, nearly twice as many as 30 years ago. This increase amounts to an extra 23 pounds a year that we're forced to work off—or carry around with us. Many of the calories come from HFCS in our drinks—especially, when it comes to kids, in our "fruit" drinks that are often nothing more than water, food coloring, and sweetener. In fact, anything you have for your kids to drink in your fridge right now—unless it's water, milk, or a diet soda—probably has HFCS in it. Go ahead—read the label.

✳ **We don't even know what's in our food.** More and more, marketers are adding new types of preservatives, fats, sugars, and other food substances to our daily meals. Indeed, there are now more than 3,000 ingredients on the FDA's list of "safe" food additives, and any one of them could end up on your plate. But often, they go unexplained (what is xanthan gum, anyway?) or, in the case of restaurant food, unmentioned. Unless we're eating it right off the tree, it's hard to know what, exactly, is in that fruity dish. (We're here to solve that problem once and for all. Turn to page 306 for the *Eat This, Not That! Food Additive Glossary*—and find out what exactly it is you're feeding yourself and your family!)

All of these disturbing trends in our food supply are a lot to chew on—but chew on them we do, often because we feel we have no choice. Yet I believe there is a better way. I believe we can enjoy all the bounty of the supermarket—and heck, some pretty good TV shows, too—and not gain weight or lose control of our bodies and our health. I believe that taking control of our food, our weight, and our lives doesn't have to be difficult. I believe that if we have the knowledge and insight we need, we can and will make the right choices.

That's why I've written **EAT THIS, NOT THAT! SUPERMARKET SURVIVAL GUIDE.**

WHAT YOU CAN GAIN FROM THIS GUIDE

If the information above is troubling—if it makes you concerned, even angry, about the way food is grown, packaged, and sold to you and your family— then let me be clear: The supermarket is filled—filled!—with great-tasting, healthy, satisfying options.

Finding them, and understanding what makes one food healthier and better for your waistline than the product sitting right next to it on the shelf, takes a lot of thought and research. Fortunately, we've done all the homework for you. All you need to do is reap the rewards. Here are just some of the ways that this guide will make your life better.

You'll save time and stress. Deciding who should get your vote for president used to be a hard decision. Nowadays, it feels easy—choice A or choice B? Compare that with the decision we make every time we sit down to watch TV—channel 1 or 2 or 10 . . . or 134 . . . or 705? Or the complex decision you have to make every time you try to decide on a new cell phone plan or a book to read or a brand of toothpaste to buy. But that's nothing compared with the challenge we all face every time we step into the supermarket: There are 50,000 different food and beverage products on sale at your local grocery store. It's no wonder shopping trips seem to take forever! With **EAT THIS, NOT THAT! SUPERMARKET SURVIVAL GUIDE,** you'll have the answers to complicated nutritional questions at your fingertips, so shopping becomes a snap!

You'll lose weight and look better. The shopping advice in **EAT THIS, NOT THAT! SUPERMARKET SURVIVAL GUIDE** is designed specifically to target belly fat—by filling you up with smart, healthy choices that rev up your resting metabolism and help keep you burning fat all day, every day— even while you sleep!

You'll reshape your body. Most "diet" plans force you to cut, cut, cut calories, until you're practically starving. And what do you get? Sure, you lose fat, but you lose muscle as well. And muscle is crucial to keeping your metabolism revving and giving you the lean, firm shape you crave. That's why I'm proud to say **EAT THIS, NOT THAT! SUPER-MARKET SURVIVAL GUIDE** is *not* a diet book. It's not going to teach you to eat less or to starve yourself or to deny your cravings. Instead, it's going to teach you to feed your cravings with smart food choices that will improve your body shape at the same time!

What Cool Hand Luke Can Teach Us about Nutrition

When Paul Newman died in September of 2008, America lost more than just a great film actor. We lost one of the pioneers of healthy eating.

Legend has it that one Thanksgiving Day in the early 1990s, Newman's daughter Nell cooked her family an all-organic dinner that Paul loved. That meal led to the founding of Newman's Own Organics, now one of the largest organic food brands in the world.

By putting his mug on organic products, Newman introduced a lot of us to the idea of eating all-natural. And his impact has been powerful.

∗ The organic food industry has grown at a rate of nearly 20 percent per year for the last seven years, according to the Agricultural Marketing Resource Center. Seventy-five percent of US grocery stores now carry at least some organic products, and in 2005 alone, American shoppers spent more than $51 billion on natural and organic products.

∗ In a 2008 survey, 66 percent of respondents said that they spent between 10 and 30 percent of their total household grocery budget on these items. Forty-six percent thought organic foods taste better.

You'll see time and again that I recommend higher-nutrition, lower-calorie organic brands over highly processed, additive-riddled options. So next time you're faced with an uncertain choice, simply ask yourself: What would Cool Hand Luke do?

You'll save money. The average family in the United States makes two trips to the supermarket each week and spends an average of $57.20 per trip. At just under $500 a month for groceries, it's no wonder we're all feeling financially pinched. But one of the advantages of **EAT THIS, NOT THAT! SUPERMARKET SURVIVAL GUIDE** is that you'll learn how to pack as much nutrition as possible into the foods you buy. As a result, you'll be wasting fewer dollars on empty calories and instead be bringing home foods that keep your family fuller longer. Fewer calories, less money, more nutrition: It's a victory on all fronts.

You'll earn more money. There's an old saying: Look the part and you'll get the part. Well, research shows that people who are leaner and fitter are viewed as being more competent and successful than those who are overweight. And when people view you as competent, they are more likely to pay you what you deserve. Don't believe me? A New York University study found that people packing on an extra 40 pounds make 9 percent less than their slimmer colleagues.

You'll gain greater health. As I said above, the number one goal of this book is to cut out empty calories and add nutrition—bringing you more nutritional bang for your buck with every bite. And by carving away belly flab, you'll cut your risk of heart disease, diabetes, stroke, and even cancer.

And who doesn't want that?

The Whine Factor
How to trick your children into never whining for sugary snacks again

Pity the poor 3-year-old. His parents tell him when to go to bed, when to wake up, even what to put on in the morning. It's a tough existence, but there's one way a child can suddenly tilt the balance of power in his favor and turn the little banana republic of his world into a superpower: He can unleash the whine.

The whine is the Weapon of Mass Destruction—it takes out not only the child's parents but everyone else in the supermarket. Five minutes of "I waaaant Crispy Sugar Mouthrot Cereal nooowwww!" and anyone in the supermarket will volunteer to buy whatever your child wants—just to stop the noise. It's embarrassing, and you can't help but feel like a bad parent when your child collapses onto the floor of the store as though he hasn't been fed in a week.

Mom, Dad: Don't panic. Here's a trick several *Men's Health* editors have learned over the years, and it's guaranteed to take even the whiniest food shopper down a peg. The next time your child whines because he wants something, pretend you can't understand what he's saying.

The logic here is so simple, it's brilliant: A child whines to get what he wants. If the child is told that you can't understand what he wants, then the whine becomes a useless tool—he might as well be asking for something in Farsi. A few bouts of "I can't understand what you're saying" and supermarket trips will become far less stressful.

Fat's Dominos

17 ways this book can improve your life if you're overweight

Slimming down to your ideal body weight will:

- Cut your risk of being hospitalized for heart disease by 25 percent, compared to overweight people (obese: 77 percent)
- Cut your risk of being hospitalized for diabetes by up to 64 percent (obese: 88 percent)
- Cut your risk of having a heart attack by 29 percent (obese: 48 percent)
- Cut your risk of having high cholesterol by 33 percent (obese: up to 29 percent)
- Cut your risk of having erectile dysfunction by 25 percent (obese: 50 percent)
- Make you appear 54 percent more attractive to the opposite sex (obese: 83 percent)
- Let you spend 27 percent less at the pharmacy each year (obese: 51 percent)
- Reduce the length of your hospital stay by 16 percent (obese: 33 percent)
- Cut your risk of having asthma by 30 percent (obese: 39 percent)
- Cut your risk of dying of any cause by up to 16 percent (obese: 38 percent)
- Cut your risk of dying in a car crash by 37 percent (obese: 40 percent)
- Cut your risk of developing stomach cancer by 10 percent (obese: 63 percent)
- Cut your risk of developing gallstones by up to 60 percent
- Cut your risk of developing esophageal cancer by 55 percent (obese: 68 percent)
- Cut your risk of developing kidney cancer by 42 percent (obese: 64 percent)
- Cut your risk of having osteoarthritis by 12 percent (obese: 25 percent)
- Cut your risk of having high blood pressure by 44 percent (obese: 66 percent)

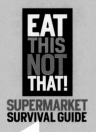

EAT
THIS
NOT
THAT!
SUPERMARKET
SURVIVAL GUIDE

Chapter 1

GETTING TO KNOW & LOVE THE SUPERMARKET

EAT THIS, NOT THAT!
RODALE
CH. 1

Master Your Market

The modern supermarket truly is a wonder, and it is by far your best tool for protecting your health and the well-being of your family. Far more than the local gym, the local supermarket is where the key to your health and fitness lies. You just need to learn how to use it.

That's another reason why I'm so excited about **EAT THIS, NOT THAT! SUPERMARKET SURVIVAL GUIDE**. Simply changing the way you look at supermarket shopping could have an enormous impact on your body—and your life! Consider this: Researchers in Australia looked at the shopping and eating habits of 1,136 women and discovered that those who said they enjoyed food shopping and eating, who made and stuck to shopping lists, and who had a "forward-planning" approach to their meals ate more fruits and vegetables and had, overall, a much healthier diet.

In other words, simply changing the way you look at a trip to the supermarket—as a chance to do something great for yourself and your family, instead of a chore to be rushed through—can make all the difference in the world.

See, buying and cooking your own food makes you the boss of your diet—not some pizza-faced kid standing over a deep fryer in the back of a chain restaurant. And it puts you in charge of your wallet as well—a recent survey found that 71 percent of Americans said they were trying to eat out less and cook in more, as a way of saving money. That's good news for our wallets, but it's even better news for our health. Nearly a third of us eat five or fewer home-cooked meals a week, and one in six of us doesn't eat even three!

Now think about it: Do you really know what's in the food you're ordering at the sports bar, the fast-food restaurant, the local diner, or the all-you-can-eat buffet? Not unless you've worked in the kitchen yourself. Do you have any idea if that burger with fries represents 200 calories or 500 or 1,000? No. (And chances are, it's more calories than you probably guessed—especially if someone in a paper hat convinced you to supersize it.)

But **EAT THIS, NOT THAT! SUPERMARKET SURVIVAL GUIDE** puts you in charge of your food intake.

Now, navigating the supermarket takes some clever thinking and a bit of insider knowledge—the kind of insider knowledge this book is packed with. To start, I want you to go forward on your next shopping trip with the following rules in mind.

RULE #1: WORK THE EDGES

In general, the healthiest food in the supermarket is found along the walls. The dairy case, produce, and meats and seafood are all found in the outlying regions of the market, while the inner aisles tend to be dominated by things that come in boxes, bags, or cans. Most of this vast nutritional dead zone is composed of highly processed foods made with plenty of corn and soy by-products as well as a veritable chemistry class worth of manufactured ingredients. The less time you spend in there, the better.

RULE #2: LOOK HIGH AND LOW

One reason why good food at the supermarket can be harder to find than Donald Trump's hairline is that big food conglomerates simply overwhelm many of the smaller companies trying to deliver healthier, more natural foods. Indeed, since the mid-1980s, supermarkets have been charging "slotting fees" to food companies who want prime real estate on the shelves. So the Krafts, the Proctor & Gambles, and the Kellogg's all have their products at eye level—or, in the cereal and candy aisles, at kids' eye level. The deeper a company's pockets, the deeper it can reach into yours. The trick: The healthier foods tend to be on the top and bottom shelves. (By the way, a great technique for cutting down on whining from hungry kids is to never let them into the center of the supermarket. If they're old enough, put them in charge of "guarding the cart"—standing sentry over the shopping cart, which you cleverly keep on the outskirts of the store. By doing this, and making targeted solo forays into the center of the market, you'll keep temptation away from their innocent eyes—at least until you get to the checkout counter.)

RULE #3: MORE PACKAGING = LESS NUTRITION

In general, the closer you can get to the earth, the better. The process of shipping, cooking, refining, and packaging foods all helps to strip out essential nutrients, leading to empty food calories—the main thing you want to try to avoid. A serving of Veggie Crisps is simply not the same as a serving of vegetables. Better to eat a carrot than carrot-flavored potato powder and soy oil. Got it?

RULE #4: LEARN THE LINGO

You have two packages in your hands. One says "whole grain." The other says "multigrain." Which do you pick? Topping the list of Most Annoying Things Food Marketers Do is their sneaky tactic of turning words that sound healthy against us. "Whole grain" means that the entire grain kernel—wheat, corn, what-have-you—has been used to make the product. That's good, because the process of refining grains, to make white bread, for example, actually strips out the vast majority of the nutrients, leaving behind only the empty calories. "Multigrain," on the other hand, only means that more than one type of grain was used.

It's entirely possible that two or more grains went into the product—after they were refined and stripped of all their nutritional value, of course.

RULE #5: FEWER INGREDIENTS MEANS HEALTHIER FOOD

You already read labels, of course, but unless you're the Stephen Hawking of foodstuffs, you'll find them pretty darn confusing. So when you must choose between two products and you're stumped, just pick the one with the shorter list of ingredients. It's almost always the right choice.

RULE #6: WATCH THE TOTEM POLE

When you're reading the ingredients list, think of it as a totem pole, with the ingredients toward the top as the most predominant and the ingredients farther down as more like bit players. So while high-fructose corn syrup may appear in just about everything, a product that lists it as ingredient number 2 is probably a lot less healthy than one listing it as ingredient number 6.

Sound good? All right, ladies and gents. Start your shopping carts—and let's move forward to a leaner, healthier, more nutritious future!

11 Secrets the Food Industry Doesn't Want You to Know

We've uncovered the truth about the products that line your supermarket's shelves.

And what we found might just surprise you.

If you want some insight into the food industry, take a stroll through your grocery store's candy aisle. There, on the labels of such products as Mike and Ike and Good & Plenty, you'll find what perhaps is a surprising claim: "Fat free." However, it's completely true—these empty-calorie junk foods are almost 100 percent sugar and processed carbs.

You see, food manufacturers think you're stupid. In fact, their marketing strategies rely on it. For instance, it may be that the aforementioned candy makers are hoping you'll equate "fat free" with "healthy" or "nonfattening"—so that you forget about all the sugar these products contain. It's a classic bait and switch.

And the candy aisle is just the start. That's why we've scoured the supermarket to find the secrets that food industry insiders don't want you to know. The very ones that deep-pocketed manufacturers use to prey on your expectations, your wallet, and most important, your health. Call it the *Eat This, Not That!* crib sheet for helping you to beat Big Food at its own game—and eat healthier for life.

1. KEEBLER DOESN'T WANT YOU TO KNOW THAT NUMBERS CAN BE DECEIVING.

On the front of a box of Reduced Fat Club Crackers—in large yellow letters—you'll find the claim, "33% Less Fat Than Original Club Crackers." Their math is accurate: The original product contains 3 grams of fat per serving (per 4 crackers), while the reduced-fat version has 2 grams (per 5 crackers). So statistically, it's a 33 percent difference, but is it meaningful? And why doesn't Keebler tout that their reduced-fat crackers have 33 percent more carbs than the original? Maybe they simply don't want you to know that when they took out 1 gram of fat, they replaced it with 3 grams of refined flour and sugar.

2. BEVERAGE MAKERS DON'T WANT YOU TO KNOW THAT SOME BOTTLED GREEN TEA MAY NOT BE AS HEALTHY AS YOU THINK.

We commissioned ChromaDex laboratories to analyze 14 different bottled green teas for their levels of disease-fighting catechins. While Honest Tea Green Tea with Honey topped the charts with an impressive 215 milligrams of total catechins, some products weren't even in the game. For instance, Republic of Tea Pomegranate Green Tea had only 8 milligrams, and Ito En Teas' Tea Lemongrass Green had just 28 milligrams, despite implying on its label that the product is packed with antioxidants.

3. FOOD COMPANIES DON'T WANT YOU TO KNOW THAT YOUR FOOD CAN LEGALLY CONTAIN MAGGOTS.

Sure, the FDA limits the amount of rodent droppings and other appetite killers in your food, but unfortunately that limit isn't zero. The regulations below aren't harmful to your health—but we can't promise that the thought of them won't make you sick.

The Wrong Kind of Protein

The little "bonus" ingredients the FDA allows in your food

FOOD	Can contain up to ...
Canned pineapple	20 percent moldy fruit
Canned tomatoes	5 fly eggs or 2 maggots per 500 grams
Frozen broccoli	60 mites per 100 grams
Ground cinnamon	400 insect fragments and 11 rodent hairs per 50 grams
Peanut butter	30 insect fragments or 1 rodent hair per 100 grams
Popcorn	1 rodent pellet in one sample or 2 rodent hairs per pound
Potato chips	6 percent rotten potatoes

4. KELLOGG'S DOESN'T WANT YOU TO KNOW THE TRUTH ABOUT CORNFLAKES.

Case in point: They've placed a "Diabetes Friendly" logo on the box's side panel. Never mind that Australian researchers have shown that cornflakes raise blood glucose faster and to a greater extent than straight table sugar. (High blood glucose is the primary symptom of diabetes.) The cereal maker does provide a link to its Web site, where nutrition recommendations are provided for people with diabetes.

5. QUAKER DOESN'T WANT YOU TO KNOW THAT A BOWL OF SOME OF THEIR "HEART-HEALTHY" HOT CEREALS HAS MORE SUGAR THAN THE SAME SERVING SIZE OF FROOT LOOPS.

One example: Quaker Maple & Brown Sugar Instant Oatmeal. Sure, the company proudly displays the American Heart Association (AHA) checkmark on the product's box. However, the fine print next to the logo simply reads that the food meets AHA's "food criteria for saturated fat and cholesterol." So it could have a pound of sugar and still qualify. But guess what? Froot Loops meets the AHA's criteria, too, only no logo is displayed. That's because . . .

6. THE FOOD INDUSTRY DOESN'T WANT YOU TO KNOW THAT COMPANIES MUST PAY TO BE AN AMERICAN HEART ASSOCIATION– CERTIFIED FOOD.

That's why the AHA logo might appear on some products but is absent from others—even when both meet the guidelines.

7. THE FOOD INDUSTRY DOESN'T WANT YOU TO KNOW THAT FOOD ADDITIVES MAY MAKE YOUR KIDS MISBEHAVE.

Researchers at the University of Southampton in the UK found that artificial food coloring and sodium benzoate preservatives are directly linked to increased hyperactivity in children. The additives included Yellow #5, Yellow #6, Red #40, and sodium benzoate, which are commonly found in packaged foods in the United States, but the researchers don't know if it's a combination of the chemicals or if there's a single one that's the primary culprit. You can find Red #40, Yellow #5, and Yellow #6 in Lucky Charms and sodium benzoate in some diet sodas, pickles, and jellies.

8. LAND O'LAKES DOESN'T WANT YOU TO KNOW THAT THERE'S NO SUCH THING AS "FAT-FREE" HALF-AND-HALF.

By definition, a half-and-half dairy product is 50 percent milk and 50 percent cream. Cream, of course, is pretty much all fat. So, technically, Fat Free Half & Half can't exist. What exactly is it? Skim milk—to which a thickening agent and an artificial cream flavor have been added. You may be disappointed in the payoff: 1 tablespoon of traditional half-and-half contains just 20 calories; the fat-free version has 10.

9. THE MEAT INDUSTRY DOESN'T WANT YOU TO KNOW THAT THE LEANEST CUTS MAY HAVE THE HIGHEST SODIUM LEVELS.

Leaner cuts by definition are less juicy. To counteract this dried-out effect, some manufacturers "enhance" turkey, chicken, and beef products by pumping them full of a liquid solution that contains water, salt, and other nutrients that help preserve it. This practice can dramatically boost the meat's sodium level.

For example, a 4-ounce serving of Shady Brook Farms Fresh Boneless Turkey Breast Tenderloin that's enhanced by a 6 percent solution contains 55 mg sodium. But the same-size serving of Jennie-O Turkey Breast Tenderloin Roast Turkey, which is enhanced by up to 30 percent, packs 840 mg—more than one-third of your recommended daily value.

10. SUPERMARKETS DON'T WANT YOU TO KNOW THAT LONG LINES WILL MAKE YOU BUY MORE.

If you're stuck in a long checkout line, you'll be up to 25 percent more likely to buy the candy and sodas around you, according to a recent study at the University of Arizona. Psychologists have found that the more exposure someone has to temptation, the more likely it is that he'll succumb to it. This may also help explain why supermarkets lay out their stores so that the common staples—such as milk, bread, and eggs—are at the very back, forcing you to run the gauntlet of culinary temptation.

11. FOOD COMPANIES DON'T WANT YOU TO KNOW THAT THEIR CALORIE COUNTS MAY BE WRONG.

That's because in order to make sure you're getting at least as much as you pay for, the FDA is more likely to penalize a food manufacturer for overstating the net weight of a product than understating it. As a result, manufacturers often either "generously" package more food than the stated net weight or make servings heavier than the stated serving size weight.

With an ordinary food scale, we put a range of products to the test by checking the actual net weight and serving size weight. Sure enough, we found that a number of popular products are heavier than the package says. And that means you may be eating more calories than you think.

The Real Calorie Counter

Our research shows you could be under-estimating your calorie intake by 10 percent or more

PRODUCT	Listed calories per serving	Calories based on actual weight of serving size
Back to Nature Granola	200	270
Bear Naked Granola	140	163
Cheerios (without milk)	100	103
Doritos	150	156
Entenmann's Chocolate Glazed Mini Donuts	150	171
Entenmann's Marble Cake	280	301
Kellogg's Nutri-Grain Bars Strawberry	130	137
Hostess Cupcakes	180	186
Oreos	160	162
SunChips Garden Salsa Flavor	140	152
Wonder Classic White Bread	60	65

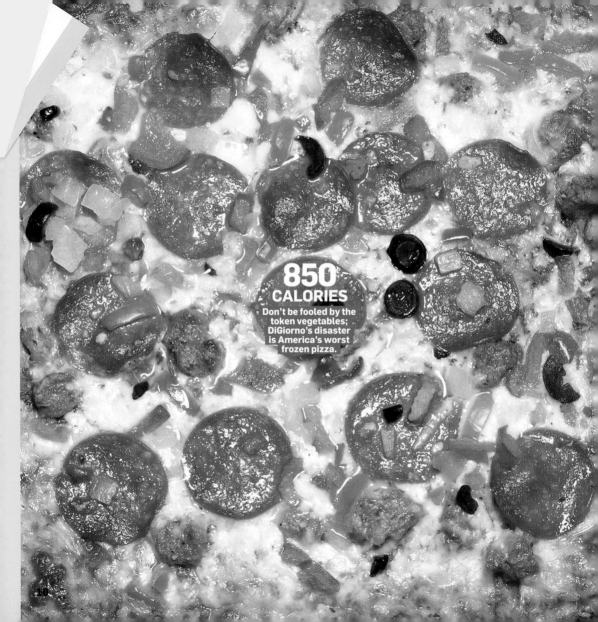

850 CALORIES

Don't be fooled by the token vegetables; DiGiorno's disaster is America's worst frozen pizza.

The 20 Worst Packaged Foods in America

The supermarket aisles are fraught with nutritional peril. Learn to disarm the food industry's industrial-strength calorie bombs and still eat the food you love.

WORST CRUNCH SNACK

20 Gardetto's Special Request Roasted Garlic Rye Chips (½ cup, 30 g)

*160 calories / 10 g fat
(2 g saturated, 2.5 g trans)
40 mg sodium*

Gardetto extracts the worst part of its Original snack mix and tries to serve it as a gourmet snack—a sneaky move that might have serious repercussions for even casual munchers. Each single serving exceeds the amount of trans fat deemed safe to consume daily by the American Heart Association.

Fat Equivalent: 3 strips of bacon

Eat This Instead:
**Snyder's of Hanover Sourdough Nibblers
(16 pieces, 30 g)**
*120 calories / 0 g fat
200 mg sodium*

WORST COOKIE

19 Pillsbury Big Deluxe Classics White Chunk Macadamia Nut
(dough; 1 cookie, 38 g)

*180 calories / 10 g fat
(3 g saturated, 2 g trans)
13 g sugars*

Stick to Nestlé Toll House when it comes to big-brand cookie dough; the people of Pillsbury have a penchant for scattering trans fats across your market's refrigerated section. This cookie has one load of dangerous oils mixed into the flour and another blended with sugar and interspersed throughout the dough as "white confectionery chunks."

Fat Equivalent: 5 "fun" size 3 Musketeers bars

Eat This Instead:
Toll House Chocolate Chip Cookie Dough (1½-inch ball, 28 g)
*130 calories
6 g fat (2.5 g saturated)
11 g sugars*

WORST YOGURT

18 Stonyfield Farm Whole Milk Chocolate Underground (6 oz)

*220 calories / 5 g fat
(3 g saturated) / 36 g sugars*

Stonyfield is notorious for being a little too generous with the sugar, but the nearly 3 tablespoons in their Chocolate Underground is bad even by their supersweet standards. Not even Ben & Jerry's makes a flavor of ice cream with this much sugar.

**Sugar Equivalent:
4 Cherry Popsicles**

Eat This Instead:
Breyers' Cookies n'Cream YoCrunch Lowfat with Oreo Pieces (6 oz)
*120 calories
2.5 g fat (1 g saturated)
11 g sugars*

WORST CANDY

17 **Twix** (1 package, 2 oz)

280 calories / 27 g sugars
14 g fat (11 g saturated)

Twix takes the already-dubious candy-bar reputation and drags it through a murky pool of saturated fat. With more than half the USDA's daily consumption recommendation for these dangerous fats in each package, this is one hazardous after-lunch snack.

Saturated Fat Equivalent:
11 strips of bacon

Eat This Instead:
100 Grand (1 package)

190 calories
22 g sugars
8 g fat (5 g saturated)

WORST CONDIMENT

16 **Eggo Original Syrup**
(¼ c)

240 calories / 40 g sugars

Breakfast is the most important meal of the day, but not when this sugar slick hits the table. Excluding water, the first three ingredients are all different forms of sugar. If you want real syrup, make sure it's 100 percent maple.

Sugar Equivalent: **Two Häagen-Dazs Vanilla & Almond ice cream bars**

Eat This Instead:
Smucker's Sugar Free Breakfast Syrup (¼ c)

20 calories / 0 g sugars

WORST ICE CREAM

15 **Häagen-Dazs Chocolate Peanut Butter**
(½ c)

360 calories / 24 g sugars
24 g fat (11 g saturated)

Häagen-Dazs makes great-tasting ice cream with an impressively short ingredient list, but that doesn't make up for the fact that their pints are consistently the fattiest in the freezer.

Fat Equivalent: **1 McDonald's Double Cheeseburger**

Eat This Instead:
Edy's Slow Churned Peanut Butter Cup (½ c)

130 calories
13 g sugars
6 g fat (3 g saturated)

WORST DRINK

14 **AriZona Kiwi Strawberry** (23.5-oz can)

353 calories / 0 g fat
82 g sugars

It claims to be blended juice, but only 5 percent of this can is any sort of real-fruit derivative. The remaining 95 percent is a blend of water and high-fructose corn syrup.

Sugar Equivalent:
4 Original Fudgsicle Bars

Drink This Instead:
Tropicana Lime Raspberry Fruit Squeeze
(15.2-oz bottle)

35 calories / 0 g fat
7 g sugars

WORST "HEALTHY" PANTRY ITEM

13 **Pop-Tarts Whole Grain Brown Sugar Cinnamon** (2 pastries)

400 calories
14 g fat (4 g saturated)
5 g fiber / 28 g sugars

Whole grain ain't the whole truth. There's also a glut of vegetable oil and seven types of sugar stuffed inside.

Sugar Equivalent: **1 Snickers bar**

Eat This Instead:
Sun-Maid Raisin English Muffins with Cinnamon
(1 muffin)

170 calories
0.5 g fat (0 g saturated)
2 g fiber / 13 g sugars

WORST FROZEN "HEALTHY" ENTRÉE

12 **Healthy Choice Complete Selections Sweet & Sour Chicken**
(340 g)

430 calories
9 g fat (1 g saturated)
600 mg sodium / 29 g sugars

Since when has fried chicken been healthy? Certainly not when it's cloaked in sugar.

Sugar Equivalent: **2 scoops Breyers Reese's Peanut Butter Cup ice cream**

Eat This Instead:
Kashi Southwest Style Chicken (283 g)

240 calories
5 g fat (0 g saturated)
680 mg sodium

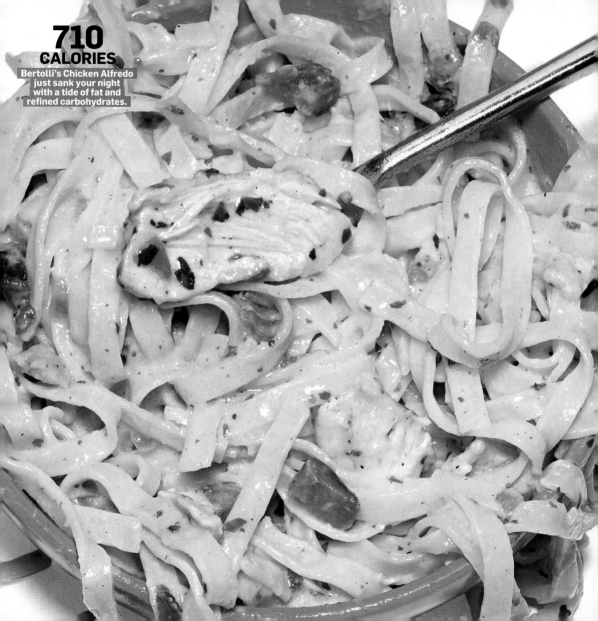

710
CALORIES

Bertolli's Chicken Alfredo just sank your night with a tide of fat and refined carbohydrates.

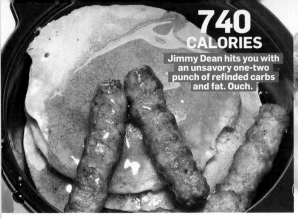

740 CALORIES

Jimmy Dean hits you with an unsavory one-two punch of refinded carbs and fat. Ouch.

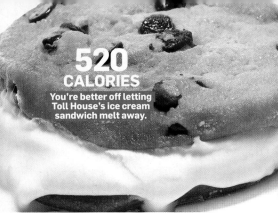

520 CALORIES

You're better off letting Toll House's ice cream sandwich melt away.

WORST CEREAL

11 Quaker 100% Natural Granola, Oats, Honey & Raisins (1 c)

420 calories
12 g fat (7 g saturated)
6 g fiber / 30 g sugars

Granola, for all its good reputation, is usually weighed down by a deluge of added sugars. In fact, for the same amount of sugar, you could have a bowl of Cocoa Pebbles more than twice the size— and you'd get more fiber and save about 60 calories in fat.

Calorie Equivalent:
8 chicken wings

Eat This Instead:
Kashi GOLEAN (1 c)

140 calories
1 g fat (0 g saturated)
10 g fiber / 6 g sugars

WORST PACKAGED SIDE

10 Pasta Roni Fettuccine Alfredo
(1 c prepared with 2% milk and margarine)

450 calories / 25 g fat
(7 g saturated, 3.5 g trans)
1,140 mg sodium

Once again Alfredo proves itself to be the biggest belt-busting option on the shelf. This side has a meal's worth of calories, and if you try to turn it into a meal in itself, expect to top 1,000 calories.

Sodium Equivalent:
4 medium orders of McDonald's French fries

Eat This Instead:
Pasta Roni Nature's Way Olive Oil & Italian Herb (1 c prepared with water and olive oil)

250 calories
8 g fat (1.5 g saturated)
800 mg sodium

WORST BAKED GOOD

9 Otis Spunkmeyer Banana Nut Muffins
(1 muffin, 114 g)

460 calories
22 g fat (3 g saturated)
2 g fiber / 32 g sugars

Despite popular belief, muffins are very rarely healthy. Case in point: The first ingredient in this muffin is sugar. The result is metabolic mayhem: Blood sugar climbs, pancreas goes into overdrive, and the body begins storing sugar as fat. Shortly after, you'll feel sluggish and crave more sugar.

Sugar Equivalent: $3\frac{1}{2}$ Rice Krispies Treats

Eat This Instead:
Vitalicious Apple Berry Muffin (1 muffin)

100 calories
0 g fat
5 g fiber / 10 g sugars

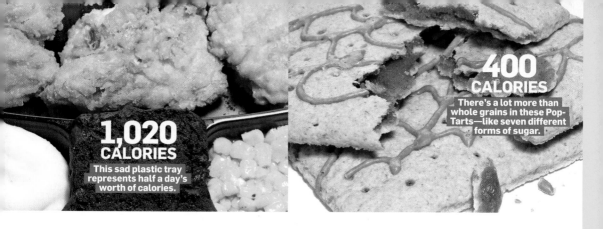

1,020 CALORIES This sad plastic tray represents half a day's worth of calories.

400 CALORIES There's a lot more than whole grains in these Pop-Tarts—like seven different forms of sugar.

WORST FROZEN TREAT

8 Toll House Ice Cream Chocolate Chip Cookie Sandwich (1 sandwich)

520 calories
23 g fat (9 g saturated)
44 g sugars

Do you really want more than a quarter of your day's calories to come from an ice-cream novelty? If you're going to take in this much fat and calories in one sitting, it better be dinner.

Calorie Equivalent: Two slices of hand-tossed pepperoni pizza from Pizza Hut

Eat This Instead:
Skinny Cow Low Fat Vanilla Ice Cream Sandwich (1 sandwich)

140 calories
2 g fat (1 g saturated)
15 g sugars

WORST INDIVIDUAL SNACK

7 Hostess Chocolate Pudding Pie (1 pie)

520 calories / 45 g sugars
24 g fat (14 g saturated,
1.5 g trans)

Skip past the enriched flour and water on the ingredient list and here's what you get: animal shortening, corn syrup, high-fructose corn syrup, sugar, modified corn starch, butter, chocolate liqueur, and so on. Any one of these ingredients alone might prompt you to raise an eyebrow, but taken together they should invoke a gag reflex and a sprint for something far healthier.

Saturated Fat Equivalent: 2 McDonald's Quarter Pounders

Eat This Instead:
Chocolatey Drizzle Rice Krispies Treat

100 calories / 8 g sugars
3 g fat (1 g saturated)

WORST PACKAGED LUNCH

6 Oscar Mayer Maxed Out Turkey & Cheddar Cracker Combo Lunchables (1 package)

680 calories / 61 g sugars
22 g fat (9 g saturated,
1 g trans) / 1,440 mg sodium

Here's your first clue that this meal has issues: The ingredient list—in its squinty small type—is a full 4 inches long. It includes just about every form of fat and sugar you can imagine. Your child deserves better.

Calorie Equivalent: 15 Chicken McNuggets

Eat This Instead:
Oscar Mayer Deli Creations Fajita Beef & Salsa Flatbread (145 g)

280 calories
9 g fat (4 g saturated)
890 mg sodium

5 Bertolli Grilled Chicken Alfredo & Fettuccine Complete Skillet Meal for Two
(½ package, 340 g)

710 calories / 1,370 mg sodium
42 g fat (22 g saturated)

A dinner for two should get your blood flowing, not stuff your arteries with more than the entire day's saturated fat.

Saturated Fat Equivalent: 22 strips of bacon

Eat This Instead:
Birds Eye Steamfresh Meals for Two Grilled Chicken in Roasted Garlic Sauce (½ bag, 340 g)

340 calories
880 mg sodium
13 g fat (5 g saturated)

4 Jimmy Dean Pancake and Sausage Links Breakfast Bowls

710 calories / 890 mg sodium
31 g fat (11 g saturated)

As if the calories, fat, and refined carbohydrates weren't bad enough, Jimmy D tops the whole thing with two Hershey's bars' worth of sugar.

Calorie Equivalent: 6 bowls of Froot Loops

Eat This Instead:
Jimmy Dean D-lights Breakfast Bowls Turkey Sausage (198 g)

230 calories
730 mg sodium
7 g fat (3 g saturated)

3 DiGiorno for One Garlic Bread Crust Supreme Pizza

850 calories / 1,450 mg sodium
44 g fat (15 g saturated, 3.5 g trans)

The bloated crust and the greasy toppings will saddle you with 60 percent of your day's sodium, 75 percent of your day's saturated fat, and nearly twice the amount of trans fats you should take in daily.

Calorie Equivalent: 6 slices Domino's Thin N Crispy Cheese Pizza

Eat This Instead:
South Beach Diet Deluxe Pizza

340 calories
660 mg sodium
11 g fat (4 g saturated)

2 Hungry-Man Classic Fried Chicken

1,020 calories / 1,570 mg sodium
57 g fat (12 g saturated)

They should rename the company Hungry-Men, because there's no way a single man needs more than a pound of fatty fried chicken, oily potatoes, and a brownie.

Calorie Equivalent: 5 Krispy Kreme Original Glazed Doughnuts

Eat This Instead:
Banquet Select Chicken Parmesan

350 calories
870 mg sodium
15 g fat (3.5 g saturated)

1 Marie Callender's Creamy Parmesan Chicken Pot Pie

1,060 calories / 1,440 mg sodium
64 g fat (24 g saturated)

Marie Callender's perpetrates the ultimate sleight of hand here: The nutrition information says this medium-size entrée has two servings, but honestly, when have you ever split a potpie? Lard-strewn pastry tops and cream-based fillings are the lowest common denominators of the nutritionally nefarious potpie, and this one, with an ingredient list that reads like an O-Chem final, beats out dozens of horrendous iterations to earn this special place on our list.

Sodium Equivalent: 8 small bags of potato chips
Fat Equivalent: 23 strips of bacon
Calorie Equivalent: 7 Taco Bell Fresco Beef Tacos

Eat This Instead:
Marie Callender's Oven Baked Chicken (369 g)

320 calories
990 mg sodium
12 g fat (3 g saturated)

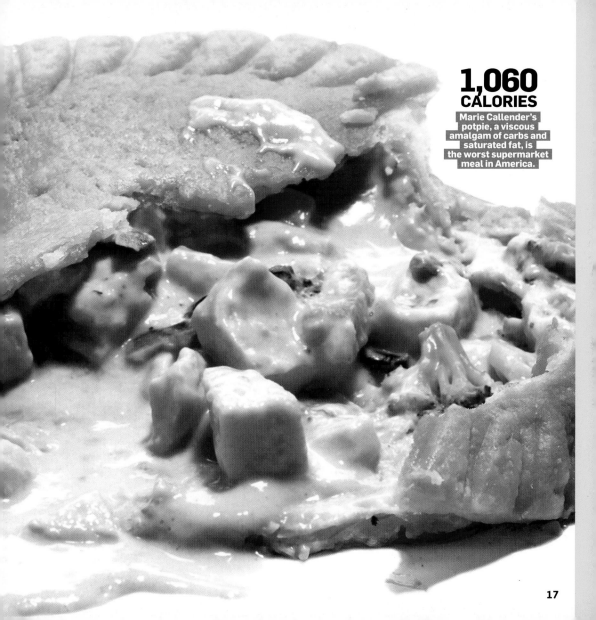

1,060 CALORIES

Marie Callender's potpie, a viscous amalgam of carbs and saturated fat, is the worst supermarket meal in America.

Chapter 2

THE PRODUCE AISLE

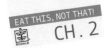

EAT THIS, NOT THAT!
CH. 2

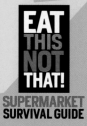

EAT
THIS
NOT
THAT!
SUPERMARKET
SURVIVAL GUIDE

Supercharge Your Meals

There's an old joke: An American mom tells her son, "Eat your broccoli. In China, kids don't even have broccoli!" Meanwhile, in China, a woman tells her son, "Eat your rice. In America, kids have to eat broccoli!"

Such is the stigma that we attach to vegetables and, to a lesser extent, to fruit: Eating them is an unpleasant chore, a duty, something we do when we aren't having the fun experience of chili-drenched nachos and cheese. And that's why the average American child eats only 25 percent of his or her daily recommended servings of vegetables and about 80 percent of the recommended servings of fruit. And that's with nagging parents looking over the kids' shoulders. What happens when the kids grow up and become . . . us?

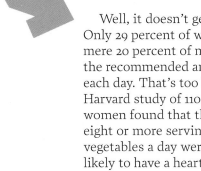

Well, it doesn't get any better. Only 29 percent of women and a mere 20 percent of men consume the recommended amount of produce each day. That's too bad, because a Harvard study of 110,000 men and women found that those who ate eight or more servings of fruit and vegetables a day were 30 percent less likely to have a heart attack or stroke than those who ate less than 1½ servings a day. You don't have to move into Mr. McGregor's garden to reap the health benefits of the produce aisle—indeed, eating just five servings of fruits and vegetables can lower your risk of coronary heart disease and stroke by 20 percent, versus those who eat three or fewer servings per day.

Now, I know what you're thinking. Five servings a day? Eight servings a day? That's a lot of kohlrabi, honcho! But it's not. Here's how you get eight servings without breaking a sweat: Have a banana with cereal and a glass of OJ for breakfast. A side salad at lunch with your sandwich and a piece of fruit. Snack on some raisins when your energy is running low around 3 p.m. At dinner, have another salad or a vegetable soup and a side of broccoli with your meat. Bang, you're at seven servings. Nosh on a couple of carrot sticks or have a V8 somewhere in your day and you've done it—how painless was that? And just look at the benefits.

- **You'll lower your blood pressure.** One study found that people with high blood pressure who ate a diet rich in fruits, vegetables, and low-fat dairy products reduced their systolic blood pressure by 11 points and their diastolic blood pressure by 6 points—as much as medications can achieve.

- **You'll protect your eyes.** A University of Texas study found that corn, orange bell peppers, kiwi, grapes, spinach, orange juice, and various

squash and leafy green vegetables were all packed with the nutrients lutein and zeaxanthin, which have been shown to protect the eyes from macular degeneration.

- **You'll build a leaner body.** Calcium (from kale, broccoli, and spinach), potassium (from Swiss chard, lima beans, yams, winter squash, and avocado), and magnesium (from potatoes, beans, and black-eyed peas) are just three of the essential muscle-building nutrients you can get from vegetables. And the fiber that's packed into most produce will help keep you fuller, longer—which means you'll stay slimmer, longer.

Trick Your Kids into Loving Vegetables
3 easy ways to help your children go green

SHAPE 'EM. A carrot is still a carrot—unless it's shaped like a ninja throwing star! A few quick turns of the knife can make vegetables into cool new edible toys. And don't forget the old trick of spelling out words with green beans.

HIDE 'EM. Toss broccoli, spinach, and other veggies into the blender, then spoon them into spaghetti sauce. Blended finely, they become almost invisible, but they still impart their magical nutritional content.

FRENCH FRY 'EM. Even kids who hate vegetables love French fries. But traditional fries are laden with grease and low in nutrition. Trick your youngsters with baked fries made from thinly cut potatoes, sweet potatoes, carrots, and parsnips. Splash the fries with a little olive oil, paprika, and salt and bake at 450°F for 30 to 40 minutes.

- **You'll have fewer sick days.**
  The essential antioxidant vitamins—E (from almonds, spinach, broccoli, and peanuts), C (from broccoli, bell peppers, papaya, and kale), and A (from carrots, cantaloupe, and apricots)—will protect you against everything from wrinkles to heart disease.

Does that get you psyched to dive into the produce aisle? It should. The USDA says that most of us need to increase our consumption of all of the vitamins, minerals, and other nutrients listed above. And eating as many vegetables and fruits as we can get our hands on is the best way to do it.

Indeed, we should probably eat even more produce than our grandparents did. USDA research has found that, because of the industrialization of farming and the need to produce larger yields, the fruits and vegetables we eat today may contain significantly fewer nutrients than those that our forebears ate. Researchers looked at 43 produce items and discovered drops in protein (6 percent), calcium (16 percent), iron (15 percent), riboflavin (38 percent), and vitamin C (20 percent).

The lesson: Eat more fruits and vegetables. Start doing it today.

Lean, Green Machines

Essentially, iceberg lettuce is the nutritional equivalent of a plastic office plant; it adds a little color, but mostly it just takes up space. Iceberg may be cheap and plentiful, but it contains almost no fiber, vitamins, or minerals. If you're going to eat salad, you might as well eat the power salad. Check out this green dream team.

The Cancer Killer:
ROMAINE
This celery-flavored green is one of the best vegetable sources of beta-carotene—712 micrograms per cup. A University of Illinois study showed that high levels of beta-carotene inhibited the growth of prostate cancer cells by 50 percent.

The Bone Builder:
ARUGULA
One cup of these mustard-flavored leaves has 10 percent of the bone-building mineral found in a glass of whole milk and 100 percent less

saturated fat. There's also some magnesium in every bite, for more protection against osteoporosis.

The Pipe Protector:
WATERCRESS
It's a pepper-flavored HEPA filter for your body. Watercress contains phytochemicals that may prevent cigarette smoke and other airborne pollutants from causing lung cancer.

The Heart Healer:
ENDIVE
It's slightly bitter and a little crisp, and it offers a good dose of fiber. A cup of endive also provides almost 20 percent of your daily requirement of folate. People who don't get enough of this essential B vitamin may have a 50 percent greater risk of developing heart disease.

The Brain Booster:
MUSTARD GREENS
These spicy, crunchy greens are packed with the amino acid tyrosine. In a recent US military study, researchers found that eating a tyrosine-rich meal an hour before taking a test helped soldiers significantly improve both their memories and their concentration.

The Antiaging Agent:
BOK CHOY
Think of it as a cabbage-flavored multivitamin. A bowl of bok choy has 23 percent of your daily requirement of vitamin A and a third of your vitamin C, along with three tongue-twisting, cancer-fighting, age-reducing phytochemicals: flavonoids, isothiocyanates, and dithiolthione.

The Sight Sharpener:
SPINACH
Spinach is a top source of lutein and zeaxanthin, two powerful antioxidants that protect your vision from the ravages of old age. A study from Tufts University found that frequent spinach eaters had a 43 percent lower risk of age-related macular degeneration.

The Pressure Punisher:
KOHLRABI
Kohlrabi tastes like the love child from a tryst between a cabbage and a turnip. Each serving contains nearly 25 percent of your daily requirement of potassium (to help keep a lid on your blood pressure), along with gluco-sinolate, a phytochemical that may prevent some cancers.

Master the Produce Aisle

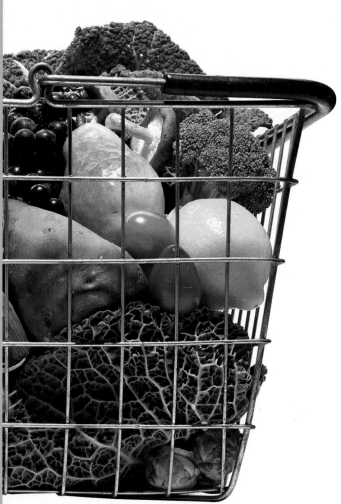

One of the reasons why Italians eat so well is that every last one of them believes it is their fundamental right to walk out of the market with the very best ingredients. They won't settle for a wrinkled eggplant, a withering artichoke, or an apple that tastes like Styrofoam. And neither should you. Problem is, finding the best, ripest, most jaw-droppingly tasty fruits and vegetables isn't as intuitive as you might think. It's a task that requires the attention of all five senses in order to pick up on the subtleties and nuances behind ultimate ripeness and utmost quality.

Regardless of what you're shopping for, start with these three rules.

1. Beautiful doesn't mean delicious. Sub-par conventional produce is bred to look waxy, glistening, and perfectly symmetrical, while prime fruits and vegetables are often irregularly shaped, with slight visual imperfections outside but a world of flavor waiting inside.

2. Use your hands. You can learn more about a fruit or vegetable from picking it up than you can from staring it down. Heavy, sturdy fruits and vegetables with taut skin and peels are telltale signs of freshness.

3. Shop with the seasons. In the Golden Age of the American supermarket, Chilean tomatoes and South African asparagus are an arm's length away when our soil is blanketed in snow. Sure, sometimes you just need a tomato, but there are three persuasive reasons to shop in season: it's cheaper, it's better, and it's better for you. So mark your calendar.

To dig even deeper in our hunt for perfect produce, we asked Aliza Green, author of *Field Guide to Produce,* and Chef Ned Elliott of Portland's Urban Farmer restaurant for the dirt on scoring the best of the bounty. Use the tips and tricks that follow and you'll bring home the best fruits and vegetables every time, just like an Italian grandma.

> **FRESH OBSESSED:** A vented lid that circulates air plus a raised tray that separates produce from moisture allows Rubbermaid's Produce Savers ($13 to $17; target.com) to keep your bounty fresh longer. Available in assorted sizes.

Apples

PERFECT PICK: Firm and heavy for its size with smooth, matte, unbroken skin and no bruising. The odd blemish (read: worm hole) or brown "scald" streaks do not negatively impact flavor. The smaller the apple, the bigger the flavor wallop.

PEAK SEASON: September to May

HANDLE WITH CARE: Keep apples in a plastic bag in the crisper away from vegetables. Here, they should remain edible for several weeks.

THE PAYOFF: Quercetin, a flavonoid linked to better heart health, plus the soluble fiber pectin, which keeps cholesterol in check.

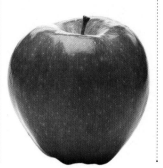

Artichokes

PERFECT PICK: Deep green and heavyset with undamaged, tightly closed leaves. The leaves should squeak when pinched together. One that is starting to open is past its best days.

PEAK SEASON: March to May

HANDLE WITH CARE: Store in the fridge in a plastic bag for up to 5 days.

THE PAYOFF: A higher total antioxidant capacity than any other common vegetable, according to USDA tests.

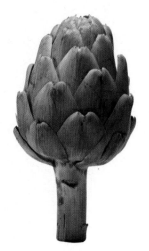

Arugula

PERFECT PICK: Emerald green leaves that are not yellowing or limp. The smaller the leaf, the less pungent its bite.

PEAK SEASON: March to November

HANDLE WITH CARE: Enclose roots in a damp paper towel and place the leaves in a plastic bag. Store in the fridge for 2 to 3 days.

THE PAYOFF: Vitamin K, which may improve insulin sensitivity, offering protection against diabetes.

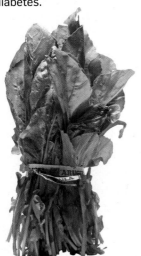

Asparagus

PERFECT PICK: Vibrant green spears with tight purple-tinged buds. Avoid spears that are fading in color or wilting. Thinner spears are sweeter and more tender.

PEAK SEASON: March to June

HANDLE WITH CARE: Trim the woody ends and stand the stalks upright in a small amount of water in a tall container. Cover the tops with a plastic bag and cook within a few days.

THE PAYOFF: Folate, a B vitamin that protects the heart by helping to reduce inflammation.

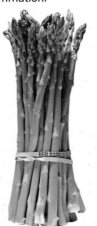

Avocados

PERFECT PICK: Firm to the touch without any sunken, mushy spots. They should not rattle when shaken—a sign the pit has pulled away from the flesh.

PEAK SEASON: Year-round

HANDLE WITH CARE: To ripen, place avocados in a paper bag and store at room temperature for 2 to 4 days. To speed up this process, add to the bag an apple, which emits ripening ethylene gas. Place ripe avocados in the fridge for up to 1 week.

THE PAYOFF: Plenty of cholesterol-lowering monounsaturated fat.

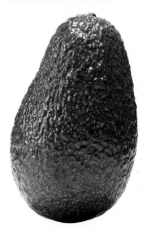

Bananas

PERFECT PICK: Ripe bananas have uniform yellow skins or small brown freckles indicating they are at their sweetest. Avoid any with evident bruising or split skins.

PEAK SEASON: Year-round

HANDLE WITH CARE: Store unripe bananas on the counter, away from direct heat and sunlight (speed things up by placing green bananas in an open paper bag). Once ripened, refrigerate; though the peel turns brown, the flavor and quality are unaffected.

THE PAYOFF: Vitamin B_6, which helps prevent cognitive decline, according to scientists at the USDA.

Beets

PERFECT PICK: Smooth, deep-red surface that's unyielding when pressed. Smaller roots are sweeter and more tender. Attached greens should be deep green and not withered.

PEAK SEASON: June to October

HANDLE WITH CARE: Remove the leaves (which are great sautéed in olive oil) and store in a plastic bag in the fridge for no more than 2 days. The beets will last in the crisper for up to 2 weeks.

THE PAYOFF: Nitrate, which may help lower blood pressure.

Bell Peppers

PERFECT PICK: Lots of heft for their size with a brightly colored, wrinkle-free exterior. The stems should be a lively green.

PEAK SEASON: July to December

HANDLE WITH CARE: Refrigerate in the crisper for up to 2 weeks.

THE PAYOFF: All bell peppers are loaded with antioxidants, especially vitamin C. Red peppers lead the pack, with nearly three times the amount of vitamin C found in fresh oranges. A single serving also has a full day's worth of vision-protecting vitamin A.

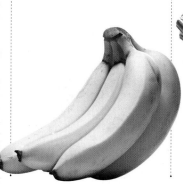

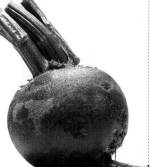

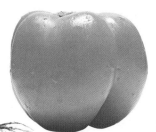

Blueberries

PERFECT PICK: Plump, uniform indigo berries with taut skin and a dull white frost. Check the bottom of the container for juice stains indicating many crushed berries. Those with a red or green tinge will never fully ripen.

PEAK SEASON: June to August

HANDLE WITH CARE: Transfer, unwashed, to an airtight container and refrigerate for 5 to 7 days. Blueberries spoil quickly if left at room temperature.

THE PAYOFF: More disease-fighting antioxidants (especially in the wild berries) than most commonly consumed fruits, according to Cornell University researchers.

Broccoli

PERFECT PICK: Rigid stems with tightly formed floret clusters that are deep green or tinged purple. Pass on any with yellowing heads—they will inevitably be more bitter.

PEAK SEASON: October to May

HANDLE WITH CARE: Place in a plastic bag and store in the refrigerator for up to 1 week.

THE PAYOFF: Sulforaphane, which activates enzymes that seek out and destroy cancerous cells.

Brussels Sprouts

PERFECT PICK: Compact, tight, and unshriveled heads that are vibrant green and feel overweight for their size. Select ones of similar size for ease of cooking, knowing that smaller sprouts pack sweeter flavor.

PEAK SEASON: October to November

HANDLE WITH CARE: Refrigerate, unwashed, in a tightly wrapped perforated plastic bag for up to 2 weeks.

THE PAYOFF: Nitrogen compounds called indoles, which have cancer-protecting efficacy.

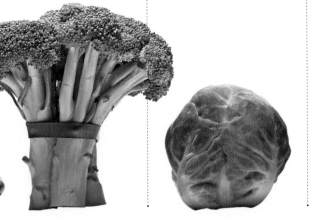

Cabbage

PERFECT PICK: Tightly packed, crisp, deeply hued leaves free of blemishes. Should feel dense when lifted; it's best that the stem not have any cracks at its base.

PEAK SEASON: Year-round

HANDLE WITH CARE: Tightly enclose cabbage in a plastic bag and store in the fridge for up to 10 days.

THE PAYOFF: More than half your vitamin K requirement in just 1 cup.

Cantaloupe

PERFECT PICK: The stem end should have a smooth indentation. Look for a sweet aroma, slightly oval shape, and a good coverage of netting. The blossom end should give slightly to pressure. Avoid those with soft spots—an indication of an overripe melon.

PEAK SEASON: May to September

HANDLE WITH CARE: Ripe cantaloupes should be stored in plastic in the fridge for up to 5 days, after which they begin to lose flavor.

THE PAYOFF: Loads of vitamin C, which may offer protection against having a stroke.

Carrots

PERFECT PICK: Smooth and firm with bright orange color. Avoid those that are bendable or cracked at the base. Bunches with bright green tops still in place are your freshest choice.

PEAK SEASON: Year-round

HANDLE WITH CARE: Store carrots in the crisper in a plastic bag with the greens removed for up to 3 weeks.

THE PAYOFF: Beta-carotene, the source of vitamin A, which helps fight off infections.

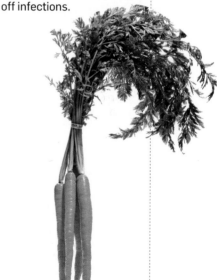

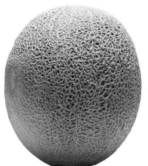

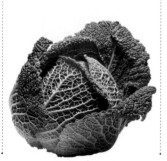

Cauliflower

PERFECT PICK: Ivory white and compact florets with no dark spotting on them or the leaves. The leaves should be verdant and perky.

PEAK SEASON: September to November

HANDLE WITH CARE: Refrigerate, unwashed, in a plastic bag for up to 1 week. If light brown spots develop on the florets, shave off with a paring knife before cooking.

THE PAYOFF: Detoxifying compounds called isothiocyanates, which offer protection against aggressive forms of prostate cancer.

Celery

PERFECT PICK: Solid, tight stalks with only a few, if any, cracks and vivid green, not yellowing leaves. The darker the celery, the stronger the flavor.

PEAK SEASON: Year-round

HANDLE WITH CARE: Sturdy celery can be stored in the fridge in a plastic bag for 2 weeks.

THE PAYOFF: Luteolin, a flavonoid linked to reduced brain inflammation, a risk factor for Alzheimer's.

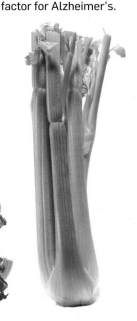

Eggplant

PERFECT PICK: Good weight to them with tight, shiny, wrinkle-free skin. When they're pressed, look for them to be springy, not spongy. The stem and cap should be forest green, not browning.

PEAK SEASON: August to September

HANDLE WITH CARE: Store eggplants in a cool location (not the fridge) for 3 to 5 days. Eggplants are quite sensitive to the cold.

THE PAYOFF: Chlorogenic acid, a phenol antioxidant that scavenges disease-causing free radicals.

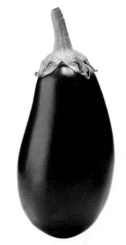

Fennel

PERFECT PICK: Bulbs should be uniform in color, with no browning and a clean, fragrant aroma. Smaller bulbs have a sweeter licoricelike flavor. Leave bulbs with wilted tops, called fronds, behind.

PEAK SEASON: Year-round

HANDLE WITH CARE: Separate the greens and bulbs and keep each, unwashed, in a plastic bag in the refrigerator for 3 to 5 days. Wilted fennel can be revived in ice water.

THE PAYOFF: Anethole, a phytonutrient that may lessen inflammation and cancer risk.

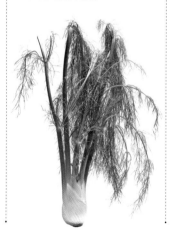

Figs

PERFECT PICK: Plump with deeply rich color; soft but not mushy to the touch. Avoid those with bruises or a sour odor.

PEAK SEASON: July to September

HANDLE WITH CARE: Place fresh figs on a plate lined with a paper towel and eat them as they ripen. They bruise easily, so gentle handling is prudent. They also ripen quickly, so eat within a few days of purchasing. If overripe, simmer with a bit of water, sugar, and balsamic vinegar for a fig jam or sauce.

THE PAYOFF: Phytosterols, which help keep cholesterol levels in check.

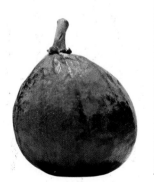

Garlic

PERFECT PICK: The bulb should feel heavy for its size, with tightly closed cloves in the bulb that remain firm when gently pressed. The skin can be pure white or have purple-tinged stripes and should be tight fitting.

PEAK SEASON: Year-round

HANDLE WITH CARE: Place bulbs in a cool, dark, well-ventilated location for up to 1 month.

THE PAYOFF: The cancer-fighting compound allicin, that can also cut down Helicobacter pylori—bacteria responsible for the development of stomach ulcers.

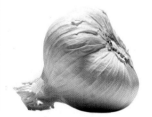

Grapefruit

PERFECT PICK: Opt for a heavy fruit (a sign of juiciness) with thin skin that is a tad responsive to a squeeze. Small imperfections in color and skin surface are not detrimental to the sweet-tart flavor. Yet, avoid any that are very rough or have soft spots. The same criteria apply for oranges.

PEAK SEASON: October to June

HANDLE WITH CARE Store refrigerated for 2 to 3 weeks.

THE PAYOFF: Anticancer lycopene and 120 percent of daily vitamin C needs in 1 cup.

Grapes

PERFECT PICK: Plump, wrinkle free, and firmly attached to the stems. There should be no browning at the stem connection, but a silvery white powder ("bloom") keeps grapes, especially darker ones, fresher longer. Red grapes are best if full-colored with no green tinge. Green grapes with a yellowish hue are the ripest and sweetest.

PEAK SEASON: June to December

HANDLE WITH CARE: Loosely store, unwashed, in a shallow bowl in the fridge for up to 1 week.

THE PAYOFF: Resveratrol, a potent antioxidant in red/purple grapes that offers protection against cardiovascular disease.

Green Beans

PERFECT PICK: Vibrant, smooth surface without any visible withering. They should "snap" when gently bent.

PEAK SEASON: April to October

HANDLE WITH CARE: Refrigerate, unwashed, in an unsealed bag for up to 1 week.

THE PAYOFF: Fiber (4 grams in 1 cup), which can reduce all-cause mortality, according to Dutch researchers.

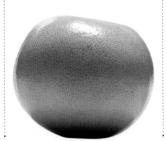

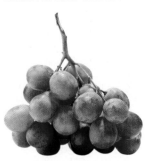

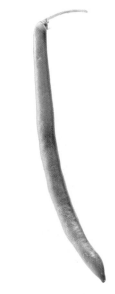

Kale

PERFECT PICK: Dark blue-green color with moist, jaunty leaves. The smaller the leaves, the more tender the kale. Avoid wilted foliage with discolored spots.

PEAK SEASON: Year-round

HANDLE WITH CARE: Peppery kale is best kept in the fridge tightly wrapped in a plastic bag pierced for aeration, where it will last 3 to 4 days.

THE PAYOFF: Lutein, an antioxidant in the retina that protects against vision loss.

Kiwi

PERFECT PICK: A ready-to-devour kiwi will be slightly yielding to the touch. Steer clear of those that are mushy, wrinkled, or bruised with an "off" smell.

PEAK SEASON: June to August

HANDLE WITH CARE: Store at room temperature to ripen. To quicken the process, place in a paper bag with an apple. Once ripened, place in the fridge in a plastic bag for up to 1 week.

THE PAYOFF: Only 56 calories for a large one and 20 percent more of the antioxidant vitamin C than an orange.

Leeks

PERFECT PICK: Green, crisp tops with an unblemished white root end. Gravitate toward small- to medium-size leeks, which are less woody and tough than larger ones. Those with spotted or yellowing leaves should be ignored.

PEAK SEASON: Year-round

HANDLE WITH CARE: Stored loosely wrapped in plastic in the fridge, they'll keep fresh for a week.

THE PAYOFF: Good amounts of eye-protecting lutein, manganese, and vitamins A, C, and K.

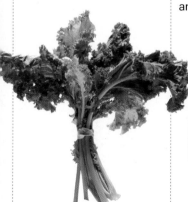

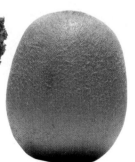

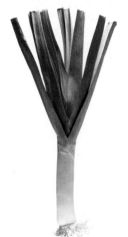

Lemons/Limes

PERFECT PICK: Brightly colored, well-shaped with smooth, thin skin. They should feel sturdy but give ever so slightly when squeezed. Small brown splotches on limes do not affect flavor (although they are a sign of deterioration and those with splotches should be consumed first). Lemons should have no hint of green.

PEAK SEASON: Lemons, year-round; limes, May to October

HANDLE WITH CARE: Store at room temperature, in a dark location, for about 1 week or refrigerate for up to 2 weeks.

THE PAYOFF: Phytonutrient liminoids, which appear to have anticancer, antiviral properties.

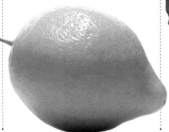

Lettuce: Romaine

PERFECT PICK: The ideal Caesar salad staple has crisp leaves that are free of browning edges and rust spots. The interior leaves are paler in color with more delicate flavor.

PEAK SEASON: Year-round

HANDLE WITH CARE: Refrigerate romaine for 5 to 7 days in a plastic bag.

THE PAYOFF: Vitamin K, which is needed for blood clotting and bone health.

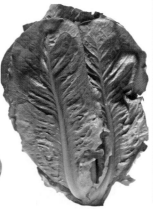

Mangoes

PERFECT PICK: Mangoes to be eaten shortly after purchase should have red skin with splotches of yellow, and the soft flesh should give with gentle pressure. Mangoes for later use will be firmer with a tight skin, a duller color, and green near the stem.

PEAK SEASON: April to August

HANDLE WITH CARE: Ripen at room temperature until fragrant and giving. Ripe mangoes can be stored in the fridge for up to 5 days.

THE PAYOFF: A good showing of vitamins A, B_6, and C, plus fiber.

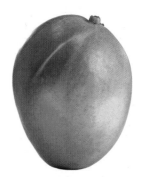

Mushrooms: Button, Cremini

PERFECT PICK: Tightly closed, firm caps that are not slimy or riddled with dark soft spots. Open caps with visible gills indicate consumption should be a priority.

PEAK SEASON: November to April

HANDLE WITH CARE: Place meaty mushrooms on a flat surface, cover with a damp paper towel, and refrigerate for 3 to 5 days.

THE PAYOFF: Immune-boosting, tumor-suppressing complex-carbohydrate polysaccharides.

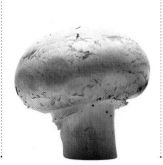

Onions

PERFECT PICK: Nicely shaped with no swelling at the neck and dry, crisp outer skin. Lackluster onions have soft spots, green sprouts, or dark patches.

PEAK SEASON: Year-round

HANDLE WITH CARE: Keep onions in a cool, dark location away from potatoes for 3 to 4 weeks.

THE PAYOFF: GPCS, a peptide shown to reduce bone loss in rats plus the cancer-fighting compound quercetin.

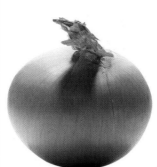

Papayas

PERFECT PICK: Beginning to turn yellow and somewhat-yielding flesh when lightly squeezed. Avoid papayas that are awash in green, have dark spots, or are shriveled. Blotchy papayas often have the most flavor.

PEAK SEASON: Year-round

HANDLE WITH CARE: Once ripe, eat immediately or refrigerate for up to 3 days. Unripe, greener papayas should be ripened at room temperature in a dark setting until yellow blotches appear.

THE PAYOFF: A complete nutritional package, including plenty of fiber and vitamins C, A, E, and K.

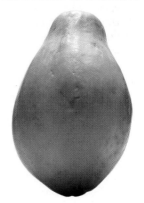

Peaches

PERFECT PICK: Fruity aroma with a background color that is a yellow or a warm cream color. Those destined for immediate consumption yield to gentle pressure along their seams without being too soft. For future intake, opt for those that are firm but not rock hard. Red blush on their cheeks is variety dependent and is not a ripeness indicator.

PEAK SEASON: June to September

HANDLE WITH CARE: Store unripe peaches at room temperature open to air. Once ripe, toss into the refrigerator and consume within 2 to 3 days.

THE PAYOFF: Vitamin C, antioxidant beta-carotene, fiber, and potassium.

Pears

PERFECT PICK: Pleasant fragrance with some softness at the stem end. The skin should be free of bruises, but some brown discoloration (russeting) is fine. Firmer pears are preferable for cooking use.

PEAK SEASON: August to February

HANDLE WITH CARE: Ripen at room temperature in a loosely closed brown paper bag. Refrigerate once they're ripe and consume within a couple days.

THE PAYOFF: Belly-busting fiber and vitamin C—as long as you eat them with the skin on.

Pineapple

PERFECT PICK: Look for vibrant green leaves with a bit of softness and a sweet fragrant aroma from the stem end. Avoid spongy fruit with brown leaves and/or a fermented odor.

PEAK SEASON: March to July

HANDLE WITH CARE: Keep a pineapple with a weak aroma at room temperature for 2 to 3 days until it softens slightly. Then refrigerate for up to 5 days.

THE PAYOFF: Bromelain, compounds with potent anti-inflammatory powers.

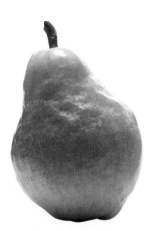

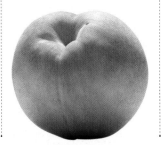

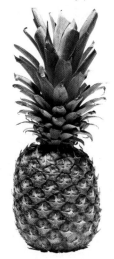

Pomegranates

PERFECT PICK: Pick pomegranates that are weighty for their size with glossy, taut, uncracked skin that is deep red. Gently press the crown end—if a powdery cloud emanates, the fruit is past its prime.

PEAK SEASON: August to December

HANDLE WITH CARE: Stored in a cool, dry location, pomegranates keep fresh for several weeks (up to 2 months in the fridge).

THE PAYOFF: Hefty amounts of antioxidants shown to improve sperm quality, thus boosting fertility.

Potatoes: Sweet, White

PERFECT PICK: Unyielding, with smooth undamaged skin. Avoid if bruised, cracked, or green tinged. Loose spuds tend to be better quality than bagged.

PEAK SEASON: Sweet, September to December; white, year-round

HANDLE WITH CARE: Outside of the fridge, in a cool, dark place separated from onions, potatoes will last for months. Sweet potatoes, however, should be used within a week.

THE PAYOFF: Potassium, which may help preserve muscle mass as we age.

Raspberries

PERFECT PICK: Plump and dry, with good shape and intense, uniform color. Examine the container carefully for mold or juice stains at the bottom. Raspberries with hulls attached are a sign of an underripe, overly tart berry.

PEAK SEASON: May to November

HANDLE WITH CARE: Place highly perishable raspberries, unwashed, on a paper towel in a single layer. Cover with a damp paper towel and refrigerate for no more than 2 to 3 days.

THE PAYOFF: More fiber (8 grams per cup) than any other commonly consumed berry. Plus, the anticancer chemical ellagic acid.

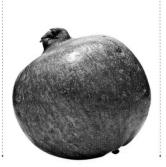

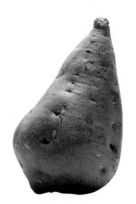

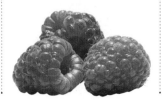

Spinach

PERFECT PICK: Opt for bunches with leaves that are crisp and verdant green, with no spots, yellowing, or limpness. Thin stems are best as thick ones are a sign of more bitter, overgrown leaves.

PEAK SEASON: March to May

HANDLE WITH CARE: Pack unwashed spinach bunches loosely in plastic bags and store in the fridge for 3 to 4 days.

THE PAYOFF: Chromium, which is involved in carbohydrate and fat metabolism and may reduce hunger and food intake.

Squash: Butternut

PERFECT PICK: Should feel dense for its size with a rind that is smooth, hard, uniformly tan, and free of splits. Being able to easily push a fingernail into the rind or scrape bits off indicates an immature, less flavorful squash.

PEAK SEASON: September to November

HANDLE WITH CARE: Butternut should be stored outside the fridge in a cool, well-ventilated, dark place, where it will stay edible for up to 3 months.

THE PAYOFF: Huge amount of vitamin A to ramp up your immune system.

Strawberries

PERFECT PICK: Seek out unblemished berries where the bright red color extends all the way to the stem. Good berries should have a strong fruity smell and be neither soft and mushy nor hard and firm. Smaller strawberries often have more flavor than the oversized megamart versions.

PEAK SEASON: June to August

HANDLE WITH CARE: Place unwashed strawberries in a single layer on a paper towel in a covered container. They will last for 2 to 3 days in the fridge.

THE PAYOFF: The most vitamin C of any of the commonly consumed berries.

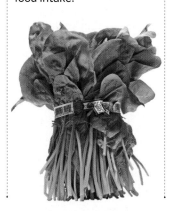

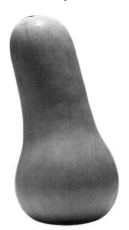

Tomatoes

PERFECT PICK: Go only for heavy tomatoes that are rich in color and free of wrinkles, cracks, bruises, or soft spots. They should have some give, unlike the rock-solid ones bred for transport. Too soft, though, and the tomato is likely overripe and watery. Off-season, select more flavorful smaller versions like Roma and cherry tomatoes.

PEAK SEASON: May to August

HANDLE WITH CARE: Never store tomatoes in the fridge; the cool temps destroy flavor and texture. Keep them at room temperature out of direct sunlight for up to 1 week.

THE PAYOFF: Lycopene, a carotenoid antioxidant that helps fend off prostate cancer.

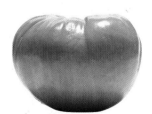

Watermelon

PERFECT PICK: Dense, symmetrical melons that are free of cuts and sunken areas. The rind should appear dull, not shiny, with a rounded creamy-yellow underside that shows where ground ripening took place. A slap should produce a hollow thump.

PEAK SEASON: May to August

HANDLE WITH CARE: Store whole in the fridge for up to 1 week. The cold prevents the flesh from drying out and turning fibrous.

THE PAYOFF: Citrulline, an amino acid that's converted to arginine, which relaxes blood vessels, thus improving blood flow.

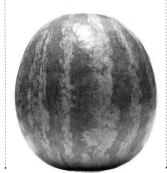

Zucchini

PERFECT PICK: Purchase heavy, tender zucchini with unblemished deep-green skins that are adorned with faint gold specks or strips. Smaller zucchini are sweeter and more flavorful.

PEAK SEASON: June to August

HANDLE WITH CARE: Refrigerate in the crisper in a plastic bag for up to 5 days.

THE PAYOFF: Riboflavin, a B vitamin needed for red blood cell production and for converting carbohydrates to energy.

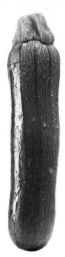

Flavor Savers

Want to boost nutrition and up your culinary game at the same time? Fresh herbs are the perfect prescription.

ROSEMARY

THE BENEFIT: Call it the smart spice. Many people swear by rosemary's ability to increase cognitive functioning, and researchers in California have identified carnosic acid as an active ingredient in rosemary that can offset cognitive degeneration, protect against Alzheimer's, and prevent stroke.

THE BLUEPRINT: Mix together minced rosemary, garlic, lemon juice, and olive oil. Use as a marinade for chicken, steak, pork, and vegetables.

BASIL

THE BENEFIT: Basil is rich in carotenoids, a class of potent antioxidants that mop up cell-damaging free radicals inside the body. This can help prevent a host of unwanted conditions, such as osteoporosis, arthritis, and high cholesterol. Basil also contains oils that prevent bacteria growth and inflammation.

THE BLUEPRINT: Make fresh pesto by blending 2 cups fresh basil leaves with 2 tablespoons pine nuts, 1/4 cup Parmesan, and 1/4 cup olive oil.

PEPPERMINT

THE BENEFIT: Thank the menthol in peppermint for the plant's ability to clear phlegm and mucus from the bronchial tract to facilitate easy breathing. And also for soothing indigestion, gas, menstrual cramps, and irritable bowel syndrome.

THE BLUEPRINT: Brighten up a batch of fruit salad with a squeeze of lime and a handful of chopped mint leaves.

SAGE

THE BENEFIT: Like rosemary, sage is known to strengthen memory. The rosemerinic acid in these plants also works to preserve your body by protecting your cells from oxidative damage and alleviating the effects of asthma and arthritis.

THE BLUEPRINT: For a quick pasta sauce, melt a pat of butter in a pan until it bubbles and turns light brown, then add a handful of whole sage leaves. Toss with store-bought cheese or pumpkin ravioli.

THYME

THE BENEFIT: This tiny herb is extremely rich in iron, which is crucial to your body's ability to transport oxygen. Just 2 teaspoons contain 20 percent of your daily intake. Plus, seasoning with thyme helps protect food from bacterial contamination.

THE BLUEPRINT: *Thyme is the ultimate utility player, pairing great with roasted meat and vegetables, tomato sauce, and scrambled eggs.*

CILANTRO

THE BENEFIT: In mice studies, coriander seeds, from the cilantro plant, encouraged the pancreas to produce more insulin—the hormone that helps shuttle glucose into the cells to be burned as energy. This prevents excess blood sugars from being stored as fat. Cilantro leaves have the same benefits.

THE BLUEPRINT: *Chop up a few tomatoes, an onion, and a jalapeño and mix with a heap of cilantro for a versatile fresh salsa.*

PARSLEY

THE BENEFIT: These dainty leaves are highly concentrated with luteolin, a powerful flavonoid with anti-inflammatory properties. Researchers at the University of Illinois found that luteolin decreased inflammation in the brain, which helps prevent decline in cognitive functions.

THE BLUEPRINT: *Chop a bushel and mix it with bulgur wheat. Add olive oil, lemon juice, and mint and you have a tasty tabbouleh salad to pair with grilled fish or meat.*

TARRAGON

THE BENEFIT: By increasing the secretion of bile and acids into the stomach, tarragon improves gastric efficiency and whets the appetite. Because of this, it's best used early in the meal as an appetizer.

THE BLUEPRINT: *Grill up a mixture of vegetables—onions, peppers, squash, asparagus—and sprinkle them with fresh goat cheese, tarragon, lemon juice, and olive oil.*

OREGANO

THE BENEFIT: A USDA study found that when adjusted for weight, it had four times the antioxidant activity of blueberries. That means big cancer-fighting potential for your next pizza or pasta sauce.

THE BLUEPRINT: *Add equal parts fresh parsley and oregano to a blender and, with the motor running, slowly drizzle in olive or canola oil. Strain and use the infused oil to top grilled fish or chicken or as a dip for toasted bread.*

The Top 10 Herbs & Spices

So how do you know how to stock the healthiest larder? Italian researchers tested several popular herbs and spices for their content of disease-fighting anti-oxidants and then ranked them. Although little-used saffron and bay leaf top the list, the scientists found that you can hardly do better than good ol' black pepper. Here's how the rest stacked up.

Antioxidant capacity (millimoles per kilogram)

Saffron: 53
Bay Leaf: 47.9
Rosemary: 44
Paprika: 40
Black Pepper: 37
Oregano: 30.7
Thyme: 30.5
Sage: 23.4
Basil: 21.8
Mint: 8.8

41

Salad Bar Survival

OIL AND VINEGAR
Your best bet, since you control the ratio. Slick your salad with equal parts oil and vinegar, but be sure to add only enough to lightly coat the greens.

VINAIGRETTES
Now you're getting warmer. Assuming the vinaigrette is based on olive oil, you'll be getting a big dose of mono-unsaturated fats. Even so, since most vinaigrettes abide by the three parts oil to one part vinegar ratio, you're still looking at 100 calories per serving.

CHICKPEAS
Like all legumes, chickpeas bring to the table both protein and fiber, the sultans of satiety. Add to that a healthy dose of antioxidants and you have the makings of a salad-topping superstar.

TUNA
Tuna fish on a salad, as opposed to tuna salad swimming in mayonnaise, will provide protein and heart-helping omega-3 fats without the heavy caloric price.

BLUE CHEESE
Delicious blue cheese comes at a caloric price. If you absolutely must have it, limit yourself to just one meat or other protein and load up on the low-cal veggies we've mentioned.

RANCH/ BLUE CHEESE/ CAESAR
The type of dressing you use is the single most important decision you make at the salad bar. These three represent the most destructive dressings, clocking in around 150 calories and 15 grams of fat per serving.

FRENCH/ CATALINA/ THOUSAND ISLAND
The trio of orange dressings are only marginally less problematic than their white counterparts. That's because they're based on low-grade oils and excess sugar. Expect at least 150 calories for 2 tablespoons of one of these.

CHICKEN
Lean protein is the key to making filling salads, and none come much leaner than chicken. If you're banking on the bird, though, remember that a healthy portion is the size of a deck of cards.

SHREDDED CHEDDAR
The worst cheese at the salad bar. Not only is it high in calories and sodium, but the minuscule shreds tend to bury themselves in the bowl, making portion control a challenge.

BACON
Bacon's gotten some bad press over the years, but one strip has only 40 calories and less than 200 milligrams of sodium. So a pinch of bacon bits is permissible; a handful, however, is not.

RAISINS OR CRAISINS
They're fruit, yes, but they're likely to be coated in sugar. Opt for fresh fruit whenever possible.

CORN
There are too many nutritionally superior vegetables at the salad bar to invest the calories on corn.

FETA CHEESE
A smarter pick than blue, being that feta provides that same crumbly bite for fewer calories and less sodium. Still, only in moderation and only with a colorful crew of vegetables to back it up.

HARD-BOILED EGG
Sick of chicken? Turn to the egg for another great source of protein. Mix with chickpeas, avocado, and red peppers for the closest thing to salad perfection.

Guide

CARROTS
You'll love them for their sweet crunch and their vision-boosting beta-carotene.

MIXED GREENS
The diversity of leaves assures you a bowl filled with a wide variety of nutrients and active compounds. The delicate nature of these little lettuces, though, means they don't hold up as well to heavy ingredients and dressings.

SPINACH
Pick darker greens for the base. Spinach, on the greenest side of the spectrum, has more vitamins and nutrients than can fit on this page, including folate, which helps ward off mental decline, and beta-carotene, which helps protect your eyes and skin.

TOMATOES
Throw some on for lycopene, which has been linked to reduced risk of cancer and heart disease. Tomatoes also provide vitamins A, C, and K.

ICEBERG
The least healthy of common salad bar lettuces. Its high water content makes for a low nutrient density. If you can't skip it, mix it in with darker, healthier greens.

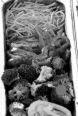

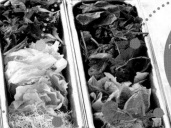

ROMAINE
Compared with iceberg, romaine contains 3 times more folate, 6 times more vitamin C, and 8 times the beta-carotene. Makes a good, sturdy bed for more substantial salads.

ALFALFA SPROUTS
These feathery salad additions have a cache of vitamins unrivaled by nearly anything else you can put in your body. Get in the habit of topping off your salad with these.

AVOCADO
Avocados provide a ton of heart-healthy fats and a rich, creamy bite to any salad. But just because monounsaturated fats are good for your heart doesn't mean they won't still make you fat. Try to choose between avocados and nuts.

CROUTONS
Think of these oil-soaked, enriched flour cubes as salad bar grenades—they'll blow your healthy salad away.

SUNFLOWER SEEDS
One of nature's finest sources of vitamin E, a fat-soluble antioxidant that helps fight inflammation and lower cholesterol.

BEETS
The scarlet crusaders help to lower blood pressure, maintain your memory, and fight cancer.

RED OR YELLOW PEPPERS
Pick red and yellow over green peppers, which contain half the amount of vitamin C. The more colorful your salad, the greater variety of nutrients you'll take in.

BROCCOLI
Vitamin C, fiber, calcium, and few calories. Need we say more?

WALNUTS
Yes, they are absolutely jacked with omega-3s and antioxidants, but they're incredibly dense with calories. Keep it down to a tablespoon or two.

CONSUMPTION KEY
- Feel free to scarf
- Show some restraint
- Avoid at all costs

43

Your Organic Primer

The 5 most important questions about organic food answered

IS ORGANIC WORTH THE EXTRA COST?

The short answer is yes, but it's complicated. As anyone who's been to Whole Foods (endearingly nicknamed Whole Paycheck by detractors and fans alike) can tell you, organic products cost more—according to a 2006 study in the *Journal of Food Science,* an average of 10 percent to 40 percent more for typical items. And while a thinner wallet is a small price to pay for protecting yourself from pesticides and fertilizers, some organic food is almost nutritionally identical to its conventional counterpart. Take, for example, onion: According to an extensive analysis by the Environmental Working Group, it's got the lowest pesticide load of all the 45 fruits and vegetables they tested. Also on the produce honor roll are avocados and asparagus. Really torn on whether or not to spend your hard-earned cash on organic? To see how your favorite fruit fares under the pressures of industrial agriculture, check out the table to the right.

IS ORGANIC BETTER FOR ME?

Yes and no. For every study that says organic food has higher concentrations of nutrients, there's another one that denies it. Researchers at the University of California at Davis found that organic kiwis had substantially more disease-fighting polyphenols than conventionally grown kiwis. Problem is, the same team of researchers found the opposite to be true of organic tomatoes—that organically grown tomatoes may have lower levels of antioxidants.

IS ORGANIC BETTER FOR THE EARTH?

In many respects, this may be the biggest reason to go organic. In fact, the certification criteria of the National Organic Standards Board specifically outline that organic food must be grown with methods that promote biodiversity, minimize pollution, and use cultural, biological, and mechanical methods of agriculture in place of synthetic materials. This goes beyond cutting out pesticides

Should you splurge on organic fruit?

Know which produce is hardest hit by pesticides

Sometimes the extra trip to the farmers' market is worth it. That's because buying organic produce can help you avoid pesticides, which may be more prevalent than you think. Case in point: The Environmental Working Group recently released its list of the pesticide levels of common fruits, ranked from 1 (lowest pesticide load) to 100 (highest load). The rankings, based on nearly 43,000 tests for pesticides conducted by the USDA, are surprising. Take a look:

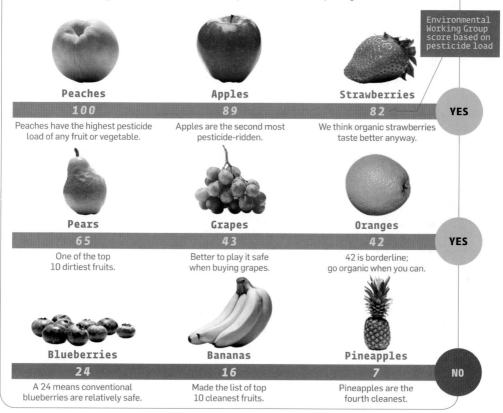

Environmental Working Group score based on pesticide load

Peaches
100
Peaches have the highest pesticide load of any fruit or vegetable.

Apples
89
Apples are the second most pesticide-ridden.

Strawberries
82
We think organic strawberries taste better anyway.

YES

Pears
65
One of the top 10 dirtiest fruits.

Grapes
43
Better to play it safe when buying grapes.

Oranges
42
42 is borderline; go organic when you can.

YES

Blueberries
24
A 24 means conventional blueberries are relatively safe.

Bananas
16
Made the list of top 10 cleanest fruits.

Pineapples
7
Pineapples are the fourth cleanest.

NO

The 21st-Century Produce Aisle

The latest in value-added produce

Far from Frankenfoods, these natural crossbreeds of traditional fruits and vegetables represent the finest in genetic ingenuity. Find these brighter, more nutritious hybrids in a grocery store or farmers' market near you.

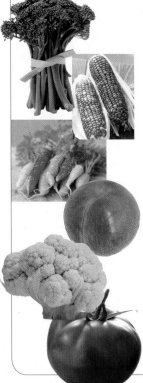

Broccolini
A hybrid of broccoli and Chinese kale
It has a peppery sweet edge that isn't overly bitter. Four stalks boost immunity with 65 percent of your day's vitamin C.

Scarlet Corn
Bred from heirloom corn seeds
Good ol' Midwestern sweet corn raised to have high levels of anthocyanin, a red-hued flavonoid that helps fight disease.

Rainbow Carrots
Kaleidoscopic carrots from heirloom yellow, purple, and red seeds
They're sweeter than the classic. Yellow heaps eye-healthy lutein, while red and purple add cancer-fighting lycopene.

Pluots
A crossbreed of plums and apricots
So sweet yet so good for you. They pack a punch of vision-protecting vitamin A.

Orange Cauliflower
A white variety mixed with an orange-tinted one from Canada
It's creamier, more tender, and bursting with cancer-fighting beta-carotene.

Rosso Bruno Tomatoes
A brown hybrid from a mix of wild varieties
A juicier, richer flavor than typical tomatoes. They also have double the fiber to help keep blood sugar stable.

and fertilizers that can be harmful to people and animals; it involves methods that actually improve the soil—for those agrophiles out there, this means using cover crops, manure, and crop rotations to fertilize; grazing animals on mixed forage pastures; using renewable resources; and conserving soil and water.

But there are two sides to that coin. Researchers at the University of Alberta found that the environmental cost of greenhouse gas emitted to transport organically grown produce was comparable to the environmental cost to transport conventional fruit and vegetables. Your best bet: Head to the farmers' market (find one in your area at ams.usda.gov/farmers-markets). While smaller farms don't always have the means to obtain official organic certification, you'll often find, after chatting with the farmers, that they use sustainable, healthy, environmentally friendly growing and transporting methods that are as good for the planet as they are for your palate.

ARE ORGANIC PACKAGED FOODS BETTER FOR ME?

When it comes to packaged and processed foods, "organic" does not equal "healthy." As Michael Pollan quips in his "eater's manifesto," *In Defense of Food,* "Organic Oreos are not a health food"—they're still a heavily processed cookie filled with fat and sugar, and your body metabolizes organic fat and sugar the same way it does conventional. In fact, some clever companies use organic as a marketing smoke screen, only to load up a cup of yogurt or a box of crackers with unhealthy amounts of organic high-fructose corn syrup (yes, HFCS made from organic corn fits under the FDA guidelines for organic).

DOES ORGANIC TASTE BETTER?

This is perhaps the most important question to discerning cooks the country over. Most chefs and organic enthusiasts would undoubtedly say so, but there is little research to back that up thus far. Part of the problem is the vast array in quality within the organic subset; while an heirloom tomato grown 10 miles from your house by a local farmer may be transcendent, an organic Roma tomato shipped in from China could leave a lot to desire. Your best bet is to find a store or a local farmer with reliably delicious products and stick to it.

Crack the Color Code

Here are the guidelines, courtesy of the USDA

The pigment of produce can provide you with information about its nutritional value. Check out how each of the five different color categories of fruits and vegetables can benefit your health. Then mix and match for a total of five servings every day. One serving equals 1 cup raw or $1/2$ cup cooked.

BLUES AND PURPLES

Blueberries, blackberries, purple grapes, plums, raisins, eggplant. *Benefits:* keep memory sharp and reduce risk of many types of cancer, including prostate cancer

GREENS

Kiwi, honeydew, spinach, broccoli, romaine lettuce, Brussels sprouts, cabbage. *Benefits:* protect bones, teeth, and eyesight

WHITES

Pears, bananas, mushrooms, cauliflower, onions, garlic. *Benefits:* lower LDL cholesterol and reduce risk of heart disease

REDS

Watermelon, strawberries, raspberries, cranberries, cherries, tomatoes, radishes, red apples. *Benefits:* help prevent Alzheimer's disease and improve blood flow to the heart

YELLOWS AND ORANGES

Oranges, grapefruit, peaches, cantaloupe, mangoes, pineapple, squash, carrots. *Benefits:* boost immune system and help prevent eye disease

THE MEAT & FISH COUNTERS

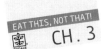

EAT THIS, NOT THAT!
CH. 3

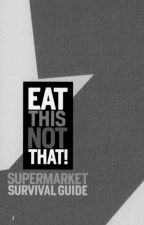

The Means for Staying Lean

Steak or seafood, chicken, pork, or lamb—for most of us, a meal isn't a meal unless it has a little meat to it. The very idea of the American meal—meat and potatoes—centers around the concept of prosperity: We're not really enjoying life, and living the American dream, unless we're tucking into a perfectly seared piece of muscle. (And then we crank up the Elvis, put the top down, and drive off into the night.)

But that relationship with meat—the American idea that the bigger your steak, the finer your life—isn't a healthy one. Many nutritionists consider a serving of meat to be about 3 ounces—about the size of a deck of playing cards. Now think about the last rib eye you ordered from Outback. Did it hang off the edge of the plate the way Jack Nicholson's belly hangs over his belt?

There's the problem: Our idea of what a piece of meat should look like leads to bellies that don't look like they should.

Now, I'm not saying that meat is bad for you—*au contraire,* my friend. Beef, pork, chicken, and fish are all terrific sources of protein, zinc, iron, and B vitamins, and fish provides exceptional amounts of heart-healthy omega-3 fatty acids. Meat is essential for building healthy bones and muscle, providing the body with long-burning energy and self-healing powers. But too much meat—and too much of the wrong kinds of meat—can wreak havoc on our bellies, our blood pressure, and our poor, hard-working arteries. Ground beef, sausage, bacon, and fattier cuts of steak, pork, and lamb can all be high in saturated fats, which raises LDL cholesterol (the bad kind) and increases your risk for heart disease. Processed meats like ham, sausage, and deli slices often contain exorbitant amounts of sodium, another heart-unhealthy risk factor. And even smart choices like poultry, fish, and lean beef can put extra air in your spare tire if they're southern fried in lard or slathered with sugary sauce.

In this chapter, I'll lead you through the smart choices in the meat and seafood aisle. But let's stop first and take a quick look at some of the ways you can make this a healthy harbor. Consider this your Eat Meat Cheat Sheet:

- **Fine-tuna your fish.** Worried about all the scary 11 o'clock news reports about contaminants in seafood? Purdue University researchers found that drinking tea with dinner may block the absorption of any toxins in your tuna. (In fact, if you're worried about toxins like mercury, then get to know your tuna: light chunk tuna is lower in mercury content than albacore.) Other low-mercury fish include shrimp, wild salmon, pollock, and catfish. Avoid higher-contaminant fish like swordfish, shark, king mackerel, marlin, and tilefish.

- **Lower your stroke risk.** The idea that eating meat is bad for your blood pressure is actually a fallacy. Researchers in Australia showed that replacing some of the carbs in your diet with red meat can actually lower blood pressure: Study participants (all of whom had hypertension) exchanged 8 percent of their daily carb calories for the same number of calories from meat—and their blood pressure dropped 4 points in just two months. That translates into as much as a 15 percent lower risk of stroke and a 6 percent lower heart disease risk. But here's the important thing to remember: It's the salt in meat products like sausage—and the extra salt that too many of us dump onto our dishes—that can make eating meat a risk for high blood pressure. Toss that salt over your left shoulder, and you're in safer waters.

- **Burn fat on your barbecue.** A British study found that men who ate a high-protein, low-carb snack after an intense exercise session burned 20 percent more fat than men who drank a sugary beverage. And meat, fish, and poultry are as solid sources of protein as you'll find!

- **Control your hunger with hanger steak.** Another British study found that high-protein foods trigger the release of a hormone that reduces hunger.

- **Bone up on T-bone.** A study in the *Journal of Nutrition* found that a diet high in protein eases bone loss over the course of 12 months relative to a diet high in carbohydrates.

- **Go wild.** Researchers at the University of Wisconsin suggest that people who want to cut down on calories, saturated fat, and cholesterol—while still indulging their inner carnivores—might want to start thinking outside the box, meat-wise. Alternative meat choices like ostrich, venison, bison, and elk typically contain as much protein and iron as traditional fare, but with lower fat and saturated content.

Bottom line? Meat is essential to the American diet—not just for flavor, not just for nutrition, but heck, for tradition. It's part of our food culture. But knowing how to buy it, how much of it to serve, and how to prepare it for maximum health benefits will take you a long way toward keeping your body in fighting trim, while still enjoying your favorite steak-and-potatoes meal.

Be the Alpha of Omegas

Tap into the healing powers of the world's finest fat

You've probably heard a lot over the past few years about omega-3 fatty acids. They've been shown to help cut our risk of heart disease while doing something even more intriguing—some scientists argue that omega-3s actually make our brains function more efficiently. Indeed, some researchers are now beginning to find that societies with the highest levels of omega-3 intake not only have the longest life spans, but they also have the lowest levels of depression and suicide.

So let's see: A nutrient that can make you smarter and happier, as well as healthier? Anybody got a problem with that?

Well, there's one problem: The biggest sources of omega-3s are either cold-water fish like salmon, tuna, mackerel, and sardines or the somewhat obscure flaxseed, which you can grind and add to cereals and salads. But what if you don't like fish, and don't happen to have a bag of flaxseed handy?

Well, there's a great alternative: Grass-fed beef. That means beef that comes from cows that have been allowed to graze at pasture, rather than being fed corn and other grains. Why is this important? Because grass, not corn, is the natural food of cattle. When they're allowed to feed naturally, cattle actually produce monounsaturated fat in their meat; and more of that fat is heart-healthy omega-3 fat. Eating grass-fed livestock also helps the environment, according to the Union of Concerned Scientists: More than 50 percent of the corn grown in the United States goes to animal feed, which can lead to water and air pollution.

Grass-fed beef isn't the same as "organic." Ask your butcher if he carries grass-fed beef, or check out one of many Web sites such as tallgrassbeef.com or panoramameats.com.

The Eat This, Not That! Fish Finder

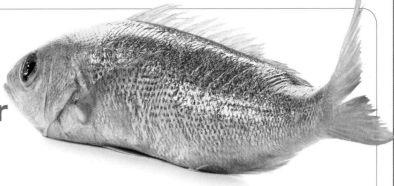

You know you should be eating more fish, but do you know which kind is healthiest? Fresh or frozen, wild or farmed, local or imported: The challenges and nuances of the industrial food complex have made choosing the right fish more complicated than string theory. To simplify matters, we've analyzed a dozen of the most popular fish choices and ranked them from first to worst. Our favorite sea creatures are rich in omega-3s; relatively low in mercury, PCBs, and dioxins; and ecologically sustainable.

HERE'S THE CATCH: A high level of mercury in your fish will undo any heart-health benefit the fish might provide, according to Finnish scientists. That's because mercury impairs arterial flexibility.

FISH	OMEGA-3S (mg per 3 oz serving)	PROTEIN (g per 3 oz serving)	CONTAMINANTS **	ENVIRONMENTAL FRIENDLINESS *
Wild Alaskan Salmon	1,253	18	low	✔✔
Farmed Rainbow Trout	838	18	low	✔✔
Pacific Halibut	444	18	low	✔✔
Farmed Catfish	391	13	medium	✔✔
Farmed Tilapia	185	17	low	✔✔
Yellowfin Tuna	207	20	medium	✔
Farmed Salmon	1,705	17	high	—
Mahimahi	104	16	low	✔
Swordfish	701	17	high	✔
Grouper	227	16	medium	—
Atlantic Cod	166	15	medium	—
Chilean Sea Bass	570	16	medium	—

*Based on each fish's sustainability, as monitored by Monterey Bay Aquarium's Seafood Watch
**Based on Environmental Defense's analysis of mercury and PCB data

Making Sense of Meat

When it comes to picking a protein, you'll find there's a lot to digest before you sit down to eat. Nearly everything you buy at the supermarket comes with a story, a collection of proclamations that are as ambiguous as they are bold. The USDA has its hands full trying to regulate these claims, leaving a gaping hole for manufacturers to fill with fluff. So whether you're planning to feast on fowl or binge on beef, be on high alert when meandering the meat section of your local market. Below are some clues to the most important—and commonly abused—terms in the industry.

BELL & EVANS AIR CHILLED BONELESS, SKINLESS CHICKEN THIGHS

THE CLAIM: "Air chilled"

THE TRUTH: Standard practice for chicken processing includes dunking the birds in a frigid bath to keep bacteria at a minimum. Air-chilling skips the cold-water treatment in favor of placing chickens in cooling chambers. Manufacturers have proclaimed its cleansing superiority, but some studies do not support the theory. Both air chilling and immersion are comparable at reducing bacteria before packaging. Flavor, however, may indeed be superior, as the slow chilling can yield a more tender, less water-saturated chicken.

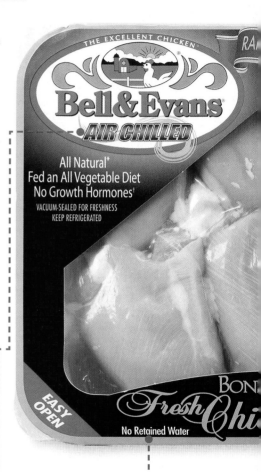

THE EXCELLENT CHICKEN

Bell&Evans

AIR CHILLED

All Natural*
Fed an All Vegetable Diet
No Growth Hormones†

VACUUM-SEALED FOR FRESHNESS
KEEP REFRIGERATED

EASY OPEN

BON
Fresh Chi

No Retained Water

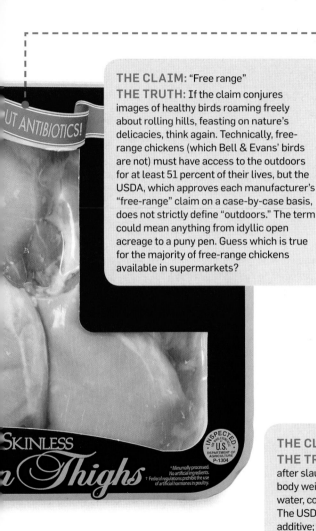

THE CLAIM: "Raised without antibiotics"

THE TRUTH: Unlike the beef industry, big chicken producers have begun to curtail the use of antibiotics in recent years, addressing concerns that bacteria dangerous to humans could be developing drug resistance. Still, Tyson, Perdue, and others have been unable to wean their birds entirely off antibiotics, so this claim is worth something. A couple extra bucks a pound? That's for you to decide.

THE CLAIM: "Free range"

THE TRUTH: If the claim conjures images of healthy birds roaming freely about rolling hills, feasting on nature's delicacies, think again. Technically, free-range chickens (which Bell & Evans' birds are not) must have access to the outdoors for at least 51 percent of their lives, but the USDA, which approves each manufacturer's "free-range" claim on a case-by-case basis, does not strictly define "outdoors." The term could mean anything from idyllic open acreage to a puny pen. Guess which is true for the majority of free-range chickens available in supermarkets?

THE CLAIM: "Organic"

THE TRUTH: The organic chicken industry has grown wildly in recent years. Big Agriculture has seen the potential profit boon of charging an average of 100% percent more for organic chickens, and they have secured the coveted (and often pricey) USDA stamp for what some activists argue are less-than-reputable practices. Look for two certification stamps—the Secretary of Agriculture seal and the USDA Organic seal—confirming that the animals were fed organic feed and had access to pasture. The chicken here was conventionally raised.

THE CLAIM: "No retained water"

THE TRUTH: When immersed in their cold-water baths after slaughter, poultry can absorb up to 8 percent of their body weight, diluting taste and nutrition. On top of added water, conventional poultry can be "enhanced" with salt. The USDA has ignored petitions to consider salt a food additive; in turn, some manufacturers have jacked up the sodium content of their chickens.

NATURE'S PROMISE USDA CHOICE BEEF

THE CLAIM: "No antibiotics administered"

THE TRUTH: Crowded feedlots are breeding grounds for bacteria, illness, and disease, which is one reason why most beef cattle are pumped full of antibiotics. The other reason: corn. Cows' stomachs are designed to digest grass, but with cheap, subsidized corn in high supply, most cows in this country live on a diet consisting of 75 percent corn, 10 percent roughage, and 15 percent animal by-products. To fight off the ulcers, heartburn, and potentially fatal liver abscesses caused by this diet, the beef industry turns to antibiotics. Not only is it bad for the cow, but it's also bad for you: Corn-fed beef is nearly twice as fatty as grass-fed beef and has lower concentrations of omega-3 fatty acids.

THE CLAIM: "No growth stimulants or added hormones"

THE TRUTH: A good thing, to be sure, and decidedly rare in the world of industrial beef. About two-thirds of cows in the United States are treated with growth hormones to speed growth and ultimately maximize profit. While the USDA has deemed growth hormones safe for cattle and the humans who consume them, the European Union (EU) isn't quite so sure. Over the years, researchers have raised concern over possible links between growth hormones and issues like premature development in girls, lower sperm count in men, and breast cancer, but the jury is still out on the final effects. The EU prohibits the use of growth hormones in the raising of cattle and has banned hormone-injected beef since 1988.

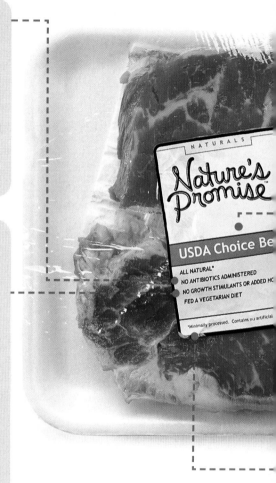

NATURALS

Nature's Promise

USDA Choice Be

ALL NATURAL*
NO ANTIBIOTICS ADMINISTERED
NO GROWTH STIMULANTS OR ADDED HO
FED A VEGETARIAN DIET

*Minimally processed. Contains no artificial

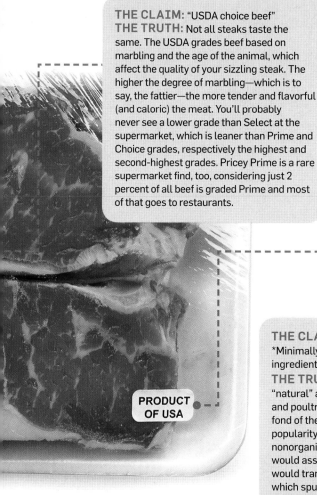

THE CLAIM: "USDA choice beef"
THE TRUTH: Not all steaks taste the same. The USDA grades beef based on marbling and the age of the animal, which affect the quality of your sizzling steak. The higher the degree of marbling—which is to say, the fattier—the more tender and flavorful (and caloric) the meat. You'll probably never see a lower grade than Select at the supermarket, which is leaner than Prime and Choice grades, respectively the highest and second-highest grades. Pricey Prime is a rare supermarket find, too, considering just 2 percent of all beef is graded Prime and most of that goes to restaurants.

THE CLAIM: "Product of the USA"
THE TRUTH: A new required label as of September 2008, this Country of Origin Labeling is designed to inform consumers about the origins of their T-bone. Fish and most produce already required an origin label. For meat, it will indicate where the meat was raised, which sometimes includes multiple countries or an indication that the meat was brought to the United States for slaughter. The food industry fought the legislation for many years to avoid the burden and expense of the extra label, and some importers fear that US consumers may be less likely to buy imported beef labeled as such. Considering we import about 2.5 billion pounds of beef a year, expect vested interests to continue to duke it out.

THE CLAIM: "All natural*
*Minimally processed. Contains no artificial ingredients."
THE TRUTH: You'll see the word "natural" all over meat packaging, both beef and poultry. The meat industry became very fond of the term "natural" with the rising popularity of organic food. Producers of nonorganic foods worried that consumers would assume that conventional meat would translate into "chemical ridden," which spurred almost all meat manufacturers to emblazon their products with the phrase "all natural." It's easy enough, since the USDA doesn't carefully regulate the term—making it all but meaningless to the consumer.

PRODUCT OF USA

57

The Meat Matrix

Not all meat was created equal. From the lean, mean bison sirloin to a heavily marbled dry-aged rib eye, the protein spectrum is populated by a vast array of characters that vary greatly in considerations both culinary and nutritional. To simplify matters a bit, we've put every major cut of beef, pork, poultry, and alternative meats through a rigorous equation to assess its core nutritional value. The criteria? We started with protein-to-fat ratio; because all the calories in your steak or your chicken breast will come from one or the other, you want to choose cuts based on as high a protein-to-fat ratio as possible. Next, we considered the density of 10 essential nutrients commonly found in proteins, from vitamins B_6 and B_{12} to zinc. We rounded out the equation by factoring in saturated fat concentrations and cholesterol levels. The result is a chart that lets you compare chicken breast with duck leg, porterhouse with pork chops, and ultimately allows you to indulge your carnivorous side with a little more strategy.

CHICKEN	TOTAL SCORE
Light meat	7.38
Dark meat	5.99
Giblets	5.97

TURKEY	TOTAL SCORE
Light meat	7.34
Dark meat	5.55
Ground	4.71

OSTRICH	TOTAL SCORE
Top loin	7.09
Ground	5.64

BISON	TOTAL SCORE
Top sirloin	6.75
Grass-fed, ground	4.63

BEEF	TOTAL SCORE
Kidney	6.79
Liver	6.22
Heart	5.82
Round	4.91
Flank	4.73
Top loin	4.25
Grass-fed, ground	4.13
T-bone	3.92
Top sirloin	3.90
Ground 90% lean	3.87
Tongue	3.77
Porterhouse	3.75
Brisket, whole	3.71
Rib eye, small end	3.60
Tenderloin	3.45
Ground 80% lean	3.38
Rib roast, whole	3.20

PORK	TOTAL SCORE
Tenderloin	6.90
Top loin/loin chops	5.92
Center loin/center rib	5.39
Sirloin	5.13
Ribs	4.72
Spareribs	4.09
Bladechops/roast	4.02
Ham, whole	3.24
Bacon (cured)	3.03

DUCK	TOTAL SCORE
Domesticated	5.22

LAMB	TOTAL SCORE
Australian, sirloin chops	4.95
Ground	3.15

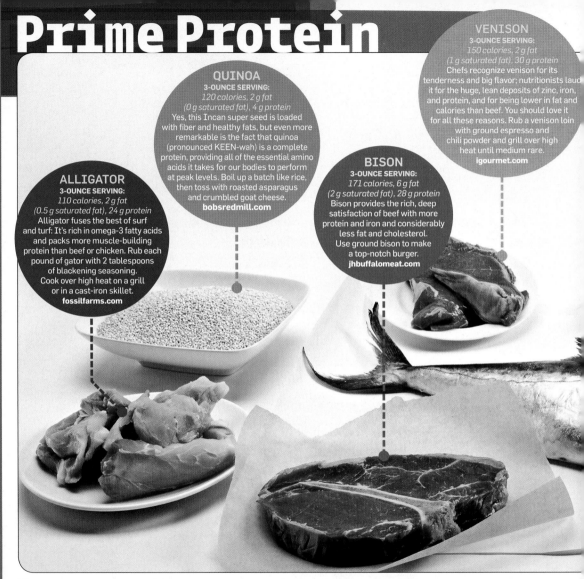

Prime Protein

QUINOA
3-OUNCE SERVING:
*120 calories, 2 g fat
(0 g saturated fat), 4 g protein*
Yes, this Incan super seed is loaded with fiber and healthy fats, but even more remarkable is the fact that quinoa (pronounced KEEN-wah) is a complete protein, providing all of the essential amino acids it takes for our bodies to perform at peak levels. Boil up a batch like rice, then toss with roasted asparagus and crumbled goat cheese.
bobsredmill.com

VENISON
3-OUNCE SERVING:
*150 calories, 2 g fat
(1 g saturated fat), 30 g protein*
Chefs recognize venison for its tenderness and big flavor; nutritionists laud it for the huge, lean deposits of zinc, iron, and protein, and for being lower in fat and calories than beef. You should love it for all these reasons. Rub a venison loin with ground espresso and chili powder and grill over high heat until medium rare.
igourmet.com

ALLIGATOR
3-OUNCE SERVING:
*110 calories, 2 g fat
(0.5 g saturated fat), 24 g protein*
Alligator fuses the best of surf and turf: It's rich in omega-3 fatty acids and packs more muscle-building protein than beef or chicken. Rub each pound of gator with 2 tablespoons of blackening seasoning. Cook over high heat on a grill or in a cast-iron skillet.
fossilfarms.com

BISON
3-OUNCE SERVING:
*171 calories, 6 g fat
(2 g saturated fat), 28 g protein*
Bison provides the rich, deep satisfaction of beef with more protein and iron and considerably less fat and cholesterol. Use ground bison to make a top-notch burger.
jhbuffalomeat.com

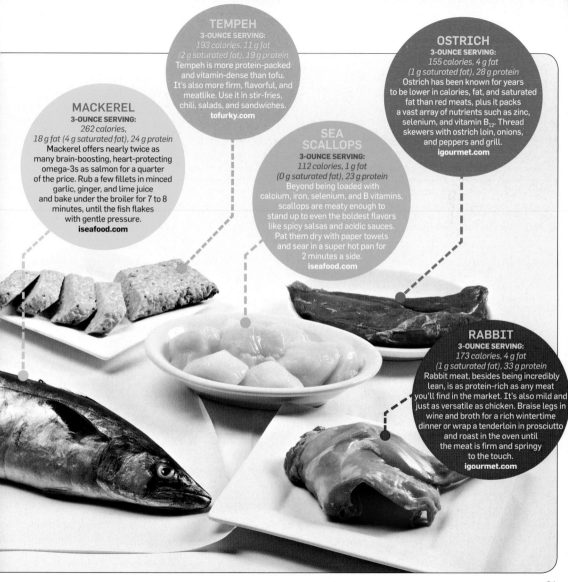

TEMPEH
3-OUNCE SERVING:
*193 calories, 11 g fat
(2 g saturated fat), 19 g protein*
Tempeh is more protein-packed
and vitamin-dense than tofu.
It's also more firm, flavorful, and
meatlike. Use it in stir-fries,
chili, salads, and sandwiches.
tofurky.com

OSTRICH
3-OUNCE SERVING:
*155 calories, 4 g fat
(1 g saturated fat), 28 g protein*
Ostrich has been known for years
to be lower in calories, fat, and saturated
fat than red meats, plus it packs
a vast array of nutrients such as zinc,
selenium, and vitamin B_{12}. Thread
skewers with ostrich loin, onions,
and peppers and grill.
igourmet.com

MACKEREL
3-OUNCE SERVING:
*262 calories,
18 g fat (4 g saturated fat), 24 g protein*
Mackerel offers nearly twice as
many brain-boosting, heart-protecting
omega-3s as salmon for a quarter
of the price. Rub a few fillets in minced
garlic, ginger, and lime juice
and bake under the broiler for 7 to 8
minutes, until the fish flakes
with gentle pressure.
iseafood.com

SEA SCALLOPS
3-OUNCE SERVING:
*112 calories, 1 g fat
(0 g saturated fat), 23 g protein*
Beyond being loaded with
calcium, iron, selenium, and B vitamins,
scallops are meaty enough to
stand up to even the boldest flavors
like spicy salsas and acidic sauces.
Pat them dry with paper towels
and sear in a super hot pan for
2 minutes a side.
iseafood.com

RABBIT
3-OUNCE SERVING:
*173 calories, 4 g fat
(1 g saturated fat), 33 g protein*
Rabbit meat, besides being incredibly
lean, is as protein-rich as any meat
you'll find in the market. It's also mild and
just as versatile as chicken. Braise legs in
wine and broth for a rich wintertime
dinner or wrap a tenderloin in prosciutto
and roast in the oven until
the meat is firm and springy
to the touch.
igourmet.com

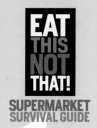

Chapter 4 **THE**
REFRIGERATOR

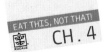

EAT THIS, NOT THAT!

CH. 4

Keep Your Cool

In researching *Eat This, Not That! Supermarket Survival Guide,* I came across something quite unexpected. Miraculous, you might say. A secret formula—a potion, an elixir, a witch's brew—that can do all of the following:

✔ **Build muscle, increase bone density, and help fight arthritis and injury.**

✔ **Protect you from heart disease, cancer, and diabetes.**

✔ **Tell your body when to store fat—and when to burn it for energy.**

✔ **Protect your body from bacteria and viruses.**

Wow. One magic potion that keeps you lean, strong, healthy, and energized? What is this incredible concoction? Simple: It's a sneaky combination of calcium and protein. And the very best place to get it is in the dairy case.

In fact, the very act of ingesting and digesting dairy foods can actually burn away calories. See, food contains energy in the form of chemical bonds, but your body can't use that energy until it first breaks those bonds. Scientists call the energy that we expend breaking those bonds the "thermic effect"—basically, the calorie-burning effect of digestion. And your body expends almost twice as many calories trying to digest protein as it does carbohydrates. In fact, when Arizona State University researchers compared the benefits of a high-protein diet with those of a high-carbohydrate diet, they found that people who ate a high-protein diet burned more than twice as many calories in the hours after their meals as those eating primarily carbs.

Now check out this real-world test: In a Danish study, researchers put 65 subjects on either a low-protein diet, a high-protein diet, or no diet. While the low-protein dieters lost an average of 11 pounds, the high-protein dieters lost an average of 20 pounds. But the more amazing statistic is this: The high-protein dieters lost twice as much abdominal fat! (One reason may be that a high-protein diet helps your body control its levels of cortisol, a stress hormone that directs fat toward the belly.)

The great news for those who love cheese, milk, yogurt, and all things dairy is that these foods come packed not only with protein but with calcium—another essential nutrient that does many of the things protein does. For example, researchers at Harvard Medical School showed that those who ate three servings of dairy a day were 60 percent less likely to be overweight! And in studies at the University of Tennessee, researchers put women on diets that were 500 calories a day less than they were used to eating. Did everyone lose weight? Of course—about a pound of fat a week. But when the researchers then put a second set of people on the same diet but added dairy to their meals, their fat loss doubled, to 2 pounds a week.

Let's say that again: You can eat the same amount of calories but double your fat loss, if you just eat enough dairy. And you can't dupli-cate the effects just by taking a calcium supplement—though good

for bone building and other bodily functions, supplements don't have the same effect as dairy—because your body doesn't burn enough calories digesting them.

Besides, there's no more affordable way to get protein and calcium into your diet than with dairy, especially good old-fashioned milk, according to a study in the *Journal of the American Dietetic Association*. What other miracles can happen in the dairy case?

● **You can beat diabetes.** Nutrients in dairy products, including calcium, may reduce the risk of insulin resistance syndrome, a precursor to diabetes, according to a research review in the *Journal of the American College of Nutrition.*

● **You can cut your risk of cancer.** Just one glass of milk per day decreases the risk of colorectal cancer by 15 percent, according to a study in the *Journal of the National Cancer Institute.*

● **You can reduce your cravings.** Cheese and eggs are both about 50 percent more satiating than white bread, according to a study in the

European Journal of Clinical Nutrition. That's in part because the protein in these foods takes longer to digest—keeping you fuller, longer.

● **You can live a healthier, happier life.** And you can do it by picking the right (read, low-fat) dairy products. No kidding: A 2002 study found that people who drink reduced-fat or skim milk take in significantly higher levels of fat-soluble vitamins, water-soluble vitamins, minerals, and dietary fiber than those who drink whole milk.

Ready to buy stock in a dairy farm? Well, not so fast: Picking the right foods from the dairy case can

Eat This, Not That Self-Test
Are you lactose intolerant?

If you think milk upsets your stomach, perhaps you should try to prove it. Researchers at the Veterans Administration Medical Center in Minneapolis found that people who described themselves as "severely lactose intolerant" responded no differently to 2 cups of milk than to a placebo beverage. Scientists think that people who've noticed discomfort after consuming dairy often eliminate it altogether, even though small amounts may not produce the same symptoms.

Step 1
Ask a friend to buy either regular or lactose-free milk and pour it into a container, labeled A.

Step 2
For 1 week, drink 2 cups a day from the container on an empty stomach and avoid all other dairy. Record any symptoms of intestinal discomfort.

Step 3
Discontinue container A for at least 1 day.

Step 4
Repeat Steps 1 and 2, but with the type of milk not used previously using a container marked B.

Step 5
Compare the results from each container.

No difference?
You aren't lactose intolerant. However, if you tested positive, you can use these strategies for better digestion of dairy products.

● **Limit your milk intake to 1 cup at a time**
And drink it with food, which slows the absorption of lactose and helps alleviate side effects.

● **Have more cheese**
It contains very little lactose. (Hint: The fewer carbohydrates a dairy product has, the less lactose it contains.)

● **Try kefir**
Ohio State University scientists found that this fermented milk beverage improves lactose digestion. Yogurt may provide similar benefits.

be a little trickier than it seems. You already know to buy reduced-fat milk and yogurt whenever possible. But did you know that some dairy products can come loaded with sugar? (Read the labels of some of those fruit-on-the-bottom yogurts if you don't believe me. They should be called "fat-on-your-bottom" yogurts!) And did you know that some of those margarine sticks claiming "reduced saturated fat" are actually worse for you than eating real butter? Just like every other aisle in the supermarket, things aren't always what they seem in the refrigerated section of your go-to grocer. The difference between a smart choice and a poor one can mean hundreds of calories per serving, which in turn could translate into dozens of extra pounds over the course of the year.

We've taken a careful spin through this section, reading labels and counting calories until our vision went blurry, all in the name of helping you make the smartest picks possible. That's why this chapter of *EAT THIS, NOT THAT! SUPERMARKET SURVIVAL GUIDE* is essential for your health, happiness—and pocketbook.

How to Use This Book

The chapters to come will walk you page by page, product by product through nearly 75 common categories in the supermarket—everything from wholesome cereals to chocolate bars. We've highlighted on these pages some of the best and worst options you'll find in the aisles, including what we consider to be the worst offenders—those packaged goods masquerading as health food that are actually damaging to your waistline and your well-being.

The product matchups that follow focus on comparisons between similar foods (strawberry yogurt versus strawberry yogurt, peanut butter cookies versus peanut butter cookies) because we know that you have specific tastes, and that you might not be willing to swap out, say, coffee ice cream for mango sorbet. With 50,000 products to choose from, we truly believe you don't have to give up your favorite types of foods in order to eat better and lose weight. Instead, you just need to seek out the healthiest versions of each, which is what this book does. Use the color-coded boxes to help you find the relevant comparisons.

Happy shopping!

The Perfect Refrigerator

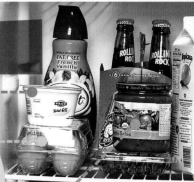

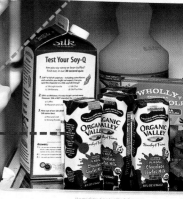

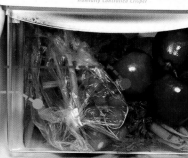

FAGE 0% PLAIN YOGURT

1 CUP: *120 calories, 0 g fat, 9 g sugars*

The watery whey is removed from this Greek-style yogurt, giving it a creamy texture and a huge dose of protein. **POWER PLAY:** Mix a cup of yogurt with minced garlic, fresh parsley, and a glug of olive oil for a healthy sauce for grilled protein.

EGGLAND'S BEST EGGS

1 EGG: *70 calories, 4 g fat (1 g saturated), 6 g protein, 0 g carbs*

No longer food taboo, protein-dense eggs should be a staple in every fridge. A recent study from Thailand found that eggs actually help raise good HDL cholesterol. **POWER PLAY:** Hard-boil half a dozen eggs at a time so they're on hand for snacks or to give salads a protein lift. They'll keep in the fridge for a week.

MUIR GLEN ORGANIC GARLIC CILANTRO SALSA

2 TABLESPOONS: *10 calories, 0 g fat*
The best-tasting 10 calories in the market. Bonus: Organic jarred tomatoes have been proven to have higher levels of the cancer-fighting antioxidant lycopene. **POWER PLAY:** Try three salsa swaps at the table: on baked potatoes (instead of sour cream), on eggs (instead of ketchup), and on salad (instead of ranch).

ORGANIC VALLEY CHOCOLATE LOWFAT MILK

1 CUP: *160 calories, 2.5 g fat (1.5 g sat), 9 g protein, 27 g carbs*

Meet your new postworkout beverage. Researchers found that not only does milk do a better job rehydrating the body than water or sports drinks but that chocolate milk repairs muscles 40 percent faster than plain milk.

RED DELICIOUS APPLES

1 MEDIUM APPLE: *95 calories, 4 g fiber*

USDA researchers found that Red Delicious apples have a higher anti-oxidant capacity than other apples. **POWER PLAY:** Leave the peeler in the drawer. The skin contains a good chunk of apple's antioxidants and fiber.

BROCCOLI SPROUTS

½ CUP: *16 calories, 0 g fat*

These diminutive broccoli sprouts have 20 times more cancer-fighting sulforaphane than their grown-up counterparts. **POWER PLAY:** Add to sandwiches, scrambled eggs, salads, and soups.

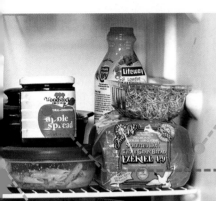

FOOD FOR LIFE 100% WHOLE GRAIN EZEKIEL 4:9 BREAD

1 SLICE: *80 calories, 0.5 g fat (0 g saturated), 4 g protein, 3 g fiber*

Sprouted grains and lentils produce a bread with a lower impact on blood sugar as well as more protein and vitamins than its whole-grain counterparts.
POWER PLAY: Toast slices and top with peanut butter and sliced banana for a solid start to your day.

ORGANIC APPLE BUTTER

1 TABLESPOON: *20 calories, 0 g fat, 4 g sugars*

A 100 percent apple spread that gives your toast a fruity bite without the sugar found in most jams.
POWER PLAY: Swirl into cottage cheese with a sprinkle of cinnamon.

RUBY RED GRAPEFRUIT JUICE

1 CUP: *90 calories, 22 g sugars*

University of Florida researchers determined that red grapefruit juice contains more nutrients per calorie than grape and apple juices. It also contains less sugar than OJ.
POWER PLAY: For a light vinaigrette, mix 2 tablespoons grapefruit juice with 1 tablespoon balsamic vinegar, and ¼ cup avocado oil.

WILD SALMON

4-OUNCE FILLET: *200 calories, 8 g fat (1 g saturated), 31 g protein*

One of the world's healthiest foods, with lots of lean protein and sky-high concentrations of omega-3s.
POWER PLAY: Place a 4-ounce fillet, some cherry tomatoes, and sliced fennel in the center of a foil sheet. Top with olive oil, salt, and pepper and seal. Bake at 400°F for 12 minutes.

RED BELL PEPPERS

1 CUP: *46 calories, 0 g fat, 1 g protein, 9 g carbs (3 g fiber)*

Red peppers supply more cancer-fighting lycopene and 60 percent extra immunity-boosting vitamin C than their green kin.
POWER PLAY: Roasting concentrates the pepper's flavor. After charring on the grill or under the broiler, put them in a sealed paper bag to sweat. When they cool, the skin will come off easily.

KALE

PER CUP: *34 calories, 0 g fat, 2 g protein, 1 g fiber*

For 18 calories a serving you get monster doses of vitamins like A, C, and K and a rush of phytonutrients.
POWER PLAY: Sauté kale over medium heat with olive oil, sliced garlic, and a pinch of red chile flakes. Finish with a splash of balsamic vinegar before serving.

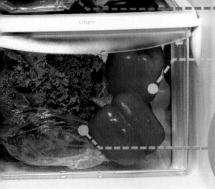

7 Life-Changing Cheeses

You don't think cheese can change your life? That's probably because you're spending too much time eating the same shredded blends and processed plastic stuff you've been devouring for years. Beyond the Jack, Cheddar, and Swiss is a whole world of diverse, delicious cheese that will satisfy more than just your taste buds. With a great combination of protein and fat, an ounce of cheese makes an incredibly satiating snack. And if you're worried about your cholesterol, chew on this: Danish scientists found that when men ate a whopping 10 daily 1-ounce servings of full-fat cheese for 3 weeks, their LDL (bad) cholesterol didn't budge. Which isn't to say you should live on the stuff—just that you don't need to fear it. Try one of these seven beauties for a taste of cheese's full potential.

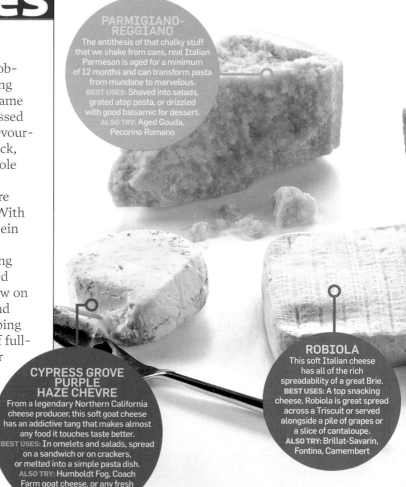

PARMIGIANO-REGGIANO
The antithesis of that chalky stuff that we shake from cans, real Italian Parmesan is aged for a minimum of 12 months and can transform pasta from mundane to marvelous.
BEST USES: Shaved into salads, grated atop pasta, or drizzled with good balsamic for dessert.
ALSO TRY: Aged Gouda, Pecorino Romano

ROBIOLA
This soft Italian cheese has all of the rich spreadability of a great Brie.
BEST USES: A top snacking cheese, Robiola is great spread across a Triscuit or served alongside a pile of grapes or a slice of cantaloupe.
ALSO TRY: Brillat-Savarin, Fontina, Camembert

CYPRESS GROVE PURPLE HAZE CHEVRE
From a legendary Northern California cheese producer, this soft goat cheese has an addictive tang that makes almost any food it touches taste better.
BEST USES: In omelets and salads, spread on a sandwich or on crackers, or melted into a simple pasta dish.
ALSO TRY: Humboldt Fog, Coach Farm goat cheese, or any fresh goat cheese

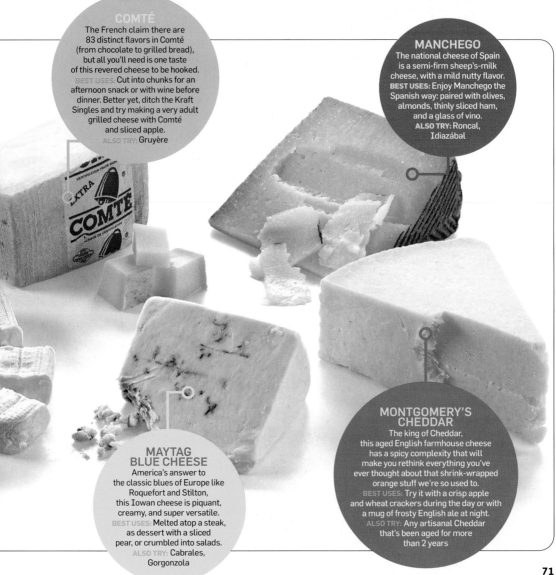

COMTÉ

The French claim there are 83 distinct flavors in Comté (from chocolate to grilled bread), but all you'll need is one taste of this revered cheese to be hooked. **BEST USES:** Cut into chunks for an afternoon snack or with wine before dinner. Better yet, ditch the Kraft Singles and try making a very adult grilled cheese with Comté and sliced apple.
ALSO TRY: Gruyère

MANCHEGO

The national cheese of Spain is a semi-firm sheep's-milk cheese, with a mild nutty flavor. **BEST USES:** Enjoy Manchego the Spanish way: paired with olives, almonds, thinly sliced ham, and a glass of vino.
ALSO TRY: Roncal, Idiazábal

MAYTAG BLUE CHEESE

America's answer to the classic blues of Europe like Roquefort and Stilton, this Iowan cheese is piquant, creamy, and super versatile. **BEST USES:** Melted atop a steak, as dessert with a sliced pear, or crumbled into salads.
ALSO TRY: Cabrales, Gorgonzola

MONTGOMERY'S CHEDDAR

The king of Cheddar, this aged English farmhouse cheese has a spicy complexity that will make you rethink everything you've ever thought about that shrink-wrapped orange stuff we're so used to. **BEST USES:** Try it with a crisp apple and wheat crackers during the day or with a mug of frosty English ale at night.
ALSO TRY: Any artisanal Cheddar that's been aged for more than 2 years

71

The Ultimate Sandwich Selector

Hoagies, heroes, grinders, subs, po'boys, zeppelins: Whatever you call them in your town, sandwiches are undeniably an American food. We may not lay claim to their invention (that vaunted distinction may belong to England's Earl of Sandwich), but we've done plenty to advance them over the years. Problem is, we've done plenty to distort them, too, turning humble creations into caloric catastrophes (see Quizno's 1,680-calorie Tuna Melt for reference) weighted down by reckless condiments, bloated breads, and an excess of ill-chosen toppings.

As our contribution to America's long-standing love affair with the sandwich, we've broken the sub down into its many components, laying out the nutritional goods on the meat, produce, cheese, and condiments you're most likely to squeeze between two slices of bread. We've even thrown in a few surprises. Consider this a blueprint for a tastier, more nutritious future.

Super Sandwiches

THE SUNRISE SAMMIE
...for energy and weight loss

Whole wheat English muffin, ham, romaine, tomato, cheddar, egg

Studies show that people who choose quality protein over refined carbohydrates for breakfast are able to burn 65 percent more calories and maintain higher levels of energy throughout the day.

THE GLADIATOR
...for muscle power

Whole-grain pita, roast beef, romaine, tomato, fresh mozz, hummus

This baby is bursting at the seams with lean protein, with the chicken, chickpeas, and mozzarella completing the trifecta. Not only is this a good postworkout option, it's great at any time of day for firing up your metabolism.

THE GOBBLER
...for cancer-fighting

Rye, avocado, turkey, Brie, arugula, cranberry sauce

Can sandwiches cure cancer? Of course not, but few fruits pack more antioxidants than cranberries, and with a dose of cell-protecting flavonols from the pile of arugula, this nutrient-dense creation certainly can't hurt the cause.

THE EINSTEIN
...for brain power

Sprouted wheat, smoked salmon, red onion, avocado, goat cheese, pesto

Omega-3 fatty acids (from the salmon) and anthocyanidins (from the red onion) are pivotal in both building and preserving our frazzled minds.

THE SURE SHOT
...for nerves

Rye, turkey, egg, arugula, red onion, grainy mustard

Big doses of magnesium from the rye and mustard, along with the calming powers of tryptophan from the turkey and egg, make for a seriously soothing sandwich.

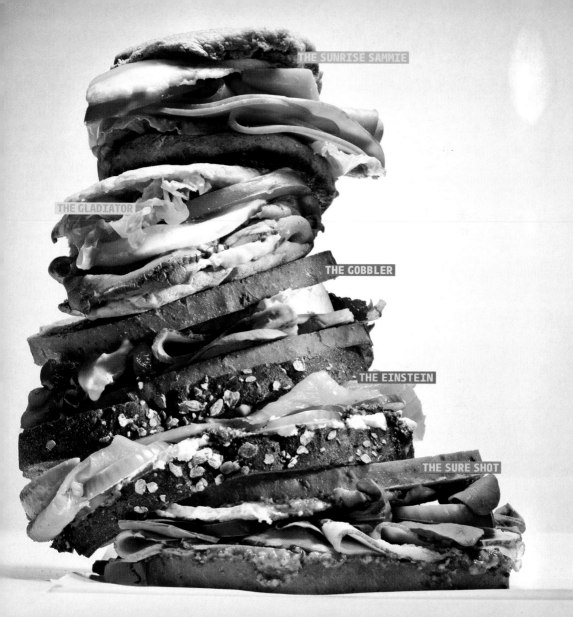

THE SUNRISE SAMMIE

THE GLADIATOR

THE GOBBLER

THE EINSTEIN

THE SURE SHOT

The Foundation

(Two 35-gram slices unless otherwise noted)

WHOLE-GRAIN PITA

(small, 28-gram pita)
74 calories
1 g fat (0 g saturated)
2 g fiber
15.5 g carbohydrates
3 g protein
149 mg sodium

What's not to love? The pita holds up well in the fiber test, and it's prime for stuffing, like a delicious piñata of meat, cheese, and veggies. It elevates your meal from a mere sandwich to a hearty salad in a thin-walled bread bowl. In the spirit of its Middle Eastern heritage, the pita cries out for hummus, cucumbers, feta, and thick-sliced tomatoes. Meat optional.

WHOLE WHEAT

182 calories
2.5 g fat (0.5 g saturated)
5 g fiber
38 g carbohydrates
7.5 g protein
264 mg sodium

High-quality wheat bread has 2 grams of fiber per ounce, which is why bread makes the single biggest fiber contribution to the American diet. Stick to 100 percent whole wheat (and make sure it says just that on the package). You'd have to eat nearly an entire loaf of white bread to earn the fiber of a few slices of 100 percent whole wheat. Wheat's mild flavor goes well with virtually any sandwich you can dream up.

SPROUTED WHEAT

160 calories
2 g fat (0 g saturated)
6 g fiber
34.5 g carbohydrates
10 g protein
330 mg sodium

No longer a loaf confined to communes and neo-hippie enclaves, even supermarkets outside of Berkeley are opening up shelf space to meet the growing demand for this bread. Thank the sprouted wheat berry for its edge over normal whole wheat in fiber, protein, and vitamins B, C, and E. The intense nuttiness pairs perfectly with roasted meats like turkey and beef and sharper spreads like grainy mustard and hummus.

FRENCH ROLL

(75-gram roll)
207 calories
3 g fat (1 g saturated)
2.5 g fiber
37.5 g carbohydrates
7 g protein
445 mg sodium

When it comes to rolls—Italian rolls, dinner rolls, hero rolls—size really does matter. If you don't keep the portions under control, these things can easily stretch to more than 300 calories. The saving grace for all this refined flour is that government mandates require it to be fortified with iron and B vitamins. Still, that's not enough to justify any regular role in your general sandwich rotation.

CIABATTA ROLL

(69-gram roll)
153 calories
2 g fat (0 g saturated)
1.5 g fiber
29 g carbohydrates
5.5 g protein
453 mg sodium

Ciabatta, the loaf named after an Italian slipper, is popping up all over the country in the form of paninis. But tread lightly around this trend, for this bread is made from refined flour and thus offers very little in the way of fiber or discernible nutrition. As with the French roll, if you're going to go ciabatta, shoot for more lean-meat and vegetables and less bread.

RYE

180 calories
2.5 g fat (0.5 g saturated)
3 g fiber
34 g carbohydrates
6 g protein
462 mg sodium

The obvious pairing for rye is pastrami, but so long as you're the chef, don't be afraid to recruit this sharp-and-sour flavor upgrade for any sandwich. Rye's distinctive bite is accompanied by a good amount of fiber and a smattering of micronutrients such as manganese, selenium, and tryptophan, an essential amino acid that helps your brain regulate serotonin levels.

SOURDOUGH

(73-gram roll)
202 calories
1.5 g fat (0.5 g saturated)
1.5 g fiber
39.5 g carbohydrates
8 g protein
454 mg sodium

Unlike rye, which is a whole grain, sourdough is refined wheat flavored with a bacteria culture—hence the lack of fiber. Eating a big hunk of this stuff has a similar effect on your blood sugar to scarfing a doughnut, so if you just can't imagine a BLT without a few sourdough slices, be sure to load it up with protein and fiber from other sources.

100% WHOLE WHEAT ENGLISH MUFFIN

(57-gram muffin)
127 calories
1 g fat (0 g saturated)
2.5 g fiber
25.5 g carbohydrates
5 g protein
315 mg sodium

This unusual suspect may be the healthiest bread you're not using to build sandwiches. Sure, it has its place on the breakfast table, but its compact size and solid fiber count make it a perfect bookend to sliced ham and cheddar or turkey and avocado. Or use it as a healthy home to America's most famous sandwich: the cheeseburger.

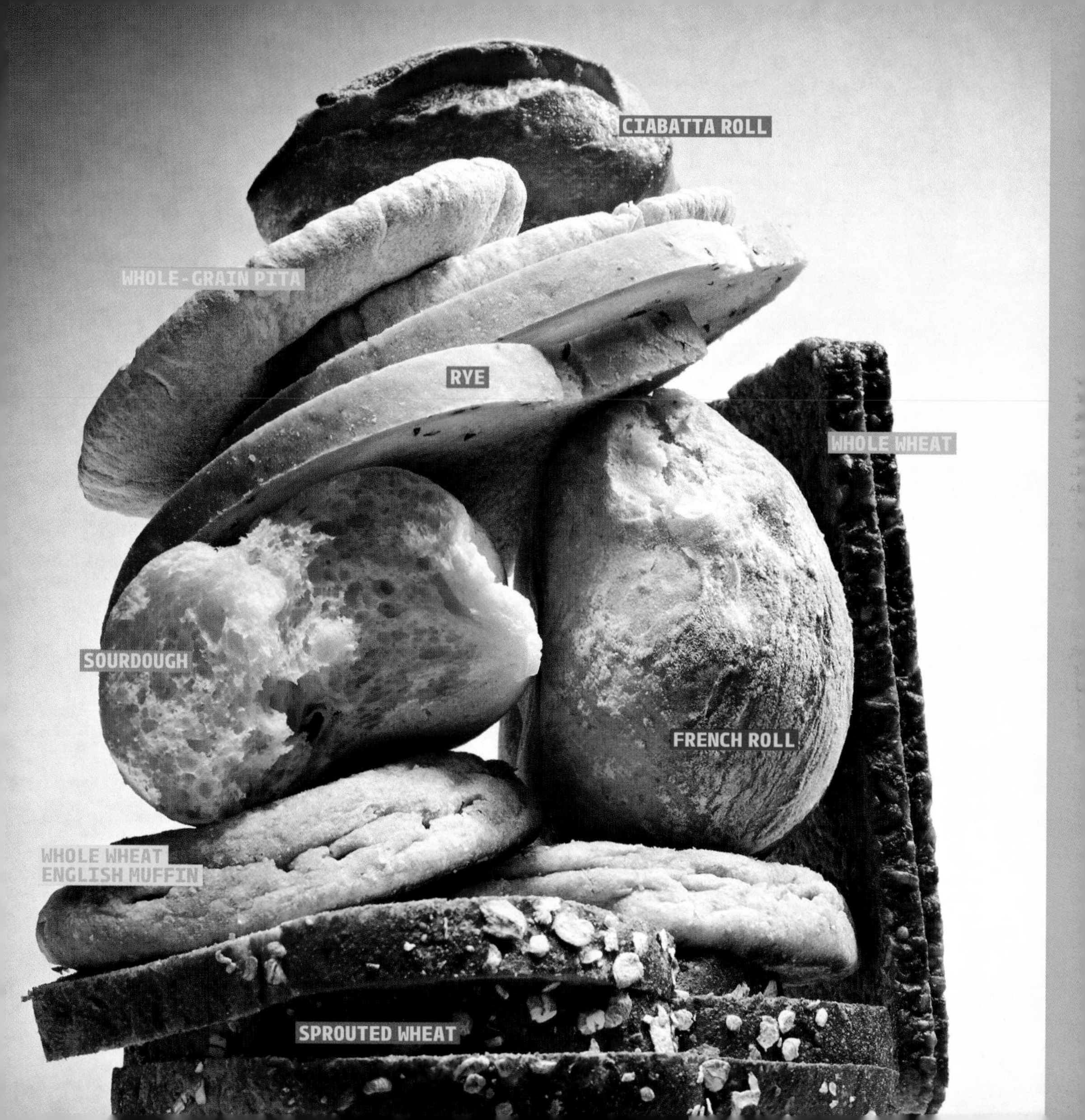

CIABATTA ROLL

WHOLE-GRAIN PITA

RYE

WHOLE WHEAT

SOURDOUGH

FRENCH ROLL

WHOLE WHEAT
ENGLISH MUFFIN

SPROUTED WHEAT

The Filling

(48-gram servings unless otherwise noted)

TURKEY BREAST

54 calories
1.5 g fat (0 g saturated)
6.5 g protein
576 mg sodium

Why do people love turkey? Well, aside from the fact that it's lean and delicious, it's replete with a serotonin-promoting amino acid, tryptophan (chicken has this, too). A 48-gram serving provides about half your day's value, which helps you fight off depression and anxiety while regulating appetite and sleep cycles. Take your sandwich to the next level by using fresh roasted turkey (instead of the processed kinds), available in many supermarket deli cases across the country.

GRILLED CHICKEN BREAST

(48 grams)
55 calories
1.5 g fat (0.5 g saturated)
10.5 g protein
285 mg sodium

In the nutritional pecking order, grilled chicken reigns supreme. Skip the processed chicken chunks in the supermarket and make up a batch of fresh grilled chicken at home. Rub a pound of boneless, skinless chicken breasts with olive oil, garlic, and dried rosemary and fire on each side for 5 minutes. Keep the results in the fridge to fill your sandwich and salad-making needs throughout the week.

ROAST BEEF

(¾ cup)
60 calories
2 g fat (0.5 g saturated)
10 g protein
450 mg sodium

Roast beef, despite suffering from unjust calorie and fat discrimination by misinformed sandwich eaters, is pretty much in the same nutritional ballpark as ham and turkey—which is to say comfortably lean and low calorie. It even boasts a protein edge on turkey and a sodium edge on ham. If roast beef is homemade or roasted by your deli, go ahead and double the fat and calories.

PASTRAMI

70 calories
3 g fat (1.5 g saturated)
10.5 g protein
425 mg sodium

Before it reaches the meat counter, the beef that will be pastrami is salted, seasoned, and smoked. The result is rich with lean protein, flavor, and phytochemicals. The seasoning blend that slathers the pastrami—garlic, peppercorns, coriander, and cloves—delivers a payload of antioxidants and micronutrients to the sandwich. Drop a pile onto rye bread with a slice of melted Swiss cheese and grilled onions for classic hot pastrami.

TUNA SALAD

(¾ cup)
360 calories
32 g fat (4.5 g saturated)
18 g protein
460 mg sodium

Tuna salad: two great foods that should never go together. They're joined in this unholy matrimony by a boatload of mayonnaise, which spikes your sandwich with more calories than a pound of turkey. Don't abandon the tuna—it's loaded with protein and healthy fat—but just try a lightened-up version at home. Mix one can with chopped celery, onion, and carrot, the juice of a lemon, and a half-tablespoon of olive oil.

HAM

63 calories
2 g fat (1 g saturated)
8 g protein
626 mg sodium

Common belief has it that turkey is the clear nutritional leader in the sandwich meat department, but most major manufacturers keep their hams very lean, yielding a product with marginally more fat and calories than the beloved white meat. But watch out for sodium, which can run high since hams are usually cured in a salty brine. For that reason, ham pairs perfectly with sweet and sharp flavors—sliced apple, Dijon mustard, and sharp cheese.

SMOKED SALMON

99 calories
3.5 g fat (1 g saturated)
17 g protein
288 mg sodium

In the last few years, salmon has come to be known as the champion of omega-3 fats. A sandwich-size slice is far smaller than a fillet, yet it still harbors more than a third of your day's omega-3 intake. And with the bagged and canned varieties being nearly as ubiquitous as canned tuna, there's no reason why you can't slip a salmon sandwich into your next lunch break. Double up on the healthy fats by covering your bread with pesto, then top with arugula and tomato.

BACON

(4 slices, 32 grams)
168 calories
13 g fat (4 g saturated)
12 g protein
767 mg sodium

The fat is a problem. So is the sodium. Yet, somehow, we can't bring ourselves to renounce its crunchy porcine goodness. At least it's no schlub in the protein department. Is that a weak justification for nearly a quarter of the day's saturated fat? Perhaps, so maybe you should limit yourself to just two or three slices, on toasted whole wheat, stacked high with lettuce and thick-sliced tomato. You could do worse.

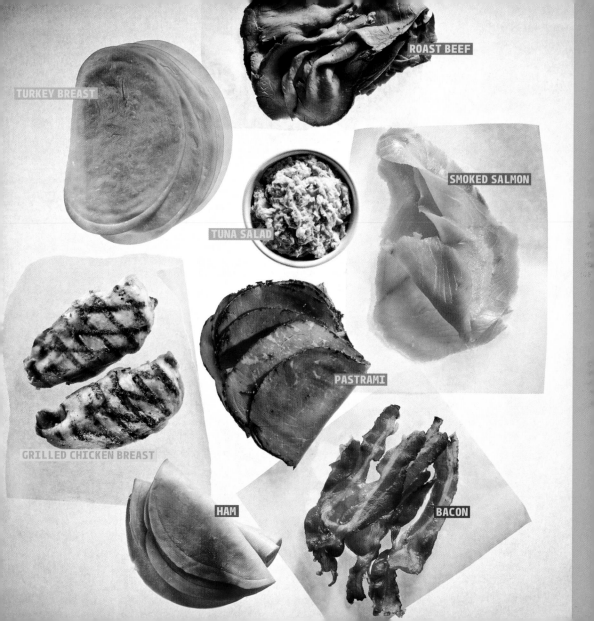

The Vegetation

(¹/₂-cup servings)

TOMATOES

16 calories
1 g fiber
1 g protein

Tomatoes are composed of about 95 percent water. That means that along with the signature sweetness comes enough moisture to allow you to cut back on or completely forgo the fattier sauces, especially in the middle of the summer tomato season. And there's also the load of lycopene—tomatoes' lauded antioxidant that fights off cancers, improves cholesterol, and protects your skin from the UV rays. Where there is bread and meat, there too should be tomato.

ROMAINE

4 calories
0.5 g fiber
0.5 g protein

Eons ago, romaine and iceberg were born into the same group of vegetables. Iceberg got the crispiest crunch, but romaine was endowed with an acute nutritional profile. Not that it's totally lacking in the crunch department; it's just balanced with massive doses of vitamins A, C, and K, manganese, and folate. Make it your go-to greenery for sandwiches.

SLICED AVOCADO

117 calories
11 g fat (1.5 g saturated)
5 g fiber
1.5 g protein

The fat's high, but these happen to be some of the healthiest fats known to man. About 63 percent of the fat imbued in the soft green flesh of California's finest fruit is monounsaturated oleic acid, the same fat that gives olive oil its power to boost your cognitive functions while lowering your blood cholesterol. Plus, avocado slices provide the necessary gloss of oil to keep you from indulging in the other, less-healthy options like mayo, cheese, and cheap sandwich oils.

RED ONIONS

9 calories
0.5 g fiber

A sweeter flavor isn't the only thing red onions have over their white cousins. Red onions are also host to potent antioxidants called anthocyanidins, the same flavonoids that give blueberries their cognitive-boosting capabilities. A slice of red onion is mild enough to eat raw, so just wedge it between a slice of tomato and a piece of turkey to replicate the long-standing classic deli sandwich.

ARUGULA

2 calories
0.5 g protein

It may not provide the satisfying crunch of romaine or a few shards of iceberg, but it does bring to the table a potent kick of cancer-fighting flavonols along with a spicy, peppery bite that other greens just can't compete with. Find bags of triple-washed arugula in the refrigerated section of the produce aisle and plant a small heap atop your next BLT or roast beef and cheddar sandwich.

PICKLES

9 calories
1 g fiber
0.5 g protein
872 mg sodium

They start out as nutritionally weak cucumbers, take a long bath in briny vinegar, and then emerge as nutritionally weak pickles with a serious sodium problem. We would renounce them completely if only their crunch wasn't so dang irresistible. Toss a couple slices onto your sandwich if you please. But don't nosh mindlessly on spears afterward—unless you're trying to pickle yourself.

ROASTED RED PEPPERS

19 calories
1 g fiber
0.5 g protein

They're light in calories but not in immune-boosting vitamins. Just toss a few on your sandwich and check off half your day's vitamin A and 150 percent of your vitamin C. Trust us, your taste buds won't mind. Actually, the boost of natural sugar can compensate for an unsweetened, whole wheat bread—yet another boon to your health. Roasted peppers pair beautifully with grilled chicken and pesto.

PEPERONCINI

18 calories
0.5 g fiber
1 g protein

Pulled from the jar and still dripping with vinegar, these sweet yellow peppers lend your sandwich a crunchy, acidic bite. They're also stacked with beta-carotene, the antioxidant precursor to vitamin A, which means that when your taste buds are done being satisfied, your cells get an army of protectors to prevent oxidative stress.

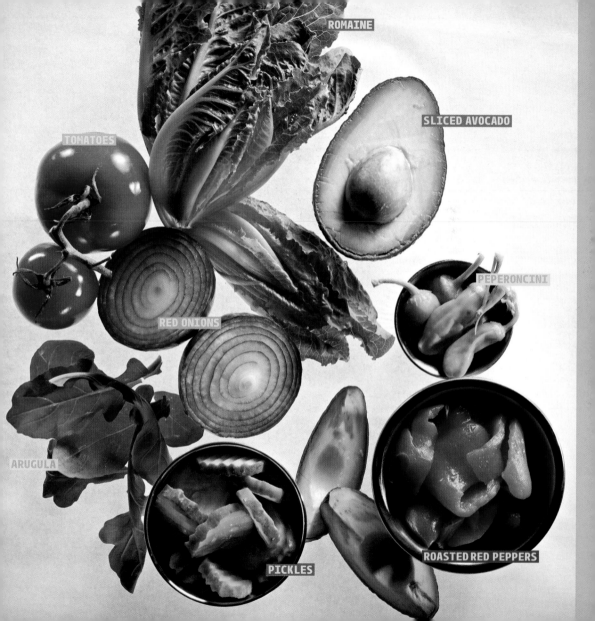

ROMAINE

SLICED AVOCADO

TOMATOES

PEPERONCINI

RED ONIONS

ARUGULA

PICKLES

ROASTED RED PEPPERS

The Dairy

(48-gram servings unless otherwise noted)

AMERICAN CHEESE

116 calories
8.5 g fat (5.5 g saturated)
7 g protein
650 mg sodium

As used here, "American" is synonymous with "processed," meaning that this product is a cheeselike puzzle with many odd dairy pieces such as milk fat, whey, and whey protein concentrate. Think of it as the distinctly American assembly line version of cheese: savings at the expense of quality. In this case, you save a few calories and lose out on flavor and that lovely intangible, wholesomeness.

BRIE

117 calories
10 g fat (6 g saturated)
7.5 g protein
220 mg sodium

Brie may have a reputation for being a fat-riddled indulgence, but its nutritional numbers tell a more tempered tale of its healthfulness. Inside its tough outer rind is a center with the consistency of thick cream, and when heated, it elevates even the blandest sandwich into a warm, buttery delicacy. Make it a meal with ham and Dijon mustard on a baguette.

FRESH MOZZARELLA

105 calories
8 g fat (4.5 g saturated)
7.5 g protein
147 mg sodium

Unlike the low-moisture mozzarella filling the coolers at most supermarkets, fresh mozzarella has a higher water content, which makes it one of the lowest-calorie sandwich cheeses out there. Look for the white balls stored in airtight packages or little plastic buckets of brine. Perfect for a vegetarian sandwich—try stacked slices of fresh mozz with heirloom tomatoes, fresh arugula, and pesto.

EGG

(medium, 44 grams)
63 calories
4.5 g fat (1.5 g saturated)
5.5 g protein
62 mg sodium

Okay, so it's not the cheese you're used to, but a sunny-side up egg makes a damn fine substitute. Beyond the fact that it brings lutein and choline to your sandwich, it can simultaneously stand in for both a slice of cheese and a slick of mayo, saving you up to 150 calories and moistening your masterpiece in the light sheen of a cracked yolk.

PEPPER JACK

138 calories
11 g fat (6.5 g saturated)
7.5 g protein
212 mg sodium

Put simply, Pepper Jack is Monterey Jack infused with jalapeño peppers. This means that along with the typical protein and calcium push of cheese comes a dose of fiery hot capsaicins, the pepper's health-promoting phytochemicals that boost metabolism and lower bad cholesterol. So long as you can stand the heat, make a wholesome meal by pairing this spirited cheese with roast beef, red onion, and salsa.

FRESH GOAT CHEESE

128 calories
10.5 g fat (7 g saturated)
7.5 g protein
180 mg sodium

The protein composition of goat milk resembles that of human breast milk, which makes it easier for us humans to digest. Its flavor is strong and acidic, so you can get by using less than other cheeses. It can be crumbled straight from the fridge into a pita with veggies and hummus or let it come to room temp before spreading it across bread like cream cheese. Try it with grilled chicken and tapenade.

CHEDDAR

141 calories
11.5 g fat (7.5 g saturated)
9 g protein
217 mg sodium

Beware: America's favorite cheese may also be one of its fattiest, with more than a third of your day's saturated fat in a serving. Cheddar is among the most calcium-packed foods on the planet, so you really need to pick and choose your cheddar moments. For our caloric buck, topping turkey and avocado on sprouted bread might make a compelling case for occasional use.

SWISS

133 calories
9.5 g fat (6 g saturated)
9.5 g protein
95 mg sodium

The bigger the holes, the better the Swiss. This is because bacteria in the cheese release carbon dioxide during the aging process, and the bigger holes signify conditions more favorable to flavorful cheese. It also means fewer calories for whatever you use it to cover. Our suggestion? Try this naturally low-sodium Alpine all-star melted over a hot open-faced turkey sandwich.

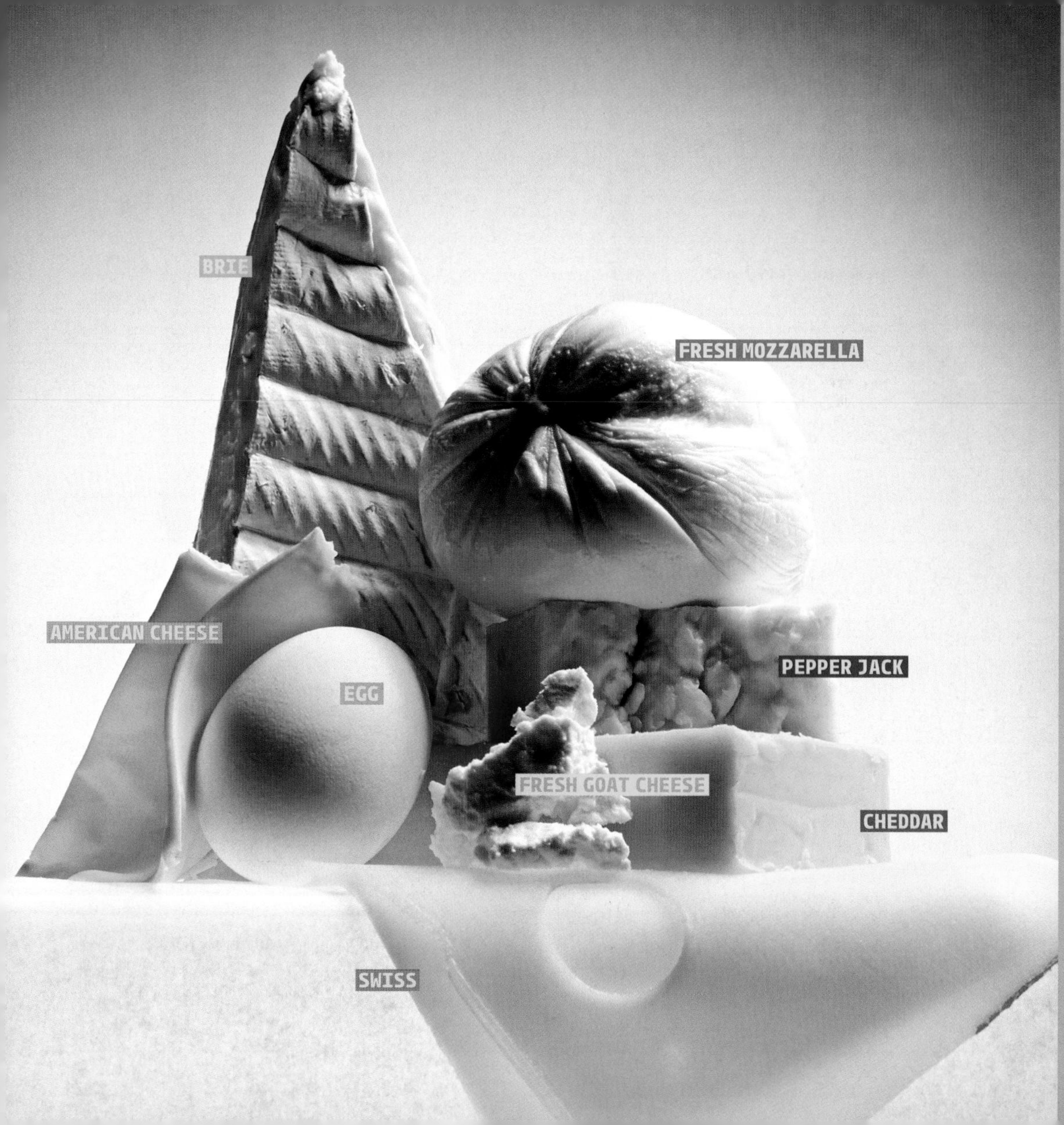

BRIE

FRESH MOZZARELLA

AMERICAN CHEESE

EGG

PEPPER JACK

FRESH GOAT CHEESE

CHEDDAR

SWISS

The Accents

(1-tablespoon servings)

SALSA

5 calories
2 g sugars
1 g fiber
60 mg sodium

It might not be a traditional sandwich topping, but it should be. After all, it combines so many of the things we love to put on our hoagies and heroes—tomatoes, onions, vinegar—in a single, delicious package. Works especially well with grilled chicken and avocado or turkey and cheddar.

TAPENADE

40 calories
4 g fat (0.5 g saturated)
290 mg sodium

The French like to spread this stuff onto everything, and why not? After all, it's made with a slew of heart-healthy ingredients: olives and their oil, capers, anchovies (you won't taste them), and garlic. A single tablespoon takes a simple turkey or grilled chicken sandwich into the upper echelons of 'wichcraft.

OIL AND VINEGAR

72 calories
8 g fat (1.5 g saturated)

The vinegar's not the problem—it's the low-grade soybean oils that wind up forming poorly distributed, soggy puddles on your bread, adding a maximal number of calories with a minimal amount of character. Try drizzling a thin layer into a stuffed pita instead. The oil and vinegar will filter through your mix to give you even distribution.

MAYONNAISE

103 calories
11.5g fat (1.5 g saturated)
73 mg sodium

There's a good reason why mayonnaise has nearly as much fat as pure vegetable oil. That's because it is nearly pure vegetable oil. With egg yolks as an emulsifying glue, the oil blends with lemon juice to become the most beastly monster in the Condiment Kingdom. Good news, though: Companies like Kraft and Hellmann's are rolling out lines of mayonnaise made from healthier oils like olive and canola.

GRAINY MUSTARD

16 calories
1 g fat (0 g saturated)
68 mg sodium

You're already familiar with mustard's distinctly mature flavor, but you might not realize that the plump seeds offer a host of health benefits as well. A scoop on your next ham sandwich will bolster your meal with selenium, magnesium, tryptophan, and omega-3 fatty acids—a group of nutrients that help your brain, muscles, and nerves function properly.

PESTO

45 calories
3.5 g fat (1 g saturated)
95 mg sodium

Yet another welcome Mediterranean contribution to the category of healthy alternative sandwich spreads. Think of pesto as oil and vinegar with nutrition, since it's made with olive oil and contains a slew of prime players like basil, garlic, and pine nuts. Layer a thin baguette with a few slices of tomato, prosciutto, fresh mozzarella, and arugula. Top it off with pesto and you're loving life.

CRANBERRY SAUCE

26 calories
6.5 g sugars
5 mg sodium

No need to wait until Thanksgiving to dig out the cranberry sauce. This flavor-packed fruit packs in 50 percent more antioxidants than blueberries (though some are lost in the cooking process), which means it preserves your cells while it explodes with tangy sweetness on your turkey sandwich. Gob it on thick to invoke the nostalgia of holidays past and good health to come or mix it into a bit of whipped cream cheese for a killer sandwich spread.

HUMMUS

25 calories
1.5 g fat (0 g saturated)
1 g fiber
1 g protein
57 mg sodium

Chickpeas, sesame tahini, olive oil, and lemon juice combine to make this spread nearly as creamy as mayonnaise but with a milder flavor and about 90 percent less fat. Plus it fights down blood sugar in two ways: with slow-digesting fiber and a load of sugar-regulating manganese. It goes with nearly anything, from pitas and pastrami to hard rolls and roast beef.

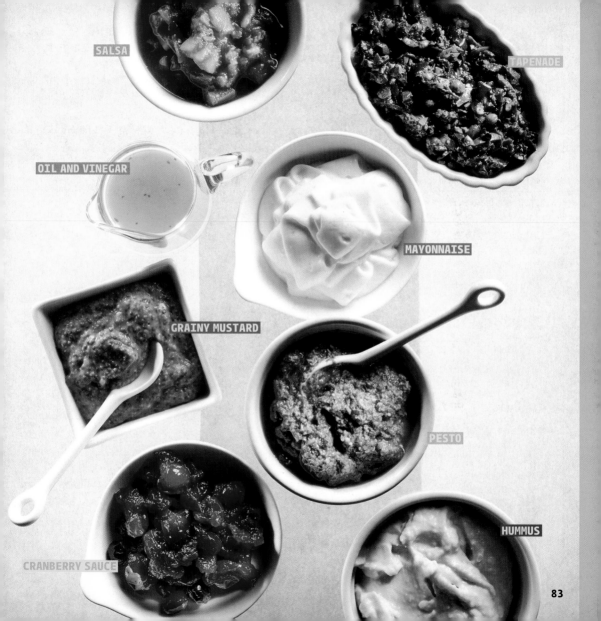

SALSA

TAPENADE

OIL AND VINEGAR

MAYONNAISE

GRAINY MUSTARD

PESTO

CRANBERRY SAUCE

HUMMUS

83

Deli Meats

Eat This

This Hormel line is one of the finest in the deli case. It's one of the only processed meats produced without nitrates, growth hormones, or other chemicals.

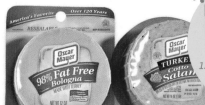

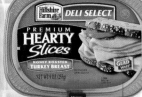

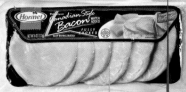

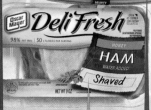

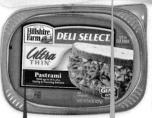

Hormel™ Natural Choice™ Carved Chicken Breast
(2 oz, 56 g)

60 calories
1.5 g fat (0.5 g saturated)
340 mg sodium

Oscar Mayer® Turkey Cotto Salami
(1 slice, 28 g)

45 calories
3 g fat
(1 g saturated)
310 mg sodium

The turkey alternative wins on calories, fat, and sodium.

Hillshire Farm Deli Select® Ultra Thin® Pastrami
(2 oz, 57 g)

60 calories
1.5 g fat
(0.5 g saturated)
620 mg sodium

This entire package has only 240 calories.

Hormel™ Canadian Style Bacon
(1 slice, 28 g)

35 calories
1.5 g fat
(0.5 g saturated)
325 mg sodium

Canadian bacon is low in fat and high in protein—this one has 5 grams per ounce.

Oscar Mayer® 98% Fat Free Bologna
(1 slice, 28 g)

25 calories
0.5 g fat
(0 g saturated)
240 mg sodium

One of the only bologna slices worth eating.

Oscar Mayer® Deli Fresh Honey Ham Shaved
(6 slices, 51 g)

50 calories
1 g fat
(0.5 g saturated)
650 mg sodium

Same protein, but with 30% fewer calories.

Hillshire Farm Deli Select® Honey Roasted Turkey Breast
(2 slices, 56 g)

50 calories
0 g fat
520 mg sodium

More than a third fewer calories than the "Heart Smart" meat.

Not That!

Thanks mostly to filler flavorings and food starch this chicken has 30% less protein than other deli chicken slices.

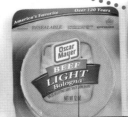
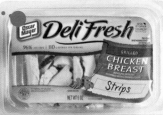

Oscar Mayer® Deli Fresh Grilled Chicken Breast Strips
(2 oz, 56 g)

73 calories
1 g fat (0.5 g saturated)
460 mg sodium

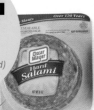
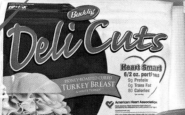
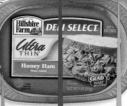
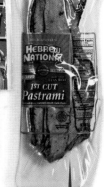

Oscar Mayer™ Hard Salami
(3 slices, 27 g)

100 calories
8 g fat
(3 g saturated)
510 mg sodium

In regular beef-and-pork salami, more than 70% of the calories come from fat.

Buddig™ Deli Cuts Honey-Roasted Cured Turkey Breast
(6 slices, 56 g)

80 calories
2.5 g fat
(1 g saturated)
460 mg sodium

Even with the "Heart Smart" line, Buddig still struggles.

Hillshire Farm™ Deli Select® Ultra Thin Honey Ham
(2 oz, 56 g)

70 calories
1.5 g fat
(0.5 g saturated)
690 mg sodium

Why give up 20 calories if they taste the same?

Oscar Mayer® Light Beef Bologna
(1 slice, 28 g)

60 calories
4 g fat
(1.5 g saturated)
240 mg sodium

Although it has 30 fewer calories than regular bologna, it's still 60% fat.

Hormel™ Original Pepperoni
(14 slices, 28 g)

140 calories
13 g fat
(6 g saturated)
490 mg sodium

Pizza lovers beware: One serving of pepperoni has about a third of your day's saturated fat.

Hebrew National® 1st Cut Pastrami
(2 oz, 56 g)

80 calories
3 g fat
(1 g saturated)
520 mg sodium

The rich color of this pastrami comes from the artificial caramel coloring.

Hot Dogs and Sausages
Eat This

You won't find a beef frank with fewer calories.

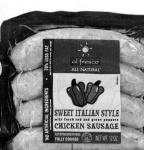

Hebrew National® 97% Fat Free Beef Franks
(1 frank, 49 g)

45 calories
1.5 g fat (0.5 g saturated)
370 mg sodium

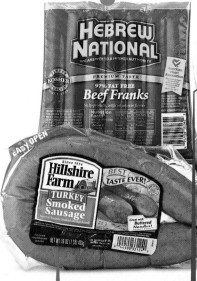

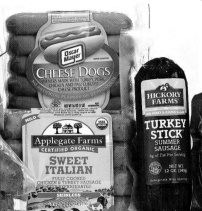

Hillshire Farm Turkey Smoked Sausage (56 g)

90 calories
5 g fat
(2 g saturated)
510 mg sodium

Turkey sausage has a third more protein than the typical beef-and-pork variety.

Oscar Mayer® Cheese Dogs
(1 link, 45 g)

140 calories
13 g fat
(4 g saturated)
540 mg sodium

You can have your cheese and eat it, too. (And you'll even save 50 calories in the process.)

Applegate Farms® Organic Sweet Italian
(1 link, 85 g)

130 calories
7 g fat
(2 g saturated)
500 mg sodium

Applegate Farms's nitrate-free poultry sausages are the best we've come across.

Hickory Farms® Turkey Stick® Summer Sausage Honey and Brown Sugar
(2 oz, 56 g)

90 calories
4 g fat (1 g saturated)
730 mg sodium

Protein accounts for more than half the calories.

Al Fresco® Sweet Italian Style Chicken Sausage
(1 link, 85 g)

130 calories
7 g fat
(2 g saturated)
480 mg sodium

This is how sausage is supposed to be made—from six very familiar ingredients.

Not That!

Ball Park® Turkey Franks
(1 frank, 57 g)

120 calories
7 g fat (2 g saturated)
550 mg sodium

Often, turkey wins the calorie battle, but it's a big mistake to assume this is an immutable law. You still have to check the numbers.

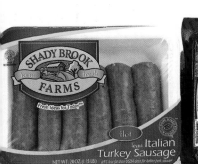

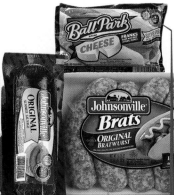

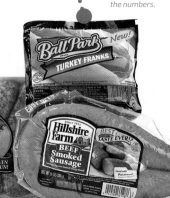

Shady Brook™ Farms Lean Italian Turkey Sausage
(1 link, 93 g)

160 calories
9 g fat
(2.5 g saturated)
620 mg sodium

Better than most beef and pork sausages, but still not ideal.

Johnsonville® Original Summer Sausage
(2 oz, 56 g)

170 calories
15 g fat
(6 g saturated, 1 g trans)
680 mg sodium

As a rule of thumb, summer sausages are the fattiest in the fridge.

Johnsonville® Brats (1 link, 85 g)

270 calories
22 g fat
(8 g saturated)
810 mg sodium

The standard brat sets you back a third of your day's fat and nearly half your saturated fat. That's assuming you stick to one.

Ball Park® Cheese Franks
(1 frank, 57 g)

190 calories
16 g fat
(7 g saturated)
580 mg sodium

Ball Park's Franks are thicker than most, which means more fat and calories per bite.

Hillshire Farm Beef Smoked Sausage (56 g)

190 calories
17 g fat
(8 g saturated, 1 g trans)
530 mg sodium

80% of the calories here come from fat. Don't expect much better from most regular sausages.

Cheese
Eat This

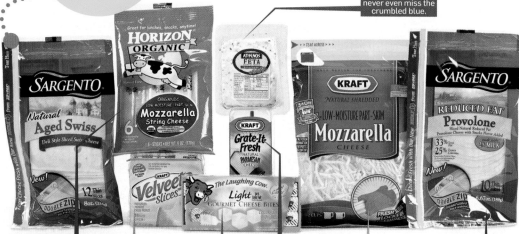

Sargento® Aged Swiss
(1 slice, 19 g)

70 calories
5 g fat (3 g saturated)
40 mg sodium

Swiss stomps cheddar by providing more calcium in fewer calories and just a quarter of the sodium.

Athenos Feta Basil & Tomato (28 g)

80 calories
6 g fat
(3.5 g saturated)
320 mg sodium

Feta is a naturally low-fat cheese. Try one flavored chunk and you'll never even miss the crumbled blue.

Horizon Organic® Mozzarella String
(1 stick, 28 g)

80 calories
5 g fat
(3 g saturated)
170 mg sodium

One of the greatest grab-and-go snacks in the market.

Kraft Velveeta
(1 slice, 21 g)

60 calories
4 g fat
(2.5 g saturated)
270 mg sodium

Velveeta is actually a blend of milk, milkfat, and milk protein, a quick-melting blend that knocks 50 calories off your sandwich.

The Laughing Cow® Light Gourmet Cheese Bites™
(5 pieces, 23.5 g)

35 calories
2 g fat
(1 g saturated)
300 mg sodium

The perfect companion to a whole-grain cracker.

Kraft Grate-It-Fresh Parmesan
(2 Tbsp, 5 g)

20 calories
1.5 g fat
(1 g saturated)
75 mg sodium

Trade in the dry powdered cheese for the real stuff.

Kraft Shredded Low-Moisture Part-Skim Mozzarella
(¼ cup, 28 g)

80 calories
6 g fat
(3.5 g saturated)
160 mg sodium

One of the great melting cheeses.

Sargento® Reduced Fat Provolone
(1 slice, 19 g)

50 calories
3.5 g fat
(2 g saturated)
140 mg sodium

A good cheese to make your go-to for all matters sandwich-related.

Not That!

Treasure Cave® Crumbled Blue Cheese (28 g)

*100 calories
8 g fat
(5 g saturated)
380 mg sodium*

Beware the concentration of sodium in crumbled blue cheese.

A single slice of this cheese provides almost a quarter of your day's saturated fat.

Kraft Deli Fresh Colby Jack
(1 slice, 23 g)

*90 calories
7 g fat (4.5 g saturated)
150 mg sodium*

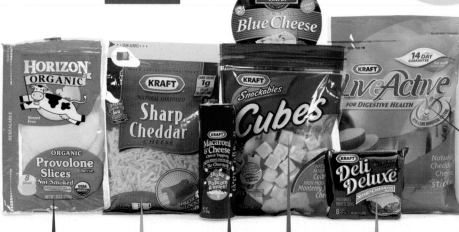

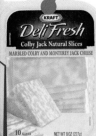

Horizon Organic® Provolone

(1 slice, 21 g)

*70 calories
6 g fat
(3.5 g saturated)
140 mg sodium*

Don't assume that organic is somehow always healthier.

Kraft Shredded Sharp Cheddar

(¼ cup, 28 g)

*110 calories
9 g fat
(6 g saturated)
180 mg sodium*

Cheddar loses nearly any head-to-head cheese comparison.

Kraft Macaroni & Cheese Topping

(2 tsp, 6 g)

*25 calories
1 g fat
(0 g saturated)
270 mg sodium*

The artificial colors here have been linked to hyperactive behavior in kids.

Kraft Snackables Cubes Colby & Monterey Jack

(5 pieces, 21 g)

*77 calories
6.5 g fat
(4 g saturated)
168 mg sodium*

Nearly 5% of your daily saturated fat in each tiny cube.

Kraft Deli Deluxe® Sharp Cheddar

(1 slice, 28 g)

*110 calories
9 g fat
(5 g saturated)
440 mg sodium*

"Deluxe"often ends up meaning "extra fat and calories."

Kraft LiveActive Natural Cheddar

(1 stick, 28 g)

*120 calories
10 g fat
(6 g saturated)
180 mg sodium*

50% more calories and twice the fat of the mozzarella.

Yogurt

Eat This

Already one of the world's healthiest yogurt producers, Fage makes their flavored versions that much more tempting by blending in more fruit than sugar.

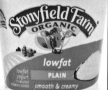
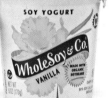
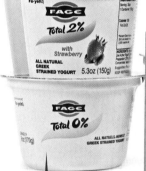
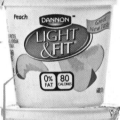
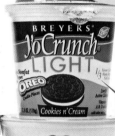

Fage 2% Strawberry
(1 container, 150 g)

140 calories
2.5 g fat (1.5 g saturated)
17 g sugars

Fage Total 0% Nonfat Greek Style
(1 container, 170 g)

90 calories
0 g fat
7 g sugars

Greek yogurt is creamier with a higher concentration of proteins. This 6-ounce cup has an astounding 15 grams.

Dannon™ Light & Fit® Peach
(1 container, 170 g)

80 calories
0 g fat
11 g sugars

The lightest cup of yogurt at your supermarket also has 15% of your calcium and 20% of your vitamin D.

Whole Soy & Co.® Vanilla
(1 container, 170 g)

150 calories
3.5 g fat
(0 g saturated)
12 g sugars

Whole Soy's Vanilla sugar levels should be considered a ceiling. Venture north of 12 grams at your own peril.

Stonyfield Farm® Lowfat Plain
(6 oz, 170 g)

90 calories
1.5 g fat
(1 g saturated)
11 g sugars

Your best option, as always, is to stick with plain yogurt and add your own fruit at home.

Breyers® YoCrunch® Light with Oreo Pieces
(1 container with pieces, 170 g)

120 calories
2.5 g fat
(1 g saturated)
11 g sugars

Make this into a harmless dessert.

90

Not That!

**Yoplait 99%
Fat Free
Cherry Orchard**
(1 container, 170 g)

*170 calories
1.5 g fat (1 g saturated)
27 g sugars*

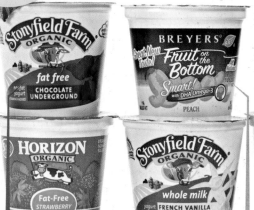

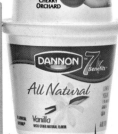

*Think this sugar comes from
the cherries? Think again:
After milk, sugar's the first
ingredient on the list.*

**Stonyfield Farm®
Organic Fat Free
Chocolate
Underground**
(1 container, 170 g)

*170 calories
0 g fat
35 g sugars*

This is the most
sugar-packed yogurt
we've ever
come across.

**Horizon Organic®
Fat-Free
Strawberry**
(1 container, 170 g)

*140 calories
0 g fat
27 g sugars*

The second ingredient
is "organic evaporated
cane juice."
Translation: sugar.

**Stonyfield Farm®
Whole Milk
French Vanilla**
(1 container, 170 g)

*170 calories
6 g fat
(4 g saturated)
22 g sugars*

Dear Stonyfield, please
cut the sugar in half
so we can enjoy your
yogurt in good
conscience.

**Breyers® Fruit
on the Bottom
Smart! Peach**
(1 container, 170 g)

*160 calories
1.5 g fat
(1 g saturated)
28 g sugars*

As much sugar as
a 5-ounce Cotton
Candy Ice Cream at
Cold Stone Creamery.

**Dannon™
All Natural
Lowfat Vanilla**
(1 container, 170 g)

*150 calories
2.5 g fat
(1.5 g saturated)
25 g sugars*

Who cares if it's
"all natural" if it packs
as much sugar
as a Kit Kat?

Butter and Butter Sub

Eat This

Breakstone's® Unsalted Whipped Butter

(1 Tbsp, 9 g)

70 calories
7 g fat (4.5 g saturated)
0 mg sodium

The butter is whipped to introduce air, making it lighter in calories and easier to spread.

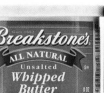

NON-HYDROGENATED • NO TRANS FATTY ACIDS

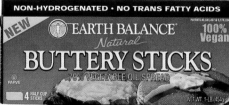

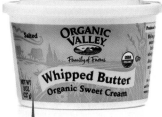

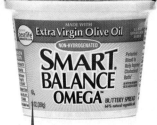

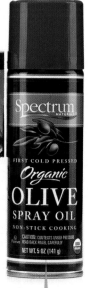

Organic Valley® Whipped Butter (1 Tbsp)

50 calories
6 g fat (3.5 g saturated)
40 mg sodium

Organic Valley employs a vast network of small family farmers to produce their nationally available dairy products. Their products tend to be honest and reliable. This butter, for example, has just two ingredients: sweet cream and salt.

Smart Balance® Omega™ Buttery Spread Made with Extra Virgin Olive Oil (1 Tbsp, 11 g)

60 calories
7 g fat (2 g saturated)
70 mg sodium

Smart Balance adds in über-healthy flaxseed oils. That's how it earns 20% of your daily intake of EPA and DHA oils, the strongest version of omega-3 fats.

Earth Balance® Natural Buttery Sticks (1 Tbsp, 14 g)

100 calories
11 g fat (4.5 g saturated)
120 mg sodium

It's higher in calories and saturated fat, but it fully eliminates the dangerous trans fats. It's a swap worth making.

Spectrum Naturals® Organic Olive Spray Oil (~⅓ second spray)

0 calories
0 g fat
0 mg sodium

Most sprays are filled with soybean oil and a long list of chemicals, colors, and artificial flavors. There's no ruse here, though—the main ingredient is extra virgin olive oil.

Not That!

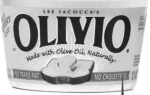

Land O Lakes® Spreadable Butter with Canola Oil
(1 Tbsp, 14 g)

100 calories
11 g fat (4.5 g saturated)
90 mg sodium

If you're looking to cut calories from real butter, this isn't the way. This blend has as many calories as full-cream butter.

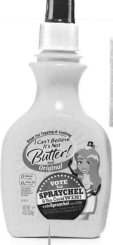

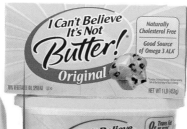

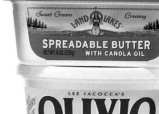

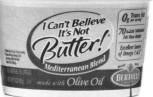

I Can't Believe It's Not Butter!™ Original Spray
(5 sprays, 1 g)

0 calories
0 g fat
15 mg sodium

Despite the label claim, this is not a calorie-free food; the fat and calories are just conveniently rounded to zero.

I Can't Believe It's Not Butter! Original
(1 Tbsp, 14 g)

90 calories
10 g fat (2 g saturated, 2.5 g trans)
90 mg sodium

Stick margarine is the absolute worst. To make it solid, it has to be stabilized with partially hydrogenated oils, the source of trans fats.

I Can't Believe It's Not Butter!® Made with Olive Oil
(1 Tbsp, 14 g)

70 calories
8 g fat (2 g saturated)
90 mg sodium

When it comes to trans fats, you just can't trust the nutrition label. Look at the ingredient list; if you see partially hydrogenated oil, leave it in the cooler.

Olivio
(1 Tbsp)

80 calories
8 g fat (1.5 g saturated)
95 mg sodium

Lee Iacocca's spread touts the benefits of olive oil on the package, but truth is, it's only one of six different oils that go into this product, including partially hydrogenated soybean oil.

93

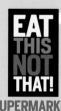

EAT
THIS
NOT
THAT!
SUPERMARKET
SURVIVAL GUIDE

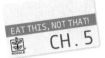

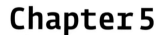

Chapter 5
PANTRY STAPLES

Power Up Your Pantry

It seems hard to imagine today, but back in the 1950s, at the height of the Cold War, many families built fallout shelters in their backyards. These snug little caverns were designed to protect the nuclear family from nuclear fallout, and during air-raid drills, people would race to their shelters to practice for the day when the Ruskies dropped The Big One.

Of course, we never actually needed bomb shelters, and in the end they were mostly used by teenagers, who snuck into them for make-out sessions and Dave Brubeck listening parties. But bomb shelters served another useful purpose: They helped teach Americans about the virtues of a well-stocked pantry. After all, you wouldn't want to survive a nuclear holocaust only to live on tomato soup and crackers, would you? The smartly turned-out bomb shelter became a status symbol of folks who wanted to live well, even in the midst of a wasteland.

Today, our pantries are still an important source of salvation, but it's not the evil Soviet Empire that threatens us—it's the obesity crisis. The bombardment of calories, the explosions of fat and carbs that are laying waste to our waistlines—these are the real threats to Americans' health. (Even if we don't worry much about nuclear winters, it's always winter if you're ashamed to take off your T-shirt at a pool party, no?) And that's why stocking up on canned and dried foods is so critical. The well-stocked pantry today is a smart way of ensuring that you and your family are always eating healthy. (And if it's a walk-in pantry and you can squeeze in a make-out session or two, more power to ya!)

Because pantry items are built to stay—I personally have a can of tomatoes that has now followed me to my third home in 5 years—it's important to spend some time thinking them over. Buy the wrong carton of juice and it's a mistake that lasts a few weeks. Buy the wrong package of noodles and those dried and twisted snakes will be laughing at you for years to come.

But if you're like most people, the pantry is the place where you expend the least amount of thought. We may wrangle with the butcher over the right cut of meat, thump and prod the produce until the perfect fruit is found, and agonize over the exact flavor of ice cream to please every fickle family taste bud. But canned goods? The spices, noodles, and condiments that make their way into our carts are most likely a mix of the products our moms used to buy of whatever's on sale, featured in a coupon, or just within easy reach.

And that's exactly the wrong approach to take. Because like it or not, it's the products you keep in your pantry that are really going to make or break your family's diet: When it's been days since you bought fresh produce and your meat supply is down to half a box of freezer-burned fish sticks, it's time to start rummag-ing through the pantry. And it's at times like that—when you haven't had the time or energy to plan a full, healthy meal—that bad stuff can start to creep into your diet.

For example, a study in the *American Journal of Public Health* compared individuals whose pantries had relatively low amounts of fat with those whose pantries had high amounts of fat. Researchers discovered that folks with low-fat pantries took in about 32 percent of their daily calories from fat. But people whose pantries were ill-considered nutritional wastelands took in 37 percent of their calories from fat, every single day. Think about it—you could cut your daily fat intake by one-seventh if you did absolutely nothing else but read the labels on cans and boxes before you bought. No dieting, no cooking, nothing. Amazing.

Now, here are what make pantry foods such terrific weapons in the war on flab and some smart strategies for updating your arsenal.

● **YOU CAN MAKE HEALTHY EATING AFFORDABLE.** Sadly, we live in a time when a bagel with cream cheese can cost less than a grapefruit. That's because a bagel can be made anywhere, but a grapefruit needs to come from tropical climes, and as economic worries continue to make us wistful for the days when all we had to worry about was the Cold War, those exotic fruits and vegetables are only getting more expensive. (And what's more dispiriting than spending big bucks on produce only to have it turn into a science experiment in your fridge because you went away for the weekend?) In fact, according to researchers at the University of Washington, high-calorie, low-nutrition foods (think bagel and cream cheese) cost an average of $1.76 for 1,000 calories, but low-cal, high-nutrition foods (think grapefruit) cost $18.16 for the same number of calories. (In fact, you could live on a junk-food diet for $3.52 a day, while a diet entirely of healthy foods would cost $36.32.) No wonder some people say that being overweight makes you look not only less physically healthy but less financially healthy as well. But canned vegetables and fruits make an intelligent and more affordable alternative.

- **YOU CAN SAVE EVEN MORE MONEY WITH SMART CHOICES.** Purchase private-label or store-brand goods whenever possible. They are almost always of the same flavor and nutritional quality as well-known, commercial brands and come at a fraction of the cost. (Just read and compare the labels, to ensure that you're still getting the nutrition you're seeking.)

- **YOU CAN CONTROL WHAT'S ADDED TO YOUR FOOD.** If there's one major pitfall to pantry foods—canned foods especially—it's sodium content and unhealthy packing additives. When buying cans, always read the labels and be diligent about eliminating the bad stuff. Look for meats like tuna that are packed in water, not oil, and choose low-sodium options whenever possible. (If you miss the added flavor that salt brings, you can boost it with pepper sauces or spices—which puts you back in charge of your food!)

- **YOU CAN INDULGE YOUR INNER NEAT FREAK.** Want to save money, improve your health, and keep your house cleaner than ever? Once every couple of months, clean your pantry. You'll almost always discover hidden foods that worked their way to the back of the cabinet, and you'll save money by not replacing what you already have. And checking packages for leaks and spills will keep food fresher and pests at bay.

The Pantry Label Decoder

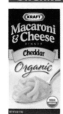

KRAFT ORGANIC MACARONI AND CHEESE

THE CLAIM: "USDA organic"
THE TRUTH: It's organic so it must be healthy, right? Not so much. For an extra 60 cents per box, consumers save 20 calories and 1 gram of fat. They also gain 2 grams of sugar, 1 gram of fiber, and 50 milligrams of sodium, and they lose 6 percent of their daily iron. The point is, even organic junk food is still junk food. Your body processes organic refined flour and powdered cheese the same way it does conventional, so at the end of the day it's still a high-calorie, low-nutrient letdown.

WHAT YOU REALLY WANT: If you must have mac, pick one with a label that reads like the recipe you'd use to fix it at home. Annie's line of macaroni and cheese contains about eight ingredients per box and cuts the fat by 72 percent over Kraft Organic.

Nutrition Facts
Serving Size 2.5 oz (70g)
(Makes about 1 cup)
Servings Per Container about 2.5

Amount Per Serving	As Packaged	As Prepared
Calories	240	310
Calories from Fat	20	80

	%Daily Value**	
Total Fat 2.5g*	4%	14%
Saturated Fat 1g	5%	25%
Trans Fat 0g		
Cholesterol <5mg	2%	8%
Sodium 630mg	26%	27%
Total Carbohydrate 49g	16%	16%
Dietary Fiber 2g	8%	8%
Sugars 8g		
Protein 10g	12%	13%
Vitamin A	0%	6%
Vitamin C	0%	0%

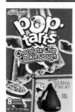

KELLOGG'S CHOCOLATE CHIP COOKIE DOUGH POP-TARTS

THE CLAIM: "Good source of 7 vitamins and minerals"
THE TRUTH: Five of the seven vitamins and minerals are derived from this product's first ingredient, enriched flour. That's the code word for "refined flour that's had nutrients added to it after it's been stripped of fiber."
WHAT YOU REALLY WANT: A breakfast without the nutritional profile of a dessert. Studies show that people who opt for high-quality protein (eggs, yogurt) over refined carbohydrates (pancakes, bagels, Pop-Tarts) lose weight faster and maintain higher levels of energy throughout the day.

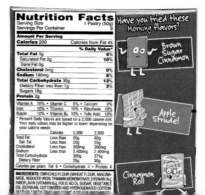

99

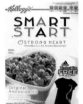

KELLOGG'S SMART START CEREAL

THE CLAIM: "Lightly sweetened"

THE TRUTH: Unregulated by the USDA, the word "lightly" gets tossed around like a Frisbee in the food packaging world. Always take it with a grain of salt; in many instances, "light" is the first sign of trouble. With this healthy-sounding cereal, "lightly" means 14 grams of sugar from 5 different sources, all of which adds up to a cereal with more added sugars per serving than Froot Loops, Frosted Flakes, or Apple Jacks.

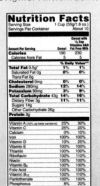

WHAT YOU REALLY WANT: A cereal with less than 10 grams of sugar per serving (and ideally less than 5), with at least 3 grams of fiber per serving. Look at cereal as a sugar-to-fiber ratio; you want a ratio no higher than two to one.

For more secrets the food industry doesn't want you to know, log on to eatthis.com

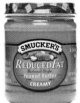

SMUCKER'S REDUCED FAT CREAMY PEANUT BUTTER

THE CLAIM: "25% less fat than regular natural peanut butter"

THE TRUTH: Smucker's has indeed removed some of the fat from the peanut butter, but they've replaced it with maltodextrin, a carbohydrate used as a cheap filler in many processed foods. This means you're trading the *healthy* fat from peanuts for empty carbs, double the sugar, and a savings of a meager 10 calories.

WHAT YOU REALLY WANT: The real stuff: no oils, fillers, or added sugars. Just peanuts and salt. Smucker's Natural fits the bill, as do many other peanut butters out there.

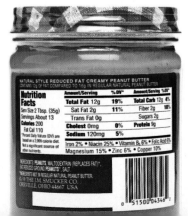

Sweeteners

BOGUS BREAD

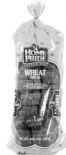

HOME PRIDE WHEAT BREAD

THE CLAIMS: "1 gram of fat per slice"; "wheat bread"

THE TRUTH: This over-trumpeted claim (since when has bread contained much fat, anyway?) tries to distract from the fact that each slice has three times more sugar than fiber. Whatever wheat that went into this bread was stripped of all of its meaningful nutrients. Perhaps most concerning, the ingredients list here is more than a dozen items long, many of them unpronounceable additives, chemicals, and preservatives. Whatever happened to the days when bread was just flour, water, and yeast?

WHAT YOU REALLY WANT: Ignore fat when it comes to bread; there's rarely enough in a slice to make a real difference. More important, seek out a bread with more fiber per slice than sugar and with as few ingredients as possible.

Nutrition Facts

Serving Size: 1 Slice (28g)
Servings Per Container: 20

Calories 70
Calories from Fat 10

Amount/Serving	%Daily Value*	Amount/Serving	%Daily Value*
Total Fat 1g	2%	**Total Carbohydrate** 13g	4%
Saturated Fat 0g	0%	Dietary Fiber 1g	4%
Trans Fat 0g		Sugars 3g	
Cholesterol 0mg	0%	**Protein** 2g	
Sodium 160mg	7%		

Vitamin A 0%	• Vitamin C 0%	• Calcium 4%	• Iron 6%
Thiamine 8%	• Riboflavin 6%	• Niacin 6%	• Folic Acid 6%

*Percent Daily Values are based on a 2,000 calorie diet. Your daily values may be higher or lower depending on your calorie needs.

INGREDIENTS: ENRICHED WHEAT FLOUR (FLOUR, BARLEY MALT, FERROUS SULFATE (IRON), "B" VITAMINS (NIACIN, THIAMINE MONONITRATE (B1), RIBOFLAVIN (B2), FOLIC ACID)), SWEETENER (HIGH FRUCTOSE CORN SYRUP OR SUGAR), YEAST, WHEAT BRAN, WHOLE WHEAT FLOUR, WHEAT GLUTEN, MOLASSES, CONTAINS 2% OR LESS OF: SOYBEAN O

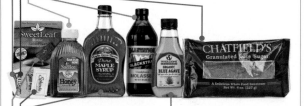

■ **Equal®** (1 packet, 1 gram)
0 calories, 0 fat, <1 g sugars
Studies on aspartame, the sweetener in both Equal and NutraSweet, indicate regular use might cause such problems as headaches, dizziness, sleep problems, and memory loss.

■ **Sweet'N Low®** (1 packet, 1 g)
0 calories, 0 g fat, <1 g sugars
Until 2000, saccharin products carried labels warning consumers about cancer risks, and recent studies link the chemical to weight gain in rats.

■ **SueBee® Clover Honey** (2 Tbsp, 42 g)
120 calories, 0 g fat, 32 g sugars
The sugars in honey are nearly a 1-to-1 ratio of glucose and fructose, which doctors say is the optimal ratio for creating the body's primary energy source, glycogen.

■ **Plantation® Blackstrap Molasses** (2 Tbsp, 42 g)
84 calories, 0 g fat 22 g sugars
Each tablespoon contains more than 10% of your daily calcium, iron, manganese, and potassium.

■ **Chatfield's® Granulated Date Sugar** (1 Tbsp, 12 g)
30 calories, 0 g fat, 9 g sugars
It's made from dried ground dates, so it's a rich source of magnesium and B vitamins.

■ **Wholesome® Sweeteners Organic Blue Agave** (2 Tbsp, 42 g)
120 calories, 0 g fat, 32 g sugars
Agave is sweeter than sugar but has a lower glycemic index than honey.

■ **Maple Grove Farms of Vermont® Pure Maple Syrup** (2 Tbsp, 30 mL)
100 calories, 0 g fat, 26 g sugars
The glycemic index of pure maple sugar is less than half that of corn syrup, which means it has less of an impact on your blood sugar. Plus it's sweeter, which means you can get by using less.

■ **Splenda®** (1 packet, 1 g)
0 calories, 0 g fat, <1 g sugars
Splenda is made from sucralose, the safest of all the artificial sweeteners on the market.

■ **SweetLeaf® Stevia Plus®** (1 packet, 1 g)
0 calories, 0 g fat, 0 g sugars
The FDA calls it a dietary supplement, but the truth is, it's an all-natural, zero-calorie sweetener, 300 times sweeter than sugar.

The Perfect Pantry

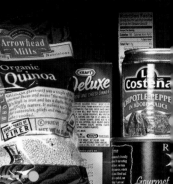
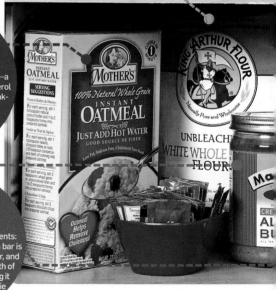

REIGHN ORIGINAL GOURMET ALBACORE TUNA

2 OUNCES: *140 calories, 6 g fat (1.5 g saturated), 22 g protein, 0 g carbs*
All the muscle-friendly protein but more kind-hearted omega-3s and less hazardous mercury than the big boys. Find a retailer at www.reighntuna.com.
POWER PLAY: Put together quick tuna burgers by mixing with an egg, bread crumbs, chopped onion, and a splash of lemon juice and forming into patties.

QUINOA

1 CUP COOKED: *222 calories, 4 g fat (0 g saturated), 8 g protein, 39 g carbs, 5 g fiber*
The Incas favored this ancient seed for a reason: Its ration of fiber, healthy fats, and protein makes it one of the healthiest foods on the planet. It makes a perfect stand-in for brown rice—and it cooks up in half the time.
POWER PLAY: Prior to cooking, rinse quinoa to remove any bitter coating. To deepen its nutty flavor, toast it in a skillet for a minute or two with a bit of oil over low heat before boiling it up.

KING ARTHUR WHITE WHOLE WHEAT FLOUR

¼ CUP: *100 calories, 0.5 g fat (0 g saturated), 4 g protein, 18 g carbs, 3 g fiber*
Has the lighter texture of white flour but all the health benefits of whole wheat like fiber and vitamin E—an antioxidant that reduces heart disease risk.
POWER PLAY: Swap it for half the white flour in any muffin, pancake, or baked good recipe.

MOTHER'S INSTANT OATMEAL

½ CUP: *150 calories, 3 g fat (0.5 g saturated), 5 g protein, 27 g carbs, 4 g fiber*
As a good source of beta-glucan—a soluble fiber that can cut cholesterol and blood sugar levels—this breakfast pick ain't old-fashioned.
POWER PLAY: Give meat loaf and burgers a nutritional lift by incorporating oats.

MARANATHA ALMOND BUTTER

1 TABLESPOON: *95 calories, 8 g fat (1 g saturated), 4 g protein, 3 g carbs, 2 g fiber*
This good alternative to peanut butter contains more bone-strengthening calcium, magnesium, and phosphorus. Plus, it's spared the sugar and hydrogenated fats added to many commercial brands of the spreadable standby.

LÄRABAR PECAN PIE

1 BAR: *200 calories, 14 g fat (1 g saturated), 16 g sugars, 4 g fiber*
Made with just three ingredients: dates, pecans, almonds. Each bar is loaded with healthy fats, fiber, and the antioxidant power of both of these first-rate nuts, making it one of the best 200-calorie snacks out there.

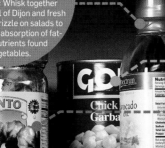

AVOCADO OIL

1 TABLESPOON: *124 calories, 14 g fat (2 g saturated)*
Mild flavor, a high smoke point, and plenty of monounsaturated fat that helps raise good HDL cholesterol.
POWER PLAY: Whisk together with a spoonful of Dijon and fresh lemon, then drizzle on salads to increase your absorption of fat-soluble nutrients found in vegetables.

CANNED CHICKPEAS (GARBANZO BEANS)

1 CUP: *286 calories, 3 g fat (0 g saturated), 12 g protein, 54 g carbs, 11 g fiber*
Chickpeas are like nature's little weight loss pills, packed full of belly-filling fiber and protein. They're also long on the magnesium, folate, iron, and zinc.
POWER PLAY: To knock out a healthy hummus, puree rinsed chickpeas in a blender with lemon juice, garlic, salt, tahini (sesame paste), and a little olive oil.

CENTO MARINATED ARTICHOKE HEARTS

1 OUNCE (3 PIECES): *25 calories*
Preparing artichokes from scratch involves a lot of spikes and thorns, but these babies are ready to eat right out of the jar. Artichokes are one of the most antioxidant-dense vegetables.

LA COSTEÑA CHIPOTLE PEPPERS

3 PEPPERS WITH SAUCE: *20 calories*
Jalapeños that have been dried, smoked, and packed into a spicy sauce called *adobo*. A single chile or a spoonful of the *adobo* lends salsas, soups, and vinaigrettes instant fire, plus a bit of capsaicin's metabolism-boosting powers.
POWER PLAY: Blend 2 chipotle peppers with 1 cup of orange juice, 2 cloves of garlic, and a handful of cilantro to make a lively marinade for chicken, pork, or steak.

SUNSWEET DRIED PLUMS

½ CUP: *209 calories, 0 g fat, 2 g protein, 56 g carbs, 6 g fiber*
Energy gels make you gag? Formally known as prunes, these delicious treats are just as portable, provide a quick carb boost, and offer up way more cancer-brawling compounds than any gooey running mate.

PUMPKIN SEEDS

1 OUNCE: *148 calories, 12 g fat (2 g saturated), 9 g protein*
Beefing up trail mix or salads with these jack-o'-lantern castoffs is a smart way to take in more magnesium. German researchers determined that consuming more of this oft-neglected mineral can slash diabetes risk by 23%.

DAGOBA XOCOLATL DARK CHOCOLATE WITH CHILIES AND NIBS

½ BAR: *158 calories, 11 g fat (6 g saturated), 4 g fiber*
Made from 74% cocoa, this fiery bar has less sugar than milk chocolate versions and is chock-full of polyphenols that have been shown to lower blood pressure and keep blood sugars in check. Can't find this bar? Look for one with at least 65% cacao on the label. Scharffen Berger and Chocolove also make great-tasting dark chocolate.

103

The Perfect Spice Rack

CAYENNE PEPPER
The heat in peppers comes from a phytochemical called capsaicin. Hot peppers have been shown to clear congestion, fight cholesterol, and raise metabolism to eliminate body fat. Taiwanese researchers also discovered that when exposed to capsaicin, cells that normally develop into fat cells die before they mature. **EAT THIS!** Sprinkle over vegetables and beans or mix with paprika, cumin, and brown sugar to make a kickin' meat rub.

MUSTARD SEEDS
Think of mustard seeds as the secret to staying calm and collected. The spice's list of essential nutrients includes magnesium to relax your nerves and muscles, omega-3 fats to keep your brain functioning, and tryptophan to promote serotonin production and keep your spirits high. **EAT THIS!** Fold a tablespoon into a pot of mashed potatoes or toss with cauliflower before roasting.

NUTMEG
Although high doses of nutmeg can lead to nausea and hallucinations, low doses have the opposite effect. Moderate amounts can calm the stomach, stop diarrhea, relieve anxiety, regulate sleep, and soothe joint and muscle pains. **EAT THIS!** Sprinkle nutmeg over sautéed spinach, French toast, or mashed sweet potatoes.

CUMIN
Historically, cumin has been used to aid digestion, and more recently, it has emerged as a powerful anticarcinogen. By boosting the liver's ability to detoxify enzymes, cumin helps decrease the incidence of colon, stomach, and liver cancers. **EAT THIS!** Spice up brown rice or couscous with cumin, coriander seeds, almonds, and dried apricots. No bowl of black beans or chili is complete without a heavy hit of this smoky spice.

CINNAMON
Researchers have linked this warm spice to increased brain functioning and blood flow, but it's most renowned for controlling blood sugar levels. This effect has been documented in several studies, with one indicating that those with type 2 diabetes could significantly lower their blood sugar with 1 to 6 grams a day. **EAT THIS!** Sprinkle on sweet potatoes, swirl into oatmeal, or make delicious Mexican-style java by adding a few pinches to ground coffee before brewing.

CORIANDER SEEDS
Studies of mice show that coriander seeds encourage the pancreas to produce more insulin—the hormone that helps shuttle glucose into the cells to be burned as energy. This prevents excess blood sugars from being stored as fat. The plant's leaves—commonly called cilantro—have the same healthful benefits. **EAT THIS!** Add ground coriander to lentil soup or mix it with black pepper and brown sugar and rub all over salmon before roasting in the oven.

CURRY POWDER
The spice rack equivalent of a greatest hits album, curry powder offers the collective benefits of cumin, dry mustard, ginger, coriander, and turmeric. **EAT THIS!** Mix a tablespoon of curry powder with a cup of plain yogurt and a few minced garlic cloves for a dipping sauce for grilled chicken, lamb, or fish.

FENNEL SEEDS

In India, fennel seeds are chewed after meals to freshen the mouth and aid digestion, but actually their benefits are much more far reaching. They play host to healthful amounts of fiber, vitamin C, potassium, folate, and other essential nutrients.

EAT THIS! Combine fennel seeds with fresh thyme, chopped garlic, and fresh-cracked pepper and rub on chicken or sprinkle on vegetables before grilling.

SMOKED PAPRIKA

This Spanish staple—often called pimentón—is ground from dried red peppers and comes in both sweet and spicy varieties. Paprika is extremely high in vitamins A and C, making it a boost to your immune system.

EAT THIS! This spice has become a secret weapon for professional chefs across the country. Try dusting it on scrambled eggs or roasted potatoes or mixing it with low-fat mayo for a smoky, colorful spread or vegetable dip.

GARLIC POWDER

A compound called allicin helps give garlic its cure-all profile. Allicin is a strong antibacterial and antifungal, linking garlic to lower cancer rates, stronger cardiovascular systems, and decreased fat storage and acne inflammation.

EAT THIS! Combine garlic powder with salt and pepper for a basic meat and vegetable rub, or add a pinch to your next pasta sauce.

BLACK PEPPER

The world's most popular spice happens to be the most potent digestive aid at your disposal. When its sharp flavor hits your tongue, it signals your brain to produce hydrochloric acid, which helps discourage unhealthy bacteria growth and may prevent symptoms such as bloating and indigestion.

EAT THIS! Try a traditional Italian way to up the pepper quotient: Mix a container of sliced strawberries with $\frac{1}{4}$ cup of balsamic vinegar and 5 or 6 grinds from the pepper mill. Trust us: healthiest dessert ever.

GROUND GINGER

Ginger's effects reach far beyond just calming uneasy tummies. Its anti-inflammatory properties make it an ideal arthritis treatment, and its antioxidant properties help it prevent such cancers as ovarian and colorectal.

EAT THIS! Sprinkle ginger and orange zest over roasted carrots or fold a teaspoon into oatmeal or pumpkin soup.

TURMERIC

Indians believe this conspicuous yellow powder to be a miracle spice. Studies show that curcumin, the plant's yellow pigment, inhibits tumor growth and can prevent a host of cancers. Turmeric has also been shown to improve cardiovascular health and prevent neurodegenerative diseases like Alzheimer's.

EAT THIS! Make a vibrant rice pilaf by adding $\frac{1}{2}$ teaspoon of turmeric to the boiling water or stock. When the rice is ready, fold in toasted cashews, raisins, and cilantro.

CLOVES

Clove oils are often used to treat pain, and the most notable of these oils is eugenol, which has antiseptic, antiviral, and anti-inflammatory properties. As a food additive, cloves are known to relieve nausea, stimulate appetite, and reduce flatulence.

EAT THIS! The sweet, woody flavor complements cinnamon well, so use the two seasonings together in apple cider or even a curry dish.

Grains

Eat This

Yes, it has a few more calories than the refined couscous, but it also has more protein and 6 times the fiber. Trust us, it's worth it.

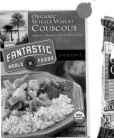

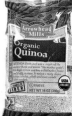

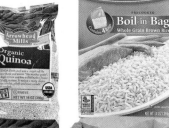

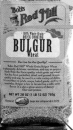

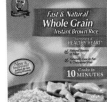

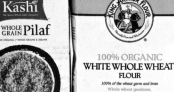

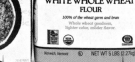

Fantastic World Foods™ Organic Whole Wheat Couscous

(¼ cup, 45 g uncooked)

170 calories
0.5 g fat (0 g saturated)
6 g fiber

Success® Boil-in-Bag Whole Grain Brown Rice

(⅓ cup dry, 43 g, ~1 cup prepared)

150 calories
1 g fat
(0 g saturated)
2 g fiber

Instant whole grains!

Bob's Red Mill® Bulgur from Hard Red Wheat (¼ cup, 40 g dry)

140 calories
0.5 g fat
(0 g saturated)
7 g fiber

Try adding this whole grain to your soups and salads.

Uncle Ben's® Fast & Natural® Whole Grain Quinoa Instant Brown Rice

(~1 cup cooked)

170 calories
1 g fat
(0 g saturated)
2 g fiber

Time is no excuse for eating white rice.

Arrowhead Mills® Organic Quinoa

(1 cup cooked)

160 calories
2.5 g fat
(0 g saturated)
3 g fiber

A true superfood, with plenty of protein, fiber, and heathy fat.

Kashi™ 7 Whole Grain Pilaf

(½ cup cooked)

170 calories
3 g fat
(0 g saturated)
6 g fiber

Compared to regular rice, Kashi's pilaf earns twice the fiber and protein with its formidable blend of whole grains.

King Arthur Flour® 100% Organic White Whole Wheat Flour

(¼ cup, 30 g)

100 calories
0.5 g fat
(0 g saturated)
3 g fiber

Three times the fiber of white flour.

Texmati® Long Grain American Basmati Rice

(¼ cup dry, 45 g)

150 calories
0.5 g fat
(0 g saturated)
0.5 g fiber

Basmati has a milder effect on blood sugar than other white rice.

Not That!

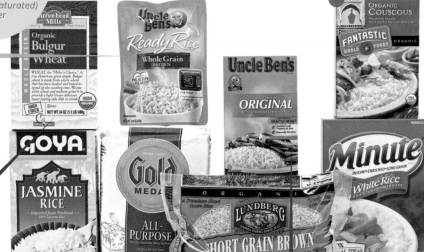

Organic is a nice touch, but whole-grain fiber is the trump.

Fantastic World Foods™ Organic Couscous
(¼ cup, 45 g uncooked)
150 calories
0.5 g fat (0 g saturated)
1 g fiber

Uncle Ben's® Ready Rice® Whole Grain Brown
(1 cup cooked)
240 calories
3 g fat
(0 g saturated)
2 g fiber
Why does Uncle Ben like to add oil to his rice?

Arrowhead Mills® Organic Bulgur Wheat
(¼ cup, 44 g dry)
160 calories
0.5 g fat
(0 g saturated)
6 g fiber
Made from white wheat, this is less nutritious than bulgur made from red wheat.

Goya® Jasmine Rice
(¼ cup dry, 45 g)
170 calories
0 g fat
0 g fiber
Of all types of rice, jasmine has the highest glycemic index—which creates blood-sugar spikes and promotes fat storage.

Gold Medal® All-Purpose Flour (¼ cup, 30 g)
100 calories
0 g fat
<1 g fiber
All-purpose flour has been stripped of the nutritious bran layers and wheat germ, leaving it with little redeeming nutrition.

Lundberg® Short Grain Brown Rice
(¼ cup, 51 g,
~¾ cup cooked)
180 calories
1.5 g fat
(0 g saturated)
3 g fiber
Brown rice is good, but blended whole grains are better.

Uncle Ben's® Original Converted Rice (~1 cup cooked)
170 calories
0 g fat
(0 g saturated)
0 g fiber
There's no room for a fiber-free grain in a healthy diet.

Minute® White Rice
(1 cup cooked)
200 calories
0 g fat
0 g fiber
With no fiber or real nutrition, white rice is decidedly not a health food.

107

Rice Sides
Eat This

This fiber-packed pilaf is completely stocked with wholesome nosh such as sweet corn, tomato paste, black beans, and bell peppers.

Kashi™
Fiery Fiesta
7 Whole Grain Pilaf
(1 cup prepared)

210 calories
5 g fat (0.5 g saturated)
400 mg sodium
7 g fiber

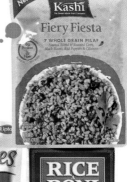

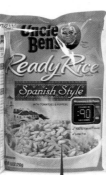
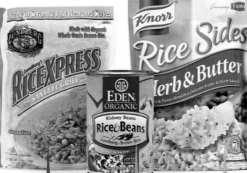
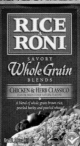

Near East® **Rice Pilaf** **Curry**	**Uncle Ben's®** **Ready Rice®** **Spanish Style**	**Lundberg®** **RiceXpress™** **Santa Fe Grill**	**Eden™** **Organic Rice** **& Beans**	**Knorr®** **Rice Sides™** **Herb & Butter**	**Rice-A-Roni®** **Whole Grain** **Chicken &** **Herb Classico**
(1 cup prepared)	(1 cup prepared)	(~1 cup prepared)	(½ cup, 130 g)	(1 cup prepared)	(1 cup prepared)
220 calories *3.5 g fat* *(2 g saturated)* *710 mg sodium* *2 g fiber*	*200 calories* *2.5 g fat* *(0 g saturated)* *680 mg sodium* *3 g fiber*	*130 calories* *2.5 g fat* *(0 g saturated)* *236 mg sodium* *1.5 g fiber*	*110 calories* *1 g fat* *(0 g saturated)* *135 mg sodium* *3 g fiber*	*280 calories* *4.5 g fat* *(2.5 g saturated)* *800 mg sodium* *1 g fiber*	*260 calories* *8 g fat* *(1 g saturated)* *760 mg sodium* *4 g fiber*
A dose of turmeric helps in the cancer fight.	Fiber + tomatoes + poblano peppers =!	Ready to eat in 60 to 90 seconds.	Nothing but brown rice and antioxidant-rich kidney beans.	Mix in some frozen peas to boost the fiber content.	Rice-A-Roni's best product.

Not That!

Choosing margarine over butter saves a few calories but adds artery-hardening trans fats. Spare your arteries and take the calories.

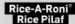

**Rice-A-Roni®
Rice Pilaf**
**(1 cup prepared
with margarine)**

*310 calories
9 g fat (1.5 g saturated,
1.5 g trans)
1,200 mg sodium
2 g fiber*

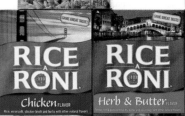

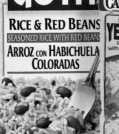

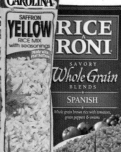

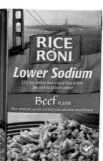

Rice-A-Roni® Chicken	**Rice-A-Roni® Herb & Butter**	**Goya® Rice & Red Beans**	**Carolina® Saffron Yellow Rice**	**Rice-A-Roni® Whole Grain Spanish**	**Rice-A-Roni® Lower Sodium Beef**
(1 cup prepared)	(1 cup prepared)	(¹⁄₂ cup prepared)	(1 cup prepared)	(1 cup prepared)	(1 cup prepared)
310 calories 9 g fat (1.5 g saturated, 1.5 g trans) 1,160 mg sodium 2 g fiber	*310 calories 9 g fat (2 g saturated, 1.5 g trans) 1,160 mg sodium 1 g fiber*	*160 calories 0 g fat 488 mg sodium 3 g fiber*	*190 calories 0 g fat 980 mg sodium 1 g fiber*	*250 calories 8 g fat (1 g saturated) 760 mg sodium 3 g fiber*	*270 calories 5 g fat (1 g saturated, 0.5 g trans) 740 mg sodium 2 g fiber*
One cup shoots half your day's sodium.	Make this with stick margarine, and you'll add 1.5 grams of trans fat.	An apple-size portion of rice will run you more than 300 calories.	The sodium glut comes from the seasoning packet.	None of Rice-A-Roni's Whole Grain Blends has less than 250 calories.	That's lower sodium?

Dry Noodles
Eat This

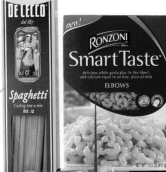

House Foods Tofu Shirataki Noodles
(113 g)

20 calories
0.5 g fat (0 g saturated)
2 g fiber

Seek out these traditional Japanese noodles at your grocery store or online at www.house-foods.com. In 2 servings—the entire bag—there are only 6 grams of carbohydrates, and 4 of them are from fiber.

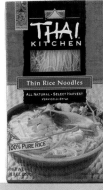

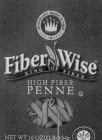

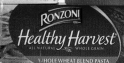

De Cecco® Spaghetti *(56 g)*	Ronzoni® Smart Taste™ Elbows *(56 g)*	Ronzoni® Healthy Harvest® Whole Wheat Blend Spaghetti *(56 g)*	Fiber Wise® High Fiber Penne *(57 g)*	Hodgson Mill® Whole Wheat Whole Grain Elbows *(57 g)*	Thai Kitchen® Thin Rice Noodles *(56 g)*
200 calories 1 g fat (0 g saturated) 2 g fiber	180 calories 1 g fat (0 g saturated) 6 g fiber	180 calories 2 g fat (0 g saturated) 6 g fiber	170 calories 1 g fat (0 g saturated) 12 g fiber	210 calories 1 g fat (0 g saturated) 6 g fiber	180 calories 0.5 g fat (0 g saturated) 1 g fiber
If you insist on white noodles, De Cecco is among the best.	As a bonus, these elbows contain 30% of your calcium.	The best-tasting wheat pasta.	As fiber-rich as any food in the supermarket.	Make your next batch of mac and cheese with these.	Made from rice and water, which provides 3 grams of protein and zero sodium.

Not That!

Don't be fooled by the flurry of health claims decorating this package. The main ingredient is still flour, making it nutritionally similar to any normal noodle.

No Yolks®
Egg White Pasta
(56 g)

210 calories
0.5 g fat (0 g saturated)
3 g fiber

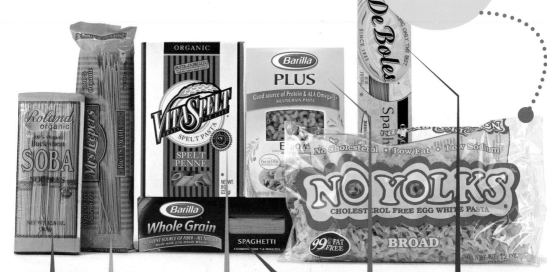

Roland® Organic Buckwheat Soba Noodles
(56 g)

200 calories
1 g fat
(0 g saturated)
1 g fiber

42% of your daily intake of sodium.

Mrs. Leeper's™ Rice Spaghetti
(56 g)

200 calories
2 g fat
(0 g saturated)
2 g fiber

Unless you're trying to avoid gluten, stick with whole-wheat pasta.

Vita-Spelt® Penne
(57 g)

210 calories
1 g fat
(0 g saturated)
2 g fiber

Spelt is nutritious and protein-rich, but not when it's refined.

Barilla® Whole Grain Spaghetti
(56 g)

200 calories
1.5 g fat
(0 g saturated)
6 g fiber

This Barilla option still beats white noodles any day.

Barilla® Plus Elbows
(56 g)

210 calories
2 g fat
(0 g saturated)
4 g fiber

Way better than normal Barilla boxes, but there are still stronger options.

DeBoles® Spaghetti Style Pasta
(57 g)

210 calories
1 g fat
(0 g saturated)
1 g fiber

Avoid noodles with fewer than 2 grams of fiber.

Packaged and Seasoned
Eat This

Kraft® Deluxe Macaroni and Cheese Dinner
(~1 cup prepared)

290 calories
4.5 g fat (2 g saturated)
850 mg sodium
2 g fiber

Go Deluxe and you can mac it up for a quarter of the fat.

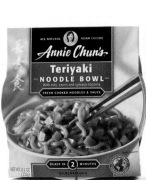

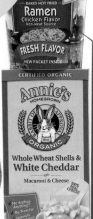

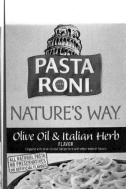

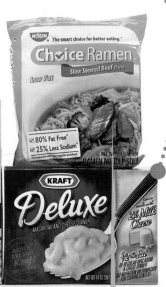

Annie Chun's® Teriyaki Noodle Bowl
(1 bowl, 232 g)

400 calories
5 g fat
(0 g saturated)
880 mg sodium

Annie Chun's gives you twice the food with only 74% of the calories.

Annie's® Organic Whole Wheat Shells & White Cheddar
(~1 cup prepared)

260 calories
5 g fat
(2.5 g saturated)
580 mg sodium

Mac and cheese made of just noodles and cheese. Imagine that.

Dr. McDougall's Ramen Chicken
(~1 cup, 60 g)

100 calories
0.5 g fat
(0 g saturated)
320 mg sodium

Dr. McDougall's will save you 100 calories of pure fat, and each cup has 10 grams of protein.

Pasta Roni® Nature's Way™ Olive Oil & Italian Herb
(1 cup prepared)

250 calories
8 g fat
(1.5 g saturated)
800 mg sodium

Nature's Way line adds no preservatives or artificial flavors.

Nissin™ Choice Ramen™ Slow Stewed Beef
(1 block, 80 g)

280 calories
2 g fat
(0 g saturated)
800 mg sodium

Since it's not fried, Nissin's Choice Ramen has 85% less fat than Maruchan Ramen.

Noodles

Not That!

**Kraft®
Macaroni &
Cheese Dinner**
(~1 cup prepared)

*410 calories
19 g fat (5 g saturated,
4 g trans)
710 mg sodium
1 g fiber*

*If you split this
box two ways, you actually
get 615 calories.
At the very least, omit the
margarine to cut out
the coating of trans fat.*

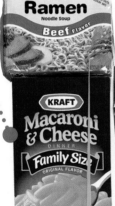

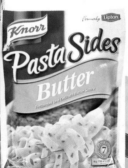

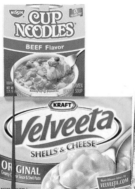

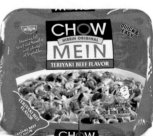

**Maruchan®
Ramen Beef**
(1 block, 86 g)

*380 calories
14 g fat
(7 g saturated)
1,580 mg sodium*

Where does all that
fat come from?
Vegetable oil is the
second ingredient
in the recipe.

**Knorr® Pasta
Sides™ Butter**
(1 cup prepared)

*270 calories
8 g fat
(3 g saturated)
810 mg sodium*

It might not seem
like much, but if you
can cut your saturated
fat in half so easily,
why not do it?

**Nissin®
Cup Noodles
Beef**
(1 cup, 64 g)

*300 calories
13 g fat
(7 g saturated)
1,110 mg sodium*

One of the cheapest
sources of empty
calories in the aisles.

**Kraft®
Velveeta
Original Shells
& Cheese**
(~1 cup prepared)

*360 calories
12 g fat
(4 g saturated)
940 mg sodium*

Why pass up an easy
opportunity to save
100 calories?

**Nissin® Original
Chow Mein
Teriyaki
Beef Flavor**
(1 container, 113.4 g)

*540 calories
22 g fat
(8 g saturated)
1,500 mg sodium*

This mini meal
has two-thirds of your
daily sodium!

113

Bread Loaves

Eat This

This unsuspecting potato bread is one of the best loaves on the shelf. It also packs an impressive 12 grams of protein.

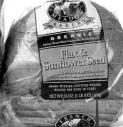

Martin's 100% Whole Wheat Potato Bread

(2 slices, 70 g)

140 calories
2 g fat (0 g saturated)
8 g fiber

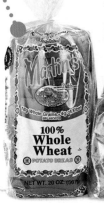

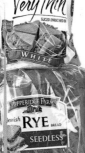

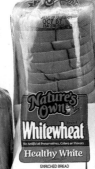

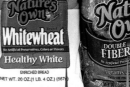

Pepperidge Farm® Very Thin White

(2 slices, 30 g)

*80 calories
0.5 g fat
(0 g saturated)
<1 g fiber*

You don't eat the thin breads for fiber—you eat them to cut carbs and calories.

Pepperidge Farm® Jewish Rye Seedless

(2 slices, 64 g)

*160 calories
2 g fat
(0 g saturated)
2 g fiber*

Not enough fiber to be your go-to bread, but good enough for the occasional pastrami sandwich.

Nature's Own® Whitewheat®

(2 slices, 52 g)

*100 calories
2 g fat
(0.5 g saturated)
5 g fiber*

The new white-wheat breads are a good compromise for finicky eaters: It carries the fiber load of whole wheat with a soft white taste.

Nature's Own® Double Fiber Wheat

(2 slices, 56 g)

*100 calories
1 g fat
(0 g saturated)
10 g fiber*

This is the most fiber you're going to find in bread less than 150 calories.

French Meadow® Organic Flax & Sunflower Seed

(2 slices, 70 g)

*180 calories
3 g fat (0 g saturated)
4 g fiber*

This nutritional powerhouse gets fiber and omega-3 fats from the flax seeds and a dose of vitamin E from the sunflower seeds.

Not That!

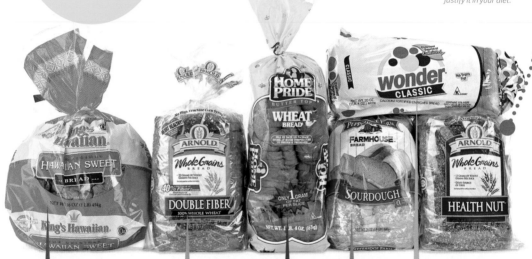

Arnold® Whole Grains Health Nut
(2 slices, 86 g)

240 calories
4 g fat (0 g saturated)
4 g fiber

Don't fall for the label braggadocio. For as calorie dense as this bread is, there's just not enough fiber to justify it in your diet.

King's Hawaiian® Hawaiian Sweet Bread (½" slice, 56 g)

200 calories
5 g fat
(3 g saturated)
2 g fiber

Aside from being absurdly loaded with sugar (12 grams), this bread lists the highly saturated palm oil as its fourth ingredient.

Arnold® Double Fiber 100% Whole Wheat (2 slices, 86 g total)

200 calories
3 g fat (0 g saturated)
10 g fiber

The fiber load is impressive, but why not get the same 10 grams for less fat and half the calories?

Home Pride® Butter Top Wheat Bread (2 slices, 56 g)

140 calories
2 g fat
(0 g saturated)
2 g fiber

It may say wheat on the label, but the vital nutrition stats don't show the benefit.

Pepperidge Farm® Farmhouse™ Sourdough (2 slices, 86 g)

240 calories
3 g fat (1 g saturated)
2 g fiber

Most sourdough is made from white flour. Either choose a whole-wheat version or switch to a better bread like rye.

Wonder® Classic (2 slices, 52 g)

120 calories
1 g fat
(0 g saturated)
0 g fiber

Wonder Bread's complete lack of fiber will have you feeling hungry for a second sandwich before you even finish the first.

115

Rolls and Buns
Eat This

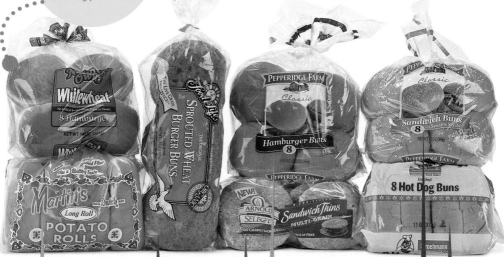

Nature's Own® Whitewheat® Hamburger Buns
(1 bun, 50 g)

100 calories
2 g fat (0.5 g saturated)
5 g fiber

To compensate for the deficiencies of enriched wheat flour, Nature's Own adds soy fiber, a good mix of soluble and insoluble.

Martin's Potato Rolls
(1 roll, 53 g)

130 calories
1.5 g fat
(0 g saturated)
4 g fiber

Four grams of fiber and 6 grams of protein could keep you from reaching for a second frank.

Food for Life® Sprouted Wheat Burger Buns
(1 bun, 62 g)

150 calories
2.5 g fat
(0 g saturated)
5 g fiber

Sprouted wheat maximizes fiber and nutrient availability.

Arnold® Select™ Multi-Grain Sandwich Thins
(1 roll, 43 g)

100 calories
1 g fat
(0 g saturated)
5 g fiber

Perfect for a burger, a turkey sandwich, or scrambled eggs.

Pepperidge Farm® Classic Hamburger Buns (1 bun, 43g)

120 calories
2 g fat
(0.5 g saturated)
1 g fiber

For those who think it's sacrilege to tarnish meat with wheat, this is your bun.

Pepperidge Farm® Classic Sandwich Buns with Sesame Seeds
(1 bun, 46 g)

130 calories
3 g fat
(0.5 g saturated)
1 g fiber

Packed with copper and magnesium.

Stroehmann® Hot Dog Buns
(1 bun, 39 g)

110 calories
1.5 g fat
(0 g saturated)
1 g fiber

Considering how many hot dogs the average American eats in a year, it's essential to have a low-cal bun on hand.

Not That!

Sara Lee® Whole Grain White Hamburger Buns
(1 bun, 43 g)

120 calories
1.5 g fat (0 g saturated)
1 g fiber

With four times as much sugar as fiber, this white-wheat hybrid fails to pass the health test.

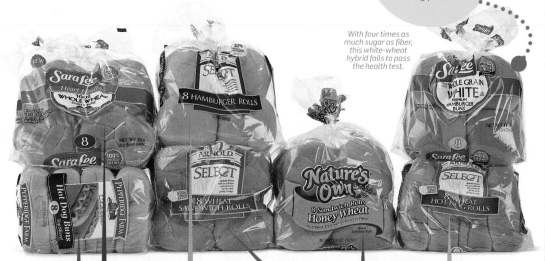

Pepperidge Farm® Classic Hot Dog Buns
(1 bun, 50 g)

140 calories
2.5 g fat
(0.5 g saturated)
<1 g fiber

Ban all buns made with partially hydrogenated oils from your pantry!

Sara Lee® Heart Healthy 100% Whole Wheat Bakery Buns (1 bun, 74 g)

210 calories
3 g fat
(1 g saturated)
4 g fiber

A 210-calorie bun is one reason careless sandwich eaters get fat.

Arnold Select® Hamburger Rolls (1 roll, 57 g)

150 calories
2 g fat
(0.5 g saturated)
1 g fiber

This bun has about the same number of calories as a very lean, 3-ounce burger.

Arnold® Select™ Wheat Sandwich Rolls (1 roll, 57 g)

150 calories
2 g fat
(0.5 g saturated)
2 g fiber

In the world of whole wheat, this is a mediocre performer at best.

Nature's Own® Honey Wheat Sandwich Rolls
(1 roll, 53 g)

130 calories
1.5 g fat
(1 g saturated)
1 g fiber

Wheat bread should always have more than 1 gram of fiber.

Arnold® Select™ Wheat Hot Dog Rolls
(1 roll, 50 g)

130 calories
2 g fat
(0 g saturated)
2 g fiber

Not bad, but Martin's are better—and they don't even taste like wheat.

Breakfast Breads
Eat This

Thomas'® Light Multi-Grain English Muffin
(1 muffin, 57 g)

100 calories
1 g fat (0 g saturated)
8 g fiber

A healthy host of fibrous and protein-rich grains with a modest caloric load makes this an exemplary breakfast bread.

Vermont Bread Company® Honey Wheat Organic English Muffins
(1 muffin, 57 g)

140 calories
1 g fat (0 g saturated)
2 g fiber

Honey provides the bulk of this muffin's modest 6 grams of sugar.

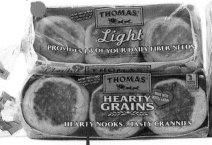
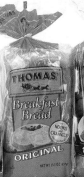
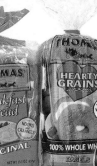

Thomas'® Hearty Grains™ Double Fiber English Muffins Honey Wheat
(1 muffin, 57 g)

110 calories
0.5 g fat (0 g saturated)
5 g fiber

A tremendous amount of fiber for such a small muffin.

Thomas'® Breakfast Bread Original
(1 slice, 37 g)

90 calories
1 g fat (0 g saturated)
1 g fiber

Not a nutritional superstar, but if you want white bread for breakfast, this is better than most.

Thomas'® Hearty Grains™ 100% Whole Wheat Bagels
(1 bagel, 95 g)

240 calories
2 g fat (0.5 g saturated)
7 g fiber

Most bagels are pure refined carbs, but this one packs a huge fiber punch.

Pillsbury Golden Layers™ Honey Butter Biscuits
(1 biscuit, 34 g)

110 calories
4.5 g fat (1 g saturated, 1.5 g trans)
290 mg sodium

Limit yourself to one biscuit; any more and you'll be flirting with a dangerous intake of trans fats.

Vermont Bread Company® Cinnamon Raisin
(1 slice, 31 g)

70 calories
0 g fat
6 g sugars
2 g fiber

If you like your breakfast to taste more like dessert, make sure there's still fiber in it.

Not That!

Thomas'® Hearty Grains™ Multi-Grain English Muffins

(1 muffin, 57 g)

150 calories
2.5 g fat
(0 g saturated)
2 g fiber

The main grain is still enriched flour (that is, white flour).

Rudi's Organic Bakery® Whole Grain Wheat English Muffins

(1 muffin, 57 g)

120 calories
1 g fat (0 g saturated)
3 g fiber

A decent choice, but if you want to see a stellar choice, see the Thomas' muffin on the opposite page.

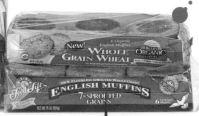

Thomas'® Swirl Cinnamon Raisin

(1 slice, 38 g)

120 calories
2 g fat
(1 g saturated)
9 g sugars
1 g fiber

Closer to dessert than breakfast with those sugar counts.

Pillsbury Grands!® Flaky Layers Biscuits

(1 biscuit, 58 g)

190 calories
9 g fat
(2.5 g saturated,
2.5 g trans)
550 mg sodium

Food manufacturers have been reluctant to replace trans fats in biscuits.

Sara Lee® Deluxe Bagels Plain

(1 bagel, 104 g)

270 calories
1.5 g fat
(0.5 g saturated)
2 g fiber

This giant wad of bleached flour will send a sugar load into your bloodstream so fast that the button might fly right off your jeans.

Pepperidge Farm® Farmhouse™ Bread Soft Oatmeal

(1 slice, 43 g)

120 calories
1.5 g fat
(0.5 g saturated)
1 g fiber

Don't assume oatmeal is always healthy.

Food for Life® 7-Sprouted Grains English Muffins

(1 muffin, 76 g)

160 calories
2 g fat
(0 g saturated)
6 g fiber

Not a bad choice, per se, but Thomas' has a much better calorie-to-fiber ratio.

119

Breakfast Pastries
Eat This

Krispy Kreme® Doughnuts Original Glazed

(1 donut, 49 g)

190 calories
11 g fat (4.5 g saturated)
10 g sugars

There is nothing nutritionally redeeming about donuts, but who would have guessed that they're less evil than blueberry muffins?

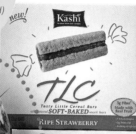

Kashi
new!
TLC
Tasty Little Cereal Bars
SOFT-BAKED snack bars
RIPE STRAWBERRY

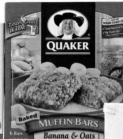

QUAKER
Tastes Great WARM!
Baked
MUFFIN BARS
Banana & Oats
Naturally Flavored
6 Bars

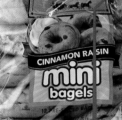

THOMAS'
CINNAMON RAISIN
mini
bagels

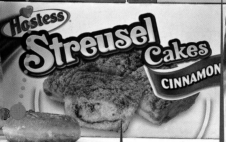

Hostess
Streusel
Cakes
CINNAMON

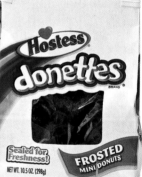

Hostess
donettes
Sealed for Freshness!
FROSTED
MINI DONUTS
NET WT. 10.5 OZ. (298g)

Kashi® TLC® Soft-Baked Snack Bars Ripe Strawberry

(1 bar, 35 g)

110 calories
3 g fat
(0 g saturated)
9 g sugars
3 g fiber

A much better fiber-to-sugar ratio.

Thomas' Mini Bagels Cinnamon Raisin

(1 bagel, 43 g)

120 calories
1 g fat
(0 g saturated)
6 g sugars

The convenience of a Little Debbie product without the tablespoon of sugar.

Hostess® Streusel Cakes Cinnamon

(1 cake, 46 g)

170 calories
6 g fat
(1.5 g saturated)
20 g sugars

It's a heavy load of sugar, so make this an occasional treat.

Quaker® Muffin Bars Banana & Oats (1 bar, 37 g)

130 calories
3.5 g fat
(1 g saturated)
11 g sugars

By trading whole oats for flour, Quaker's Muffin Bars manage more fiber with a fraction of the calories.

Hostess® Donettes® Frosted

(4 donuts, 57 g)

240 calories
14 g fat
(10 g saturated)
16 g sugars
<1 g fiber

In the world of donuts, nobody wins, but these are the lesser evils.

Not That!

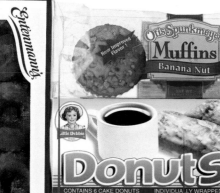
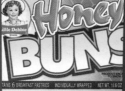
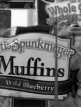
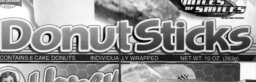

The serving size on back is half a muffin, but who eats just half a muffin?

**Otis Spunkmeyer®
Muffins Wild
Blueberry**
(1 muffin, 114 g)

*420 calories
22 g fat (3 g saturated)
30 g sugars*

**Entenmann's®
Frosted Devil's
Food Donuts**
(1 donut, 67 g)

*310 calories
18 g fat
(12 g saturated)
24 g sugars
2 g fiber*

You'd save 100 calories eating most donuts from Dunkin Donuts.

**Otis
Spunkmeyer®
Muffins
Banana Nut**
(1 muffin, 114 g)

*460 calories
22 g fat
(3 g saturated)
32 g sugars*

Sounds healthy, right? Think again.

**Little Debbie®
Donut Sticks**
(1 donut, 47 g)

*230 calories
14 g fat
(7 g saturated)
15 g sugars*

One stick brings nearly a day's saturated fat to the breakfast table.

**Little Debbie®
Honey Buns**
(1 pastry, 50 g)

*220 calories
12 g fat
(6 g saturated)
13 g sugars*

Each sticky bun is a mix of flour, sugar, palm oil, and partially hydrogenated vegetable oil.

**Kellogg's®
Pop-Tarts®
Whole Grain
Strawberry**
(1 pastry, 50 g)

*190 calories
5 g fat
(1.5 g saturated fat)
15 g sugars
3 g fiber*

Even whole-wheat flour can't save the Pop-Tart.

121

Eat This

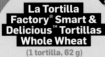

La Tortilla Factory® Smart & Delicious™ Tortillas Whole Wheat

(1 tortilla, 62 g)

80 calories
3 g fat (0 g saturated)
12 g fiber

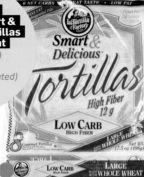

This giant tortilla is easily the best on the shelf. In addition to lower calories and more fiber, it has more protein and less sodium than the Mission tortilla.

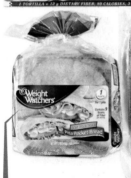

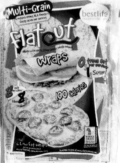

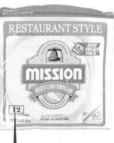

Weight Watchers® Pita 100% Whole Wheat

(1 pita, 57 g)

100 calories
1 g fat
(0 g saturated)
9 g fiber

It's not the low calories and fat that's impressive, it's the massive load of fiber.

Flatout® Wraps Multi-Grain

(1 flatbread, 53 g)

100 calories
2.5 g fat (0 g saturated)
8 g fiber

These soft flatbreads have even more protein than fiber, and their stretchy consistency makes them perfect for overstuffing with hummus and salads.

Mission® White Corn Tortillas

(2 tortillas, 51 g)

110 calories
1.5 g fat
(0 g saturated)
3 g fiber

Corn tortillas will always trump flour tortillas. That's because they're made with whole grain corn and little else.

Tumaro's® Low in Carbs Tortillas Salsa

(1 tortilla, 39 g)

100 calories
2.5 g fat (0 g saturated)
8 g fiber

This tortilla carries 7 grams of protein and is packed with healthy oat fiber.

Wraps

Not That!

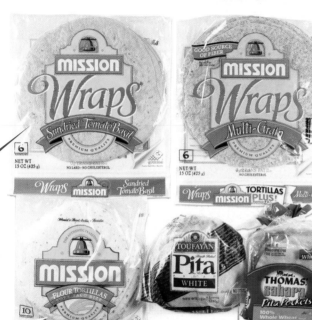

Mission® Wraps Multi-Grain
(1 tortilla, 70 g)

210 calories
6 g fat (1.5 g saturated)
7 g fiber

Mission's big tortillas are nearly a full meal before you even start filling them.

Mission® Wraps Sundried Tomato Basil
(1 tortilla, 70 g)

210 calories
5 g fat (2 g saturated)
2 g fiber

Even in the flavored varieties, you just can't trust Mission's flour tortillas. They're just massive vehicles for refined carbs.

Mission® Flour Tortillas Soft Taco Size
(1 tortilla, 49 g)

150 calories
3.5 g fat (1.5 g saturated)
1 g fiber

Corn tortillas carry a far lighter caloric load than their wheat flour counterparts. Watch for "vegetable shortening" on the ingredients list. That usually means there's a secret stash of trans fats inside.

Toufayan Bakeries Pita White
(1 loaf, 56 g)

160 calories
0 g fat
1 g fiber

Any bread that says "white" on it is bound to do a number on your blood sugar.

Thomas' Sahara® Pita 100% Whole Wheat
(1 loaf, 57 g)

140 calories
1.5 g fat
(0 g saturated)
4 g fiber

A better sandwich option than many sliced breads, but not the best pita on the shelf.

123

Bread Mixes

Eat This

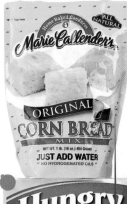

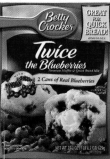

Hungry Jack® Complete Buttermilk Pancake and Waffle Mix

(½ cup prepared, 4 3" pancakes)

150 calories
1.5 g fat (0 g saturated)
7 g sugars

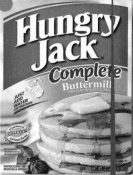

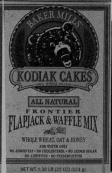

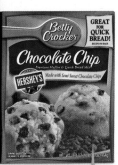

If you're making a carb-heavy breakfast, buttermilk trumps Belgian, but please, use the condiments in moderation.

Marie Callender's® Original Corn Bread Mix

(¼ cup prepared)

150 calories
3 g fat
(0 g saturated)
9 g sugars

About as good as it gets with corn muffins.

Betty Crocker® Twice the Blueberries Muffin and Quick Bread Mix

(39 g mix & blueberries prepared)

160 calories
4.5 g fat
(1 g saturated)
16 g sugars

Baker Mills® Kodiak Cakes Frontier Flapjack & Waffle Mix

(⅓ cup prepared with water, 40 g)

130 calories
1 g fat
(0 g saturated)
2 g sugars

Made from whole grain wheat and oat flour.

Betty Crocker® Premium Muffin & Quick Bread Mix Chocolate Chip

(¼ cup prepared)

212 calories
9 g fat
(3 g saturated)
17 g sugars

25% less sugar than Ghirardelli's.

Not That!

Krusteaz® Belgian Waffle Mix
(½ cup prepared)

*400 calories
4 g fat (0.5 g saturated)
12 g sugars*

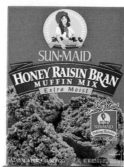

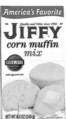

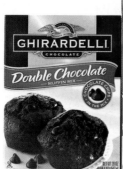

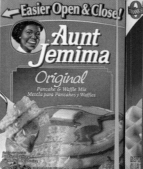

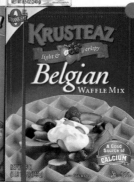

Ghirardelli® Double Chocolate Muffin Mix
(¼ cup prepared)

*250 calories
10 g fat
(3.5 g saturated)
24 g sugar*

Aunt Jemima® Original
(4 4" pancakes prepared with oil and egg)

*250 calories
9 g fat
(2.5 g saturated)
10 g sugars*

Avoid pancakes that can't boast more than a single gram of fiber.

Sun-Maid® Honey Raisin Bran Muffin Mix
(⅓ cup prepared with egg and vegetable oil, 45 g)

*266 calories
7.5 g fat
(2 g saturated, 0.5 g trans)
27 g sugars*

The first ingredient is sugar.

Jiffy® Corn Muffin Mix
(¼ cup prepared, 38 g)

*170 calories
6 g fat
(3 g saturated)
7 g sugars*

Jiffy manages to stuff quite a bit of fat into such a small package.

Add butter and syrup and you're looking at 600 calories of sweet, fatty, and fiber-free bread dough.

125

Wholesome Cereals
Eat This

Kashi™ Vive™ Toasted Graham & Vanilla
(1 cup, 44 g)

136 calories
2 g fat (1 g saturated)
8 g sugars
9.5 g fiber

This unique and healthful powerhouse includes ginger and broccoli extract.

Nature's Path Heritage® Heirloom Multigrain
(1 cup, 40 g)

160 calories
1.5 g fat
(0 g saturated)
5.5 g sugars
8 g fiber

A mix of 7 different whole grains.

General Mills® Cheerios®
(1 cup, 28 g)

100 calories
2 g fat
(0 g saturated)
1 g sugars
3 g fiber

Low calories and a great fiber-to-sugar ratio for this American icon.

General Mills® Fiber One® Raisin Bran Clusters®
(1 cup, 55 g)

170 calories
1 g fat
(0 g saturated)
13 g sugars
11 g fiber

More fiber at breakfast means fewer calories over the rest of the day.

Kellogg's® All-Bran® Original
(1 cup, 62 g)

160 calories
2 g fat
(0 g saturated)
12 g sugars
20 g fiber

As fiber-rich as it gets, which is great news for your blood sugar levels.

Post® Shredded Wheat Original Spoon Size
(1 cup, 49 g)

170 calories
1 g fat
(0 g saturated)
0 g sugars
6 g fiber

One ingredient: whole grain wheat. It just doesn't get any better.

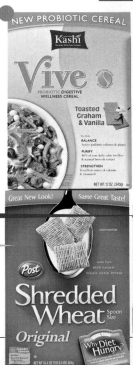

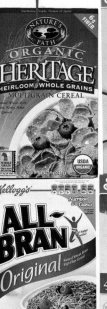

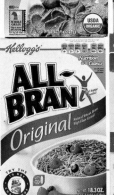

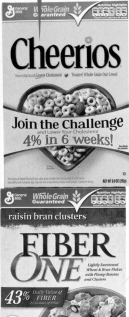

Not That!

Kellogg's® Raisin Bran® (1 cup, 59 g)

190 calories
1.5 g fat
(0 g saturated)
19 g sugars
7 g fiber

Be wary of Raisin Bran. The sugar-saturated cereal is like a wolf in sheep's clothing on the supermarket shelf.

Quaker® Life® (¾ cup, 32 g)

120 calories
1.5 g fat
(0 g saturated)
6 g sugars
2 g fiber

Not a bad choice, but there are too many better ones to make this part of your daily regimen.

General Mills® Basic 4® (1 cup, 55 g)

200 calories
2.5 g fat
(0.5 g saturated)
13 g sugars
3 g fiber

The box looks healthy, but the recipe says otherwise. It includes partially hydrogenated oils and a huge helping of sugar.

Kellogg's® Smart Start® Original Antioxidants
(1 cup, 50 g)

190 calories
0.5 g fat (0 g saturated)
14 g sugars
3 g fiber

Despite Kellogg's loaded health claims about this cereal, sugar and other sweeteners show up no fewer than 10 times on the ingredient list.

Quaker® Natural Low Fat Granola with Raisins
(1 cup, 78 g)

315 calories
4.5 g fat
(2.5 g saturated)
4.5 g fiber
27 g sugars

This granola has more sugar than a pack of Peanut M&M's.

General Mills® Chex® Multi-Bran
(1 cup, 59 g)

210 calories
2 g fat
(0 g saturated)
13 g sugars
8 g fiber

"Hint of Sweetness" means as much sugar as a scoop of vanilla ice cream.

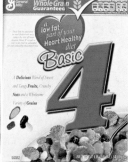

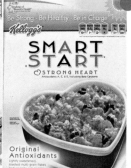

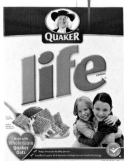

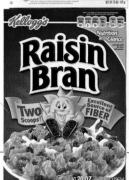

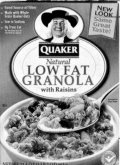

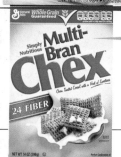

127

Sweet Cereals

None of these cereals are ideal for daily consumption, but if you must have sugary stuff in your pantry, stick to this page.

Eat This

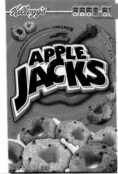

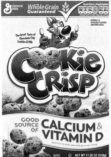

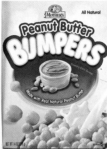

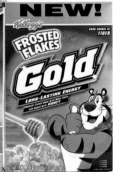

Kellogg's® Apple Jacks®
(1 cup, 28 g)
110 calories
0.5 g fat (0 g saturated)
12 g sugars
<1 g fiber

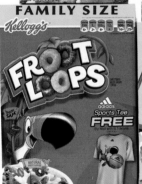

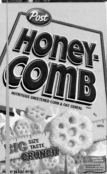

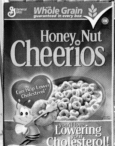

**Kellogg's®
Froot Loops®**
(1 cup, 29 g)

110 calories
1 g fat
(0.5 g saturated)
12 g sugars
<1 g fiber

In the world of sugary cereals, this is a surprisingly sober pick.

**General Mills®
Cookie Crisp®**
(1 cup, 35 g)

133 calories
1.5 g fat
(0 g saturated)
15 g sugars
1.5 g fiber

Don't look at this as breakfast; look at it as dessert.

**Post®
Honey-Comb**
(1 cup, 21 g)

87 calories
0.5 g fat
(0 g saturated)
7 g sugars
1.5 g fiber

Not particularly nutritious, but as a treat, this one is relatively harmless.

**General Mills®
Honey Nut
Cheerios®**
(1 cup, 36 g)

147 calories
2 g fat
(0 g saturated)
12 g sugars
2.5 g fiber

Blend with regular Cheerios to cut down on the sugar.

**Kellogg's®
Frosted Flakes
Gold**
(1 cup, 40 g)

147 calories
0.5 g fat
(0 g saturated)
13 g sugars
4 g fiber

High in sugar, but high in fiber as well.

**Mother's®
Peanut Butter
Bumpers™**
(1 cup, 33 g)

130 calories
2.5 g fat
(0.5 g saturated)
10 g sugars
1 g fiber

Made with real peanut butter, honey, and molasses.

Not That!

Regular Cheerios are great, but whenever General Mills tries to tinker, the outcome is always a fat-inducing glob of wheat and sugar.

General Mills® Apple Cinnamon Cheerios®

(1 cup, 40 g)

160 calories
2 g fat (0 g saturated)
16 g sugars
1.5 g fiber

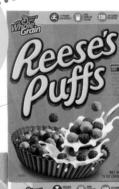

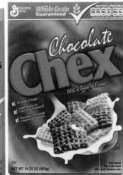

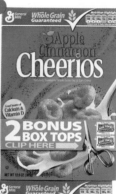

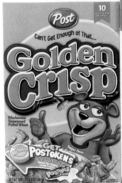

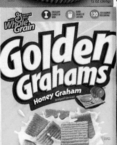

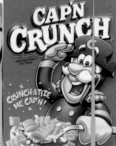

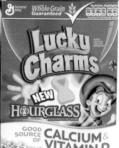

General Mills® Reese's® Puffs®

(1 cup, 38 g)

160 calories
4 g fat
(1 g saturated)
16 g sugars
1.5 g fiber

One cup has 20% more sugar than a peanut butter cup.

Post® Golden Crisp®

(1 cup, 36 g)

147 calories
0 g fat
19 g sugars
<1 g fiber

More than 50% of the calories come from sugar.

General Mills® Golden Grahams®

(1 cup, 40 g)

160 calories
1.5 g fat
(0 g saturated)
15 g sugars
1.5 g fiber

"Golden" is not a redeeming quality in breakfast cereals.

Cap'n Crunch®

(1 cup, 36 g)

147 calories
2 g fat
(1.5 g saturated)
16 g sugars
1.5 g fiber

Cap'n includes a liberal dose of yellow #5, which has been linked to hyperactive behavior in children.

General Mills® Chocolate Chex®

(1 cup, 42 g)

174 calories
3.5 g fat
(1 g saturated)
11 g sugars
1 g fiber

Don't choose a sweetened cereal with more than 150 calories per cup.

General Mills® Lucky Charms®

(1 cup, 36 g)

147 calories
1.5 g fat
(0 g saturated)
15 g sugars
1.5 g fiber

Marshmallows are bad news—especially in cereal.

129

Hot Cereals
Eat This

Quaker® Oats Quick-1 Minute
(½ cup dry, 40 g)

150 calories
3 g fat
(0.5 g saturated)
1 g sugars
4 g fiber

A sprinkle of cinnamon will help your body regulate your blood sugar.

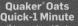

Quaker® High Fiber Cinnamon Swirl
(1 packet, 45 g)

160 calories
2 g fat (0.5 g saturated)
6 g sugars
10 g fiber

This has just what you want in a presweetened instant oatmeal: high fiber and low sugar.

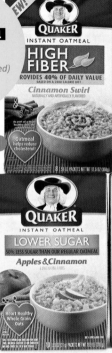

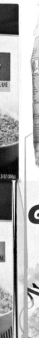

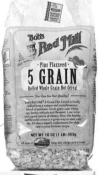

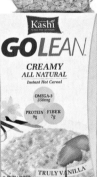

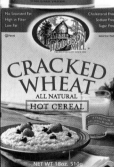

Quaker Lower Sugar Apples & Cinnamon
(1 packet, 31 g)

110 calories
1.5 g fat
(0.5 g saturated)
6 g sugars
3 g fiber

Half the sugar of Quaker's regular Apples & Cinnamon oatmeal.

Bob's Red Mill® 5 Grain Rolled Whole Grain
(½ cup, 35 g)

120 calories
1.5 g fat
(0 g saturated)
0 g sugars
5 g fiber

Bob's grains are some of the most reliable products in the market.

Kashi™ GoLean™ Creamy Instant Truly Vanilla™
(1 packet, 40 g)

150 calories
2 g fat
(0 g saturated)
6 g sugars
7 g fiber

Kashi has a third of Simple Harvest's sugar with triple the fiber.

Hodgson Mill® Cracked Wheat
(¼ cup, 40 g)

110 calories
1 g fat
(0 g saturated)
0 g sugars
5 g fiber

The entire wheat berry cracked open, boxed, and delivered to your supermarket.

Not That!

Quaker® Instant Grits Original
(2 packets, 56 g)

200 calories
0 g fat
2 g fiber

The processed corn from which grits are made has a high concentration of starches, which bumps the calories but not the fiber.

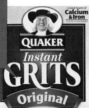

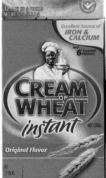

Quaker® Instant® Oatmeal Cinnamon & Spice
(1 packet, 46 g)

170 calories
2 g fat (0.5 g saturated)
15 g sugars
3 g fiber

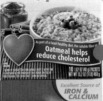

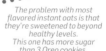

The problem with most flavored instant oats is that they're sweetened to beyond healthy levels. This one has more sugar than 3 Oreo cookies.

Cream of Wheat Instant Maple Brown Sugar
(1 packet, 35 g)

120 calories
0 g fat
12 g sugars
1 g fiber

Who cares if it's fat-free with this much sugar and this little fiber?

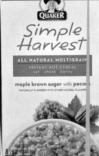

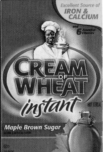

Cream of Wheat Instant
(3 Tbsp, 33 g)

120 calories
0 g fat
0 g sugars
1 g fiber

Cream of Wheat loses its fiber when the bran and germ are removed. Either stick to oatmeal or switch to a less-processed wheat cereal.

Quaker® Simple Harvest® Multigrain Maple Brown Sugar with Pecans
(1 packet, 42 g)

160 calories
3.5 g fat (0.5 g saturated)
9 g sugars
2 g fiber

Quaker® Oatmeal Express™ Golden Brown Sugar
(1 cup, 54 g)

200 calories
2.5 g fat (0.5 g saturated)
18 g sugars
3 g fiber

You'll need a lot more fiber to curtail the sugar surge.

Breakfast Condiments
Eat This

Land O Lakes® Whipped Butter Salted
(1 Tbsp, 7 g)

50 calories
6 g fat (3.5 g saturated)
50 mg sodium

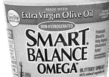

"Whipped" is the key word here—it means air has been introduced into the butter so that it's lighter and easier to spread.

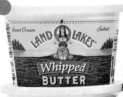

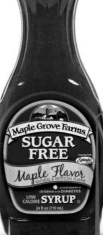

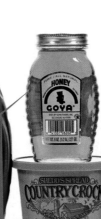

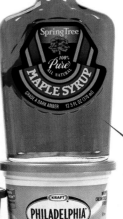

Smart Balance® Omega™ Buttery Spread with Extra Virgin Olive Oil
(1 Tbsp, 11 g)

60 calories
7 g fat
(2 g saturated)
70 mg sodium

Packs a big boost of omega-3s.

Maple Grove Farms® Sugar Free Syrup Maple Flavor
(¼ cup, 60 mL)

30 calories
0 g fat
0 g sugars

Maple Grove uses safer sugar alternatives than the standard aspartame.

Goya® Honey
(2 Tbsp, 42 g)

120 calories
0 g fat
32 g sugars

Honey's antiviral, antibacterial, and antifungal properties help explain why full books are written on the natural sweetener's healing powers.

Shedd's Spread Country Crock® Spread
(1 Tbsp, 14 g)

60 calories
7 g fat
(1.5 g saturated)
110 mg sodium

If you're going to buy margarine, pick up a trans fat-free tub.

Kraft® Philadelphia® Whipped Cream Cheese Spread
(2 Tbsp, 21 g)

60 calories
6 g fat
(3.5 g saturated)
<1 g sugars

Lower in calories and easier to spread.

Spring Tree® 100% Pure Maple Syrup
(¼ cup, 60 mL)

210 calories
0 g fat
50 g sugars

The benefit is more than a few calories. The big dose of manganese boosts energy and stabilizes blood sugar levels.

132

Not That!

I Can't Believe It's Not Butter!® Original
(1 Tbsp, 14 g)

70 calories
8 g fat (2 g saturated)
90 mg sodium

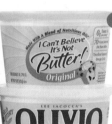

Margarine is a scientist's amalgamation of chemicals and artificial flavors, and most still contain trace amounts of trans fats. Your best choice, as always, is real butter in moderation.

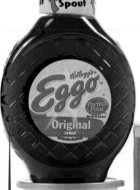

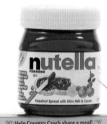

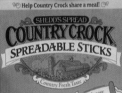

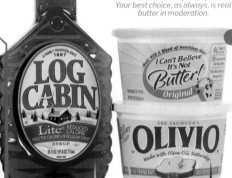

Kellogg's® Eggo™ Original Syrup	Kraft® Philadelphia Cream Cheese	Shedd's Spread Country Crock® Spreadable Sticks	Nutella®	Log Cabin® Lite™ Syrup	Olivio®
(¼ cup, 60 mL)	(2 Tbsp, 31 g)	(1 Tbsp, 14 g)	(2 Tbsp, 37 g)	(¼ cup, 60 mL)	(1 Tbsp, 14 g)
240 calories *0 g fat* *40 g sugars*	*90 calories* *9 g fat* *(5 g saturated)* *1 g sugars*	*80 calories* *8 g fat* *(1.5 g saturated; 2 g trans)* *90 mg sodium*	*190 calories* *11 g fat* *(3.5 g saturated)* *21 g sugars*	*100 calories* *0 g fat* *24 g sugars*	*80 calories* *8 g fat* *(1.5 g saturated)* *95 mg sodium*
This is the worst syrup at your grocery store. Three of the first four ingredients are forms of sugar.	Save 30 calories and 3 grams of fat per slather with the whipped.	Never buy margarine in stick form.	Contains "modified palm oil," an interesterified fat that may spike bad cholesterol levels more than trans fats do.	This is just watered-down Log Cabin Original. At least save some money and water it down yourself.	In small amounts, trans fats don't have to appear on the label, but Olivio is made with partially hydrogenated oils.

133

Condiments

Eat This

Olive oil mayo cuts fat by more than half, and of that remaining, there's a higher percentage of the monounsaturated kind, which improves the fluid movement of the blood.

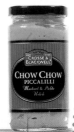

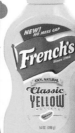

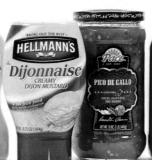

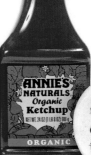

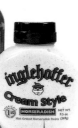

Kraft®
Mayo with Olive Oil
(1 Tbsp, 15 g)

45 calories
4 g fat (0 g saturated)
95 mg sodium

**Crosse & Blackwell®
Chow Chow Piccalilli Mustard & Pickle Relish**
(2 Tbsp, 32 g)

20 calories
0 g fat
400 mg sodium

A versatile blend of mustard and cauliflower.

**French's®
Classic Yellow Mustard**
(1 Tbsp, 15 g)

0 calories
0 g fat
165 mg sodium

Mustard seeds contain the amino acid tryptophan, which boosts serotonin production in the brain.

**Hellmann's®
Dijonnaise®**
(1 Tbsp, 15 g)

15 calories
0 g fat
210 mg sodium

The nutritional boon of mustard, the rich flavor of mayo, and fewer than half the calories of the homemade combination.

**Pace®
Pico De Gallo**
(2 Tbsp, 30 mL)

10 calories
0 g fat
150 mg sodium

Never underestimate the versatility of pico. Make it your go-to condiment to accompany omelets, salads, crackers, and quesadillas.

**Annie's
Naturals®
Organic Ketchup**
(1 Tbsp, 17 g)

15 calories
0 g fat
150 mg sodium

Researchers found that organic ketchup has close to double the lycopene.

**Inglehoffer®
Cream Style Horseradish**
(1 tsp, 5 g)

10 calories
*0.5 g fat
(0 g saturated)*
20 mg sodium

A good horseradish sauce will list horseradish root as the first ingredient.

Not That!

Mayonnaise is like the evil villain of the condiment world. One tablespoon—an incredibly small amount—eats up 15% of your daily fat intake.

Kraft® Real Mayo
(1 Tbsp, 13 g)

90 calories
10 g fat (1.5 g saturated)
70 mg sodium

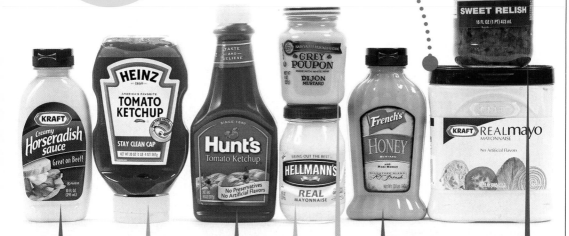

Kraft® Creamy Horseradish Sauce
(1 tsp, 5 g)

15 calories
1.5 g fat
(0 g saturated)
40 mg sodium

Horseradish appears 9 items down the ingredients list, just behind high-fructose corn syrup.

Heinz Tomato Ketchup
(1 Tbsp, 17 g)

15 calories
0 g fat
190 mg sodium

Ketchup is rich in the antioxidant lycopene, but you can do better than Heinz; each tablespoon has 4 grams of sugar.

Hunt's® Tomato Ketchup
(2 Tbsp, 34 g)

40 calories
0 g fat
380 mg sodium

Salsa is now America's most used condiment. Go with it.

Hellmann's® Mayonnaise and Grey Poupon Dijon Mustard
(½ Tbsp each, 14 g)

53 calories
5 g fat
(0.75 g saturated)
205 mg sodium

More calories and more work than Dijonnaise.

French's® Honey Mustard
(1 Tbsp, 15 g)

30 calories
0 g fat
90 mg sodium

This "honey mustard" has more high-fructose corn syrup than mustard seed or honey.

Mt. Olive Sweet Relish
(2 Tbsp, 30 g)

40 calories
0 g fat
160 mg sodium

Sweet relish is little more than nutritionally weak pickles spiked with high-fructose corn syrup.

Asian Sauces

Eat This

Watch the sodium in your soy sauce; some brands pack in more than 1,000 mg per tablespoon.

Kikkoman® Less Sodium Soy Sauce
(1 Tbsp, 15 mL)

10 calories
0 fat
575 mg sodium

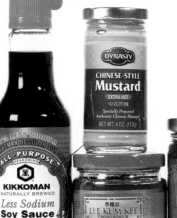

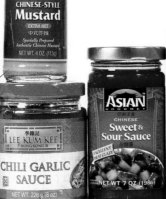

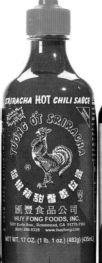

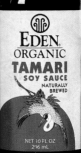

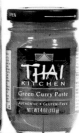

Dynasty® Chinese-Style Mustard Extra Hot (1 Tbsp, 15 g)

15 calories
0 g fat
135 mg sodium
0 g sugars

Contains an array of seasonings like garlic, licorice root, and ginger.

Lee Kum Kee Chili Garlic Sauce
(1 Tbsp, 18 g)

15 calories
0 g fat
810 mg sodium
2 g sugars

One scoop adds instant flavor and the benefits of garlic and chili to a stir-fry.

Asian Gourmet™ Sweet & Sour Sauce (2 Tbsp, 35 g)

45 calories
0 g fat
170 mg sodium
10 g sugars

The main ingredient is apple cider vinegar, and it also includes tomato paste, diced apricots, and crushed pineapple.

Huy Fong Sriracha Hot Chili Sauce
(1 Tbsp, 15 g)

15 calories
0 g fat
300 mg sodium
3 g sugars

Capsaicin in chile peppers helps boost metabolism and burn body fat.

Eden® Organic Tamari Soy Sauce
(1 Tbsp, 15 mL)

15 calories
0 g fat
860 mg sodium

Tamari is a darker, more flavorful soy sauce. Use it in place of all the high-sodium, high-sugar Japanese sauces.

Thai Kitchen Green Curry Paste
(2 Tbsp, 42 g)

20 calories
0 g fat
1,000 mg sodium

They keep the calories down by replacing the oils with pureed chiles, garlic, and lemongrass.

136

Not That!

Leave the La Choy on the shelf. In terms of sodium, this is the worst of all the major soy-sauce brands.

La Choy® Soy Sauce
(1 Tbsp, 15 mL)

10 calories
0 fat
1,160 mg sodium

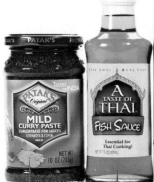

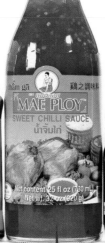

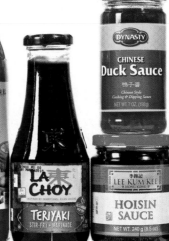

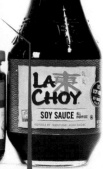

Patak's® Mild Curry Paste
(2 Tbsp, 30 g)

180 calories
16 g fat
(1 g saturated)
910 mg sodium

Steer clear of curries with a vegetable oil base like this one.

A Taste of Thai® Fish Sauce
(1 Tbsp, 19 g)

15 calories
0 g fat
1,730 mg sodium

One splash of this briny liquid eats up more than 70% of your recommended daily sodium intake.

Mae Ploy™ Sweet Chilli Sauce
(1 Tbsp, 15 g)

35 calories
0 g fat
200 mg sodium
7 g sugars

Sweet comes before spice here, which is probably why sugar is the first ingredient.

La Choy® Teriyaki Stir-Fry Sauce and Marinade
(2 Tbsp, 34 g)

60 calories
0 g fat
640 mg sodium
8 g sugars

This teriyaki sauce is like liquid sugar.

Lee Kum Kee Hoisin Sauce
(1 Tbsp, 21 g)

50 calories
0 g fat
580 mg sodium
10 g sugars

More than 3 times the calories and 5 times the sugar of the Chili Garlic Sauce.

Dynasty® Chinese Duck Sauce
(1 Tbsp, 18 g)

40 calories
0 g fat
49 mg sodium
5 g sugars

Duck sauce might sound fancy, but its first ingredient is corn syrup.

137

Nut and Seed Butters
Eat This

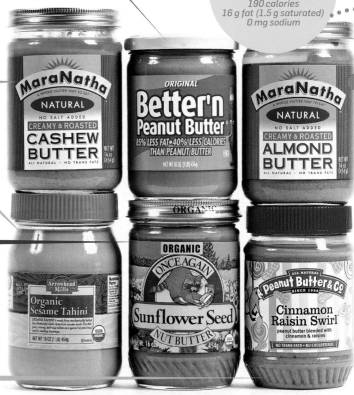

Better'n Peanut Butter®
(2 Tbsp, 32 g)

100 calories
2 g fat (0 g saturated)
190 mg sodium

The taste may not be the same as peanut butter, but you'll cut calories.

MaraNatha Cashew Butter No Salt Added (2 Tbsp, 32 g)

190 calories
15 g fat (3 g saturated)
0 mg sodium

Loaded with copper—good for healthy bones and connective tissue.

Arrowhead Mills Organic Sesame Tahini (2 Tbsp, 32 g)

190 calories
18 g fat (2.5 g saturated)
10 mg sodium

The only ingredient is hulled sesame seeds. Tahini is essential in authentic hummus.

Once Again Nut Butter Sunflower Seed (2 Tbsp, 30 g)

170 calories
15 g fat (1.5 g saturated)
90 mg sodium

A great, healthy alternative for people with peanut allergies.

Peanut Butter & Co. Cinnamon Raisin Swirl (2 Tbsp, 32 g)

160 calories
11 g fat (2 g saturated)
35 mg sodium

Spread it on whole-wheat toast in place of your normal dessert.

Instead of trying to score health points with reduced-fat peanut butters, switch to a butter from a better nut. Vitamin E-rich almonds are as good as they get.

MaraNatha® Almond Butter No Salt Added
(2 Tbsp, 32 g)

190 calories
16 g fat (1.5 g saturated)
0 mg sodium

Not That!

You're better off taking the fat. To get it out, reduced-fat peanut butters add corn syrup solids, soy protein, and a cache of unpronounceable chemicals.

Jif® Crunchy Reduced Fat
(2 Tbsp, 36 g)

190 calories
12 g fat (2.5 g saturated)
210 mg sodium

Soy Wonder® Creamy Soy Nut Butter (2 Tbsp, 32 g)

180 calories
12 g fat (2.5 g saturated)
170 mg sodium

If you're going to lose the peanuts, there are better ways to go than this.

MaraNatha® Macadamia Butter No Salt Added (2 Tbsp, 32 g)

230 calories
24 g fat (4 g saturated)
0 mg sodium

Macadamias are the fattiest nuts.

Peter Pan® Creamy Peanut Butter (2 Tbsp, 32 g)

190 calories
17 g fat (3.5 g saturated)
140 mg sodium

Peter Pan carries the mark of a low-quality peanut butter: partially hydrogenated oils.

Simply Jif® Creamy Peanut Butter (2 Tbsp, 31 g)

190 calories
16 g fat (3 g saturated)
65 mg sodium

It takes 2 ingredients to make peanut butter. This one has 7.

Skippy® Creamy Peanut Butter Roasted Honey Nut™ (2 Tbsp, 32 g)

190 calories
16 g fat (3 g saturated)
125 mg sodium

Skip Skippy—they use partially hydrogenated oils to prevent separation.

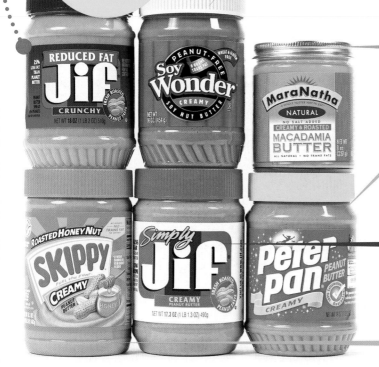

Jellies, Jams, and Pres

Eat This

Here's a rule to follow: Buy only fruit spreads that have real fruit as the first ingredient.

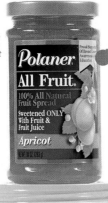

Polaner® All Fruit® Fruit Spread Apricot
(1 Tbsp, 18 g)

40 calories
0 g fat
8 g sugars

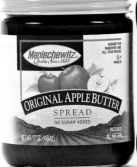

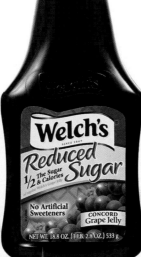

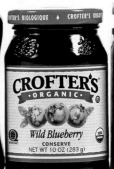

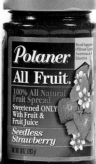

Manischewitz® Original Apple Butter
(1 Tbsp, 16 g)

20 calories
0 g fat
4 g sugars

It's not usually considered a jam, but apple butter is a fruit spread in the truest sense. It contains only two ingredients: apples and apple cider.

Welch's® Concord Grape Jelly Reduced Sugar Squeezable
(1 Tbsp, 17 g)

20 calories
0 g fat
5 g sugars

Since most jellies get their calories from added sugars, you can halve the calories by using half the sugar.

Crofter's® Organic Wild Blueberry Conserve
(1 Tbsp, 18 g)

35 calories
0 g fat
8 g sugars

Crofter's lightly sweetened organic conserves are among the best, and compared to cultivated blueberries, wild blueberries contain 26% more antioxidants.

Polaner® All Fruit® Fruit Spread Seedless Strawberry Spread
(1 Tbsp, 18 g)

40 calories
0 g fat
9 g sugars

Instead of using nutrient-free sweeteners, Polaner's All Fruit line sweetens with pear and grape juice from concentrate.

erves

Not That!

Smucker's® Organic Apricot Preserves
(1 Tbsp, 20 g)

50 calories
0 g fat
12 g sugars

The main ingredient in Smucker's organic preserves is organic sugar, which spikes your blood sugar just as quickly as regular, nonorganic sugar.

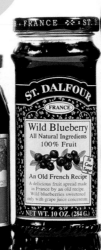

Smucker's® Red Raspberry Jam
(1 Tbsp, 20 g)

50 calories
0 g fat
12 g sugars

It's the source of the sugar that makes Smucker's a nutritional loser—it comes from a blend of corn syrup and high-fructose corn syrup.

St. Dalfour 100% Fruit Wild Blueberry Preserves
(1 Tbsp, 23 g)

70 calories
0 g fat
13 g sugars

Plenty of nutrients to go around, but the excessive use of concentrated grape juice pushes the calorie count beyond the norm.

Smucker's® Squeeze™ Grape Jelly
(1 Tbsp, 20 g)

50 calories
0 g fat
12 g sugars

Admit it: You'll squirt more than 1 tablespoon on your peanut butter and bread. Those sugar calories add up quickly.

Crosse & Blackwell® Mint Flavored Apple Jelly
(1 Tbsp, 20 g)

50 calories
0 g fat
12 g sugars

Mint isn't listed anywhere on the ingredients list. High-fructose corn syrup, on the other hand, is the second ingredient.

Pasta Sauces
Eat This

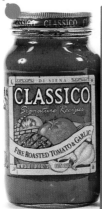
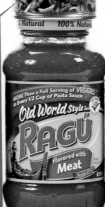
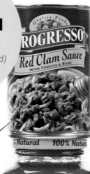
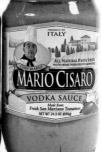
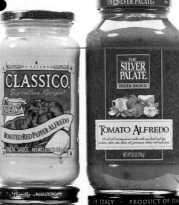
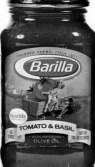

**Classico®
Fire Roasted
Tomato & Garlic**

(½ cup, 125 g)

*50 calories
0.5 g fat (0 g saturated)
320 mg sodium*

**Classico®
Roasted Red
Pepper
Alfredo**

(¼ cup, 60 g)

*60 calories
5 g fat
(3 g saturated)
310 mg sodium*

One of the best
Alfredos
in the aisles.

**The Silver
Palate® Tomato
Alfredo**

(½ cup, 125 g)

*80 calories
5 g fat
(1.5 g saturated)
750 mg sodium*

This buffers
troublesome Alfredo
with a healthy
tomato-sauce base.

Look to
Classico first;
it's the most
trustworthy brand
on the shelf.

**Progresso®
Red Clam
Sauce**

(½ cup, 125 g)

*60 calories
1 g fat
(0 g saturated)
350 mg sodium*

Clams are always
healthiest in red,
tomato-based
sauces.

**Ragú® Old
World Style
Flavored
with Meat**

(½ cup, 125 g)

*70 calories
3 g fat
(0.5 g saturated)
570 mg sodium*

Ragú wins over
Prego in nearly
every matchup.

**Barilla®
Tomato & Basil**

(½ cup, 125 g)

*60 calories
1 g fat
(0 g saturated)
460 mg sodium*

Exactly what you
want: a simple
marinara that goes
light on the sugar
and oil.

**Mario Cisaro
Vodka Sauce**

(½ cup, 125 g)

*80 calories
5 g fat
(2 g saturated)
530 mg sodium*

This sauce
maintains a creamy
texture with a
third fewer calories
than Classico's
version.

142

Not That!

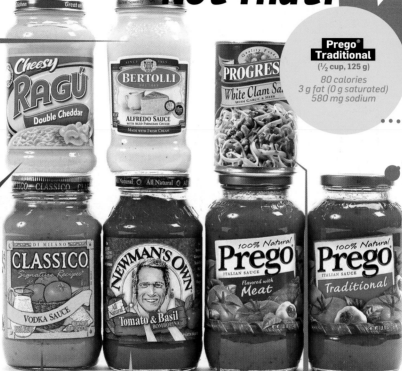

Bertolli® Alfredo Sauce
(¹⁄₄ cup, 61 g)

*110 calories
10 g fat
(5 g saturated)
460 mg sodium*

The fat and calorie glut comes from the heavy mix of cream, cheese, butter, and soybean oil.

Ragú® Double Cheddar
(¹⁄₂ cup, 128 g)

*200 calories
18 g fat
(6 g saturated)
900 mg sodium*

One half cup of this liquefied fat constitutes more than 25% of your daily fat and 40% of your sodium.

Prego® Traditional
(¹⁄₂ cup, 125 g)

*80 calories
3 g fat (0 g saturated)
580 mg sodium*

Classico® Vodka Sauce
(¹⁄₂ cup, 125 g)

*120 calories
7 g fat
(3 g saturated)
510 mg sodium*

This is Classico's biggest mistake; each half cup relies on 63 calories from fat in cream and cheese.

Newman's Own® Tomato & Basil Bombolina™
(¹⁄₂ cup, 125 g)

*90 calories
4.5 g fat
(0.5 g saturated)
620 mg sodium*

Twice the sugar and more than four times the fat.

Prego® Flavored with Meat
(¹⁄₂ cup, 125 g)

*100 calories
4 g fat
(1 g saturated)
580 mg sodium*

Pass on the Prego: It's consistently worse than other major brands.

Progresso® White Clam Sauce
(¹⁄₂ cup, 124 g)

*130 calories
10 g fat
(1.5 g saturated)
880 mg sodium*

A soybean oil base means 10 times more fat than the red sauce.

Prego wrecks this sauce by blending in 10 grams of sugar and a hefty slosh of vegetable oil.

143

Barbecue Sauces and

Eat This

As low in calories and sugar as you're going to find in the supermarket. Make this your all-purpose barbecue sauce.

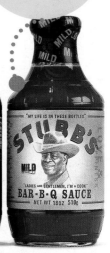

**Stubb's®
Bar-B-Q Sauce
Mild**

(2 Tbsp, 32 g)

*15 calories
0 g fat
210 mg sodium*

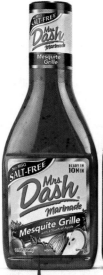

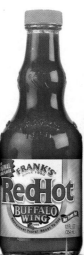

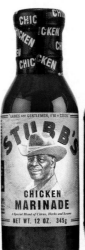

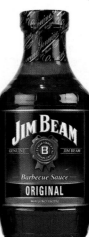

**Mrs. Dash®
Marinade
Mesquite Grille**

(2 Tbsp, 30 g)

*50 calories
3 g fat
0 mg sodium*

Kudos to Mrs. Dash for setting the standard on sodium-free seasoning.

**Frank's® RedHot®
Buffalo Wing Sauce**

(2 Tbsp, 30 mL)

*10 calories
0 g fat
920 mg sodium*

The sodium is high, but with this much heat, half a tablespoon is all you'll need. And in terms of calories, you're not going to spoil your meal with this cayenne-seasoned hot sauce.

**Stubb's®
Chicken Marinade**

(2 Tbsp, 32 g)

*20 calories
0 g fat
420 mg sodium*

More than just vintage-looking labels, Stubb's also serves up some of the safest meat marinades at the supermarket.

**Jim Beam®
Original Barbecue
Sauce**

(2 Tbsp, 33 g)

*30 calories
0 g fat
120 mg sodium*

The classic booze battle extends beyond the bar and into the barbecue pit. This one's no contest, though.

Marinades
Not That!

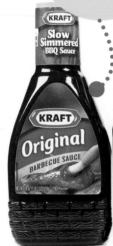

Kraft® Original Barbecue Sauce
(2 Tbsp, 36 g)

50 calories
0 g fat
440 mg sodium

Ever wonder why your barbecue chicken burns so easily on the grill? It's because your sauce is loaded with sugar—just like this one.

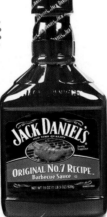

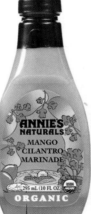

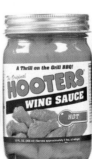

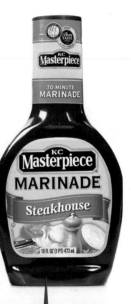

Jack Daniel's Original No. 7 Recipe™ Barbecue Sauce
(2 Tbsp, 34 g)

50 calories
0 g fat
290 mg sodium

No whiskey in Jack's No. 7 Recipe, just a smattering of natural and artificial flavors that are supposed to mimic the taste.

Annie's Naturals® Mango Cilantro Marinade (2 Tbsp, 30 mL)

40 calories
1 g fat (0 g saturated)
240 mg sodium

We love Annie's products, but this isn't our favorite. Higher calorie levels indicate higher sugar levels, which promote excessive charring on grilled food. If you do use a marinade, choose a light one.

Hooters® Wing Sauce Hot
(1 oz, 28 g)

80 calories
8 g fat (2 g saturated)
520 mg sodium

Wings already get one oil bath—why add another?

KC Masterpiece® Marinade Steakhouse
(2 Tbsp, 30 mL)

80 calories
3 g fat (0 g saturated)
620 mg sodium

Apparently the steakhouse is a great place for high-fructose corn syrup (first ingredient) and a towering mound of salt (26% of your recommended daily intake).

Salad Dressings
Eat This

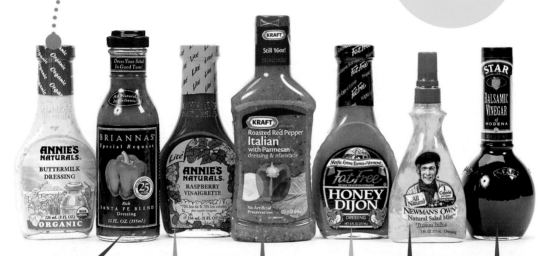

Ranch's rich flavor and creamy texture, but with fewer than half the calories.

Annie's Naturals® Organic Buttermilk
(2 Tbsp, 30 g)
60 calories
6 g fat (1 g saturated)
230 mg sodium

Briannas® Sante Fe Blend
(2 Tbsp, 30 mL)
25 calories
0 g fat
480 mg sodium
The flavor comes from a savory mix of seasonings blended into vinegar without a hefty dose of fat.

Annie's Naturals® Lite Raspberry Vinaigrette
(2 Tbsp, 31 g)
40 calories
3 g fat
(0 g saturated)
60 mg sodium
Annie's makes simple, delicious, wholesome dressings. Load up.

Kraft Roasted Red Pepper Italian with Parmesan
(2 Tbsp, 32 g)
40 calories
2 g fat
(0 g saturated)
440 mg sodium
This is about as low-cal as Italian gets.

Maple Grove Farms of Vermont® Fat Free Honey Dijon
(2 Tbsp, 30 mL)
40 calories
0 g fat
200 mg sodium
Not one in this great line of fat-free dressings has more than 40 calories per serving.

Newman's Own® Natural Salad Mist™ Tuscan Italian
(10 sprays, 8 mL)
10 calories
1 g fat
(0 g saturated)
100 mg sodium
Spraying ensures minimum calories and maximum distribution.

Star® Balsamic Vinegar of Modena
(1 Tbsp, 15 mL)
5 calories
0 g fat
0 mg sodium
Turn the classic oil-and-vinegar ratio on its head by mixing 2 parts balsamic with only 1 part olive oil.

Not That!

**Hidden Valley®
The Original Ranch®**
(2 Tbsp, 30 g)
140 calories
14 g fat (2.5 g saturated)
260 mg sodium

Ranch is one of the most dangerous things you can keep in your kitchen.

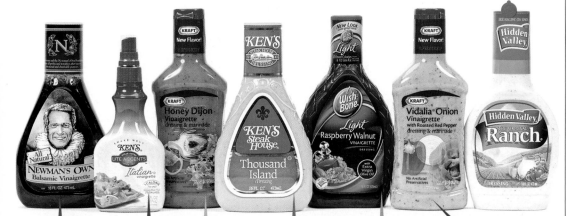

Newman's Own® Balsamic Vinaigrette
(2 Tbsp, 30 g)

90 calories
9 g fat
(1 g saturated)
350 mg sodium

Most vinaigrettes have an oil-to-vinegar ratio of 3 parts to 1.

Ken's Steak House® Lite Accents™ Italian Vinaigrette
(10 sprays, 8 mL)

15 calories
1 g fat
(0 g saturated)
110 mg sodium

Contains a chemist's list of ingredients.

Kraft Honey Dijon Vinaigrette
(2 Tbsp, 32 g)

90 calories
7 g fat
(0.5 g saturated)
340 mg sodium

About what you can expect from any full-fat vinaigrette in the market.

Ken's Steak House® Thousand Island
(2 Tbsp, 30 g)

140 calories
13 g fat
(2 g saturated)
300 mg sodium

This dubious dressing cancels out a salad's benefits.

Wish-Bone® Light Raspberry Walnut Vinaigrette
(2 Tbsp, 30 mL)

80 calories
5 g fat
(0.5 g saturated)
260 mg sodium

Better than most full-fat varieties, but still not all that light.

Kraft Vidalia® Onion Vinaigrette
(2 Tbsp, 32 g)

80 calories
5 g fat
(1 g saturated)
320 mg sodium

Just because it's a vinaigrette doesn't mean it's safe.

Add-Meat Meals

Eat This

Campbell's Lemon Chicken Supper Bakes®
(1 cup prepared)

260 calories
3.5 g fat (1 g saturated)
750 mg sodium

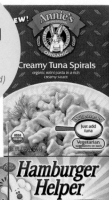

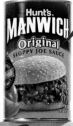

Hunt's® Manwich® Original Sloppy Joe Sauce
(¼ cup with 3 oz cooked ground turkey and wheat bun)

300 calories
10.5 g fat (1 g saturated)
630 mg sodium

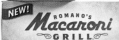

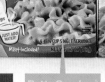

The garlic chicken version is even leaner, with just 190 calories per serving.

Annie's® Organic Creamy Tuna Spirals
(1 cup prepared)

260 calories
7 g fat (4 g saturated)
650 mg sodium

Use light tuna and cut an extra 50 calories.

Betty Crocker® Hamburger Helper® Microwave Singles® Stroganoff
(1 pouch)

170 calories
3 g fat (1 g saturated, 0.5 g trans)
660 mg sodium

Betty Crocker® Chicken Helper® Chicken Fried Rice (1 cup prepared, 30 g)

250 calories
9 g fat (2 g saturated)
550 mg sodium

The leanest of the Chicken Helper line.

Annie's® Organic Cheesy Lasagna
(1 cup prepared)

280 calories
9 g fat (4 g saturated)
670 mg sodium

Annie's beats Hamburger Helper in every category.

Romano's Macaroni Grill® Garlic & Herb Chicken Penne
(1 cup prepared, 83 g)

240 calories
7 g fat (1.5 g saturated)
390 mg sodium

Loaded with 21 grams of protein.

Not That!

Betty Crocker® Hamburger Helper® Double Cheeseburger Macaroni
(1 cup prepared)

*320 calories
13 g fat
(5 g saturated,
1 g trans)
730 mg sodium*

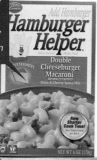

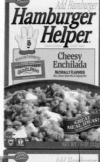

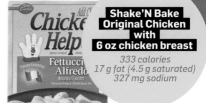

Shake'N Bake Original Chicken with 6 oz chicken breast

*333 calories
17 g fat (4.5 g saturated)
327 mg sodium*

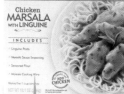

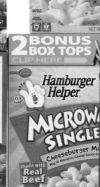

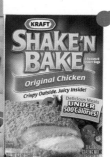

Romano's Macaroni Grill® Chicken Marsala with Linguine (1 cup prepared, 53 g)

*330 calories
13 g fat
(3.5 g saturated)
450 mg sodium*

Save 90 calories with the garlic & herb variety.

Betty Crocker® Hamburger Helper® Three Cheese (1 cup prepared, 34 g)

*320 calories
13 g fat
(5 g saturated,
0.5 g trans)
770 mg sodium*

Twice the ingredients used in Annie's.

Betty Crocker® Hamburger Helper® Cheesy Enchilada (1 cup prepared with lean hamburger, 40 g)

*320 calories
12 g fat
(5 g saturated,
1 g trans)
690 mg sodium*

Betty Crocker® Hamburger Helper Microwave Singles® Cheeseburger Macaroni (1 pouch, 52 g)

*210 calories
7 g fat (2 g saturated, 2 g trans)
610 mg sodium*

Betty Crocker® Chicken Helper® Fettuccine Alfredo (1 cup prepared)

*340 calories
12 g fat
(3.5 g saturated,
1.5 g trans)
840 mg sodium*

A half chicken breast with vegetables on the side would be a more sensible approach than Shake'N Bake.

Quick Sides
Eat This

Manischewitz® Matzo Ball Mix
(2 Tbsp mix, 16 g)

50 calories
0 g fat
(0 g saturated)
700 mg sodium

Try eating these low-calorie, wheat-based matzo balls from a shallow bowl of broth.

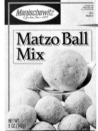

Kraft Pasta Salad Classic Italian
(¾ cup prepared with Kraft Zesty Italian Dressing)

230 calories
7 g fat (1 g saturated)
620 mg sodium

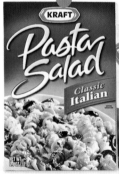

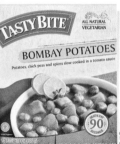

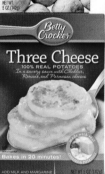

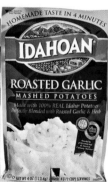

Sides based on refined carbohydrates are never ideal, but if you must do pasta salad, this may be your best option.

Tasty Bite® Bombay Potatoes
(½ pack, 5 oz)

100 calories
4 g fat
(0.5 g saturated)
410 mg sodium

Check out the ethnic foods section to find dishes that depend on healthy spice blends instead of oils and butter.

Near East® Taboule Mix
(~⅔ cup prepared)

120 calories
0 g fat
270 mg sodium
5 g fiber

This side packs stuffing with more fiber and protein and no dangerous fats.

Betty Crocker® Three Cheese Potatoes
(⅔ cup prepared)

120 calories
3.5 g fat
(1 g saturated,
0.5 g trans)
590 mg sodium

These have 50 fewer calories than the roasted garlic & cheddar variety.

Idahoan® Roasted Garlic Mashed Potatoes
(½ cup prepared)

110 calories
3 g fat
(1 g saturated)
590 mg sodium

You're always better off making a homemade mash, but in a pinch, these will work.

Not That!

**Manischewitz®
Potato Pancake
Mix** (3 Tbsp mix, 24 g)

*80 calories
1 g fat
(0.5 g saturated)
500 mg sodium*

Blame the extra fat
calories on the partially
hydrogenated
cottonseed oil holding
these patties together.

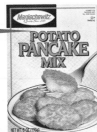

**Betty Crocker®
Suddenly Pasta
Salad® Creamy
Parmesan**

(¾ cup prepared)

*350 calories
23 g fat (3 g saturated)
440 mg sodium*

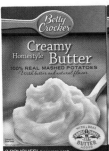

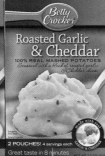

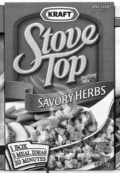

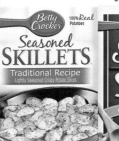

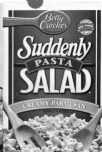

*With numbers
like these,
you'd be better off
eating a hefty helping
of French fries.*

**Betty Crocker®
Creamy
Homestyle Butter
Mashed Potatoes**

(½ cup prepared)

*170 calories
7 g fat (2 g saturated,
1 g trans)
360 mg sodium*

Since when did home-
style include partially
hydrogenated oil?

**Betty Crocker®
Roasted Garlic
& Cheddar
Mashed Potatoes**

(½ cup prepared)

*170 calories
7 g fat (2 g saturated,
1 g trans)
480 mg sodium*

Roasting is normally
a healthy cooking
technique. Not so here.

**Kraft Stove Top
Stuffing Mix
Savory Herbs**

(½ cup prepared)

*160 calories
7 g fat
(1.5 g saturated,
1.5 g trans)
530 mg sodium*

Use butter or tub
margarine to keep out
the trans fats.

**Betty Crocker®
Seasoned
Skillets™
Traditional
Recipe Potatoes**

(½ cup prepared)

*180 calories
9 g fat (1 g saturated)
500 mg sodium*

When preparing
boxed meals, cut the
added oil by half.

151

Soups
Eat This

**Campbell's®
Soup at Hand®
Vegetable Beef**

(1 container, 305 g)

*60 calories
1 g fat (0.5 g saturated)
930 mg sodium*

*One of the healthiest
lunches ever to
come from a can.
Just add a salad or
a piece of fruit.*

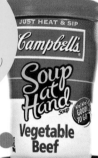

**Campbell's®
Chunky™ Slow
Roasted Beef**

(1 cup, 240 mL)

*120 calories
1.5 g fat
(1 g saturated)
830 mg sodium*

A great mix of fiber
(3 grams), protein
(7 grams), and
immune-boosting
vitamin A (40%).

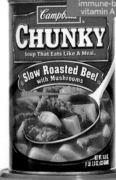

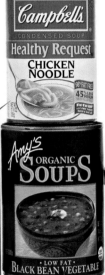

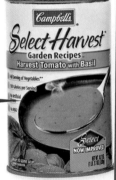

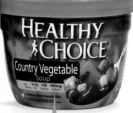

**Campbell's®
Select Harvest™
Harvest Tomato
with Basil**

(1 cup, 240 mL)

*100 calories
0 g fat
480 mg sodium*

Basil brings with it a
cache of antioxidants.

**Campbell's®
Healthy Request®
Condensed
Chicken Noodle**

(1 cup prepared)

*60 calories
2 g fat
(0.5 g saturated)
470 mg sodium*

The new classic.

**Amy's® Black
Bean Vegetable**

(1 cup, 240 mL)

*130 calories
1.5 g fat
(0 g saturated)
430 mg sodium*

Black beans offer
the nutritional
trifecta—they're packed
with protein, fiber,
and antioxidants.

**Healthy Choice®
Country
Vegetable**

(1 cup, 246 g)

*100 calories
0.5 g fat
(0 g saturated)
480 mg sodium*

Nutrient-dense and
teeming with fiber.

Not That!

Campbell's® Chunky™ Fully Loaded Turkey Pot Pie
(1 cup, 240 mL)

200 calories
8 g fat
(1.5 g saturated)
800 mg sodium

The whole can will cost you 700 calories.

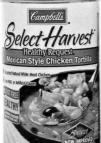

Campbell's® Soup at Hand® Creamy Tomato
(1 container, 305 g)

190 calories
4 g fat (1 g saturated)
940 mg sodium

Why does Campbell's feel the need to spike this soup with 24 grams of sugar? That's about as much as you'll find in a candy bar.

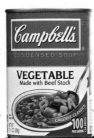

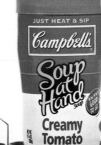

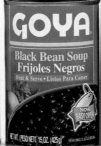

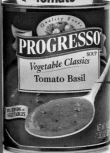

Progresso® Tomato Basil
(1 cup, 244 g)

160 calories
3 g fat
(0.5 g saturated)
960 mg sodium

With each cup comes 16 grams of sugar—the same amount as you'll get from a scoop of ice cream.

Campbell's® Select Harvest™ Healthy Request® Mexican Style Chicken Tortilla
(1 cup, 240 mL)

130 calories
2 g fat
(1 g saturated)
480 mg sodium

Still a fine pick when compared to other lines.

Goya® Black Bean
(1 cup, 246 g)

210 calories
1.5 g fat
(0.5 g saturated)
1,050 mg sodium

One serving of this soup has more sodium than 6 single-serving bags of Ruffles potato chiips.

Campbell's® Condensed Vegetable
(1 cup prepared)

100 calories
0.5 g fat
(0.5 g saturated)
890 mg sodium

More than a third of your recommended daily sodium intake in 1 cup.

Beans and Chili
Eat This

Van Camp's Pork and Beans
(½ cup, 130 g)

110 calories
1 g fat
(0 g saturated)
390 mg sodium

Don't let your beans have any more than 10 grams of sugar. Van Camp's keeps it very reasonable at only 7.

Hormel® Chili Meals Chili'n Mac
(1 tray)

260 calories
6 g fat (2.5 g saturated)
950 mg sodium

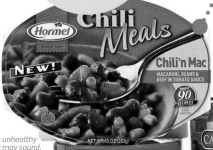
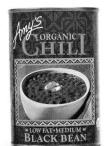
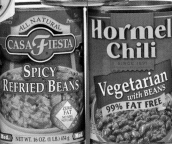
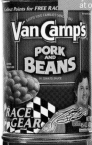
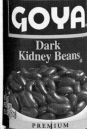

As unhealthy as it may sound, 17 grams of protein, 6 grams of fiber, and very reasonable calorie and fat counts make this a commendable pick for lunch on the run.

Campbell's Chunky™ Roadhouse Chili Beef & Bean
(1 cup, 240 mL)

230 calories
8 g fat
(3.5 g saturated,
0.5 g trans)
870 mg sodium

Casa Fiesta® Spicy Refried Beans
(½ cup, 113 g)

130 calories
0 g fat
370 mg sodium

"Zero Fat" means "made without the lard most companies dump in beans."

Amy's Organic Chili Black Bean (1 cup, 260 g)

200 calories
2 g fat
(0 g saturated)
680 mg sodium

The wealth of black beans in this can contributes 26 grams of protein, so you won't even miss the turkey.

Hormel® Chili Vegetarian with Beans
(1 cup, 247 g)

190 calories
1 g fat
(0 g saturated)
780 mg sodium

Vegetarian chili trades protein for fiber—not a bad swap.

Goya® Dark Kidney Beans
(½ cup, 125 g)

90 calories
0.5 g fat
(0 g saturated)
380 mg sodium

Beans should be a staple in your diet. They're packed with protein, fiber, and disease-fighting antioxidants.

Not That!

Campbell's® Pork & Beans
(½ cup, 130 g)

140 calories
1.5 g fat
(0.5 g saturated)
440 mg sodium

Extra calories,
extra salt,
extra fat,
extra sugar.

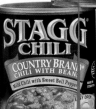

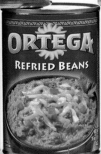

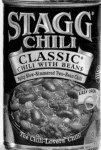

Hormel® Chili with Beans
(1 container)

520 calories
14 g fat (6 g saturated)
2,380 mg sodium

Do you really want to waste an entire day of sodium intake on a bowl of chili?

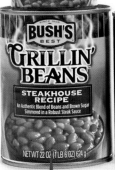

**Bush's® Grillin'
Beans™
Steakhouse
Recipe**
(½ cup, 130 g)

130 calories
0.5 g fat
(0 g saturated)
510 mg sodium

Each half cup has
a staggering
21 grams of sugar.

**Stagg® Chili
Country
Brand® Chili
with Beans**
(1 cup, 247 g)

330 calories
17 g fat
(7 g saturated,
1 g trans)
1,140 mg sodium

Gobbles up half your
day's sodium.

**Hormel® 98%
Fat Free
Turkey with
Beans**
(1 cup, 247 g)

210 calories
3 g fat
(1 g saturated)
1,250 mg sodium

Low in fat, but
more than half your
day's sodium.

**Ortega®
Refried Beans**
(½ cup, 131 g)

150 calories
2.5 g fat
(1 g saturated)
570 mg sodium

There are too
many great fat-free
versions out there
to settle for this.

**Stagg®
Classic® Chili
with Beans**
(1 cup, 247 g)

330 calories
17 g fat
(7 g saturated,
0.5 g trans)
810 mg sodium

Way too high in
saturated fat.

155

Canned and Cupped Fru

Eat This

100% juice is the best you can hope for— it means you eat only real fruit and their juices.

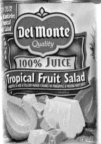

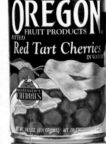

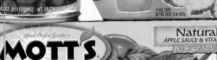

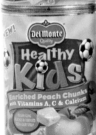

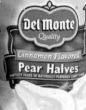

Del Monte® 100% Juice Tropical Fruit Salad
(½ cup, 122 g)

60 calories
0 g fat
14 g sugars

Del Monte® Healthy Kids Enriched Peach Chunks
(½ cup, 124 g)

30 calories
0 g fat
14 g sugars

Fortified with 100% of the recommended daily intake of vitamin C.

Oregon® Pitted Red Tart Cherries
(⅓ cup, 70 g)

30 calories
0 g fat
6.5 g sugars

Free from the syrupy sugar solution that accompanies most packaged cherries.

Mott's® Natural Apple Sauce No Sugar Added
(1 container, 111 g)

50 calories
0 g fat
11 g sugars

This cup is nothing but blended apples, water, and 20% of your vitamin C.

Dole® Pineapple Tidbits in 100% Pineapple Juice
(1 container, 122 g)

70 calories
0 g fat
15 g sugars

Naturally occurring sugars from fruit break down slower, ensuring an easy ride for your blood sugar.

Del Monte® Cinnamon Flavored Pear Halves in Naturally Flavored Light Syrup
(½ cup, 126 g)

80 calories
0 g fat
19 g sugars

its

Not That!

Dole® Tropical Mixed Fruit in Passion Fruit Nectar
(½ cup, 122 g)

90 calories
0 g fat
20 g sugars

This recipe is augmented with a gob of sugar, which adds unnecessary calories to the can.

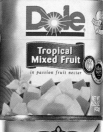

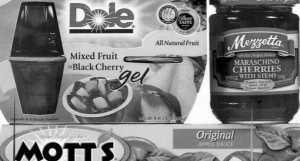

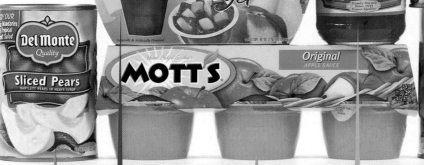

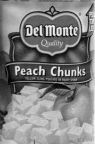

Del Monte® Sliced Pears in Heavy Syrup
(½ cup, 127 g)

100 calories
0 g fat
23 g sugars

A blend of corn syrup and sugar add more than a tablespoon of unnecessary sugar to this can.

Dole® Mixed Fruit in Black Cherry Gel (1 container, 123 g)

90 calories
0 g fat
22 g sugars

No black cherries in the gel, but there is cochineal extract, a red dye drawn from the body and eggs of a beetlelike, cactus-dwelling insect.

Mott's® Original Apple Sauce
(1 container, 113 g)

100 calories
0 g fat
22 g sugars

These abused apples have doubled their caloric load by soaking in a bath of high-fructose corn syrup.

Mezzetta® Maraschino Cherries
(11 cherries, 66 g)

110 calories
0 g fat
22 g sugars

Maraschino means the cherry is basting in an unhealthy mix of sugar, preservatives, and artificial coloring.

Del Monte® Peach Chunks in Heavy Syrup
(½ cup, 127 g)

100 calories
0 g fat
23 g sugars

Translation for Heavy Syrup: overly sweetened goo that turns otherwise healthy fruit into sugar-loaded candy.

Canned and Jarred Veg

Eat This

Go figure. Green Giant adds sugar to their Corn Niblets, but the only sugar in the Extra Sweet Corn Niblets is au natural.

Green Giant® Extra Sweet Corn Niblets
(⅓ cup, 75 g)

50 calories
0.5 g fat (0 g saturated)
200 mg sodium

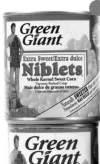

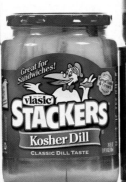

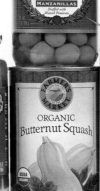

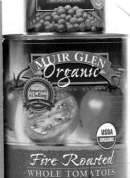

Green Giant® Cut Green Beans 50% Less Sodium
(½ cup, 120 g)

20 calories
0 g fat
200 mg sodium

Green beans have one of the best calorie-to-nutrient ratios of any veggie.

Vlasic® Stackers® Kosher Dill
(2 slices, 56 g)

10 calories
0 g fat
410 mg sodium

Keep a cap on the pickle snacking or the sodium will add up quickly.

Farmer's Market™ Butternut Squash
(½ cup, 100 g)

50 calories
0 g fat
5 mg sodium

A great product. Each cup provides 90% of your day's vitamin A.

Star Spanish Olives

15 calories
1 g fat
(0 g saturated)
260 mg sodium

Olives are a great quick snack, loaded with vitamin E, iron, fiber, and the same heart-healthy fats found in their oil.

Muir Glen® Organic Fire Roasted Whole Tomatoes
(½ cup, 122 g)

25 calories
0 g fat
290 mg sodium

Cooked tomatoes contain more cancer-fighting lycopene.

Del Monte® Fresh Cut® Sweet Peas No Salt Added
(½ cup, 125 g)

60 calories
0 g fat
10 mg sodium

Try seasoning with lemon juice and pepper and you'll never miss the salt.

etables

Not That!

**Green Giant®
Corn Niblets**
(⅓ cup, 77 g)

*80 calories
0.5 g fat (0 g saturated)
230 mg sodium*

*How Green Giant
manages to make
such a caloric corn
is a mystery.
This can contains
320 calories.*

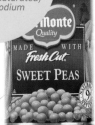

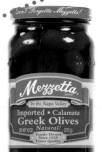

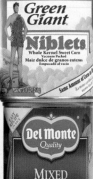

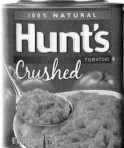

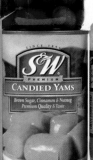

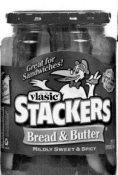

**Del Monte®
Fresh Cut®
Sweet Peas**
(½ cup, 125 g)

*60 calories
0 g fat
390 mg sodium*

Avoid briny
veggies like these,
which pile on
unnecessary
amounts of sodium.

**Hunt's®
Crushed
Tomatoes**
(½ cup, 121 g)

*35 calories
0 g fat
320 mg sodium*

Hunt's tomatoes
emerge from
processing with
less vitamin C and
A than Muir Glen's.

**Mezzetta
Calamata
Greek Olives**
(4 olives, 15 g)

*40 calories
4 g fat
(0 g saturated)
240 mg sodium*

One jar has 720 cal-
ories and virtually
no trace of the
vitamins found in the
Star alternative.

**S&W®
Candied Yams**
(½ cup, 141 g)

*170 calories
0 g fat
360 mg sodium*

Candied yams
should be reserved
for dessert; three
different sweeteners
in this can con-
tribute to the
63 grams of sugar.

**Vlasic®
Stackers®
Bread & Butter**
(2 slices, 56 g)

*60 calories
0 g fat
340 mg sodium*

"Bread & butter"
means that these
pickles have been
injected with high-
fructose corn syrup.

**Del Monte®
Mixed
Vegetables**
(½ cup, 124 g)

*40 calories
0 g fat
360 mg sodium*

Be wary of such
unspecified
vegetable blends.

159

Canned and Packaged
Eat This

**StarKist®
Low Sodium
Chunk Light
Tuna in Water**

(½ can, 56 g)

*50 calories
0.5 g fat (0 g saturated)
60 mg sodium*

Easy To Open • No Messy Draining!

Premium Quality

BUMBLE BEE.
• FRESH TASTE
• FIRM TEXTURE

Premium Wild PINK SALMON
SKINLESS & BONELESS

NET WT 6.0 OZ (170g)

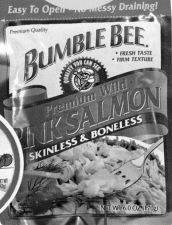

Hormel
Premium Quality
CORNED BEEF
PRODUCT OF BRAZIL

NET WT 18 OZ (340g)

*Choose light over
white or albacore and
you'll cut calories,
sodium, and mercury
levels in one smart
decision.*

StarKist
LOW SODIUM
Chunk Light
Tuna   IN WATER

White
PREMIUM CHUNK
Chicken Breast IN WATER
by Protein Per Serving

SWANSON

KING OSCAR
Finest Brisling
SARDINES
IN PURE SPRING WATER
ONE LAYER
NET WT 3.75 OZ (106g)

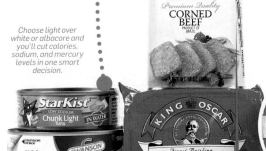

BUMBLE BEE.
Easy Peel
Sensations
SUNDRIED TOMATO & BASIL
SEASONED TUNA MEDLEY
NET WT 5 OZ (142g)

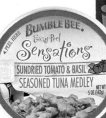

Swanson® White Premium Chunk Chicken Breast in Water	**King Oscar® Sardines in Pure Spring Water**	**Hormel® Corned Beef**	**Bumble Bee® Sensations™ Seasoned Tuna Medley Sundried Tomato & Basil**	**Bumble Bee® Premium Wild Pink Salmon Skinless & Boneless**
(~½ can, 112 g)	(1 can, 106 g)	(⅙ can, 56 g)	(1 can, 142 g)	(⅔ package, ~½ cup, 112 g)
100 calories 2 g fat (1 g saturated) 520 mg sodium	*140 calories 10 g fat (2.5 g saturated) 200 mg sodium*	*120 calories 6 g fat (3.5 g saturated) 490 mg sodium*	*130 calories 5 g fat (1 g saturated) 360 mg sodium*	*120 calories 2 g fat (0 g saturated) 360 mg sodium*
While it's always better to cook it fresh, this is a great source of lean, instant protein.	Sardines are packed with coenzyme Q10, a powerful immune-boosting antioxidant.	A full can of corned beef instead of Spam saves 360 calories and 1,800 mg sodium.	Peel back the lid and eat straight from the can.	This salmon mixes well into salads and pastas.

Protein
Not That!

StarKist® Solid White Albacore Tuna in Water
(½ can, 56 g)

75 calories
2 g fat (<0.5 g saturated)
225 mg sodium

Due to high levels of methylmercury in albacore, the Center for Science in the Public Interest recommends limiting consumption to no more than 6 ounces per week. Children and pregnant women shouldn't even touch the stuff.

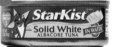

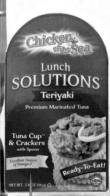

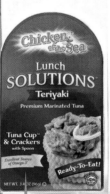

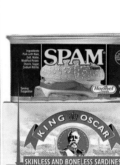

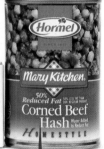

Bumble Bee® Prime Fillet™ Pink Salmon Steak Lightly Marinated with Lemon & Dill
(1 pouch)

150 calories
4.5 g fat
(1 g saturated)
600 mg sodium

Bumble Bee's marinade is soybean oil.

Chicken of the Sea Lunch Solutions™ Teriyaki
(1 package, 98 g)

190 calories
5 g fat
(3 g saturated)
470 mg sodium

There's little point in eating tuna if it's packed with sugar.

Spam®
(⅛ can, 56 g)

180 calories
16 g fat
(6 g saturated)
790 mg sodium

For 70 years Spam has been a poor-choice pantry staple; each 2-ounce slice provides a third of your recommended daily sodium intake and 25% of your fat.

King Oscar® Skinless and Boneless Sardines in Soya Oil
(1 can, 110 g)

240 calories
14 g fat
(3 g saturated)
700 mg sodium

Sardines contain healthy fish oils—so they don't need the soya.

Hormel® 50% Reduced Fat Homestyle Corned Beef Hash
(½ cup, 118 g)

145 calories
6 g fat (3 g saturated)
535 mg sodium

Replace the beef hash with chicken and you'll save 180 calories per can.

Chapter 6
SNACKS & SWEETS

EAT THIS, NOT THAT!
CH. 6

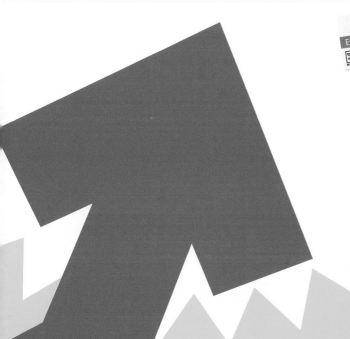

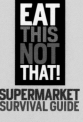

EAT THIS NOT THAT!
SUPERMARKET SURVIVAL GUIDE

The Only Way to Snack

Ahh, the snack aisle—the place so many diets and New Year's resolutions have come to know as their final resting place.

The problem is that most of us snack the way that we twirl our hair, bite our cuticles, or watch *Hannity & Colmes*—mindlessly. But while those habits are only mildly bad for us, snacking is a different story altogether. Indeed, between the years 1977 and 1996, a simple snack of a bag of chips and a Coke has increased a whopping 142 calories. Yeah, it's the same snack as 30 years ago, but eat it just two or three times a week and you'll gain up to 6 more pounds this year than you would have back when the Captain & Tennille were crooning "Muskrat Love."

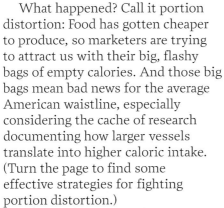

What happened? Call it portion distortion: Food has gotten cheaper to produce, so marketers are trying to attract us with their big, flashy bags of empty calories. And those big bags mean bad news for the average American waistline, especially considering the cache of research documenting how larger vessels translate into higher caloric intake. (Turn the page to find some effective strategies for fighting portion distortion.)

Even those of us trying to pick "healthy" snacks are often fooled by packaging. For example, Cornell University researchers found that people tend to eat an average of 28 percent more calories when snacking on low-fat foods. After all, flavor has to come from somewhere, and when food marketers eliminate the fat, they often make up for it with sugar.

What we all need in response is a completely different approach to snacking. We need to leave the mindlessness behind and begin snacking with a sense of purpose. Each snack ought to be considered not an indulgence but rather an opportunity to do something great for our health, our weight, and our energy level.

You see, as Gordon Gekko might

have put it, Snacking is good. Snacking works.

Consider the phenomenon known as "energy balance." Researchers at Georgia State University developed a technique to measure hourly energy balance—that is, how many calories we burn versus how many calories we take in. They found that if you keep your hourly surplus or deficit within 300 to 500 calories at all times, you will maintain lean muscle while burning fat. But if you take in 500 more calories in an hour than you're burning—by snacking on a high-calorie food—you begin to put on weight. Similarly, if you burn 500 more calories in an hour than you take in—by sticking to your three squares a day and never snacking—you lose lean muscle mass, which sets you up for gaining flab. But in the same study, subjects who added three snacks a day to three regular meals a day balanced out their energy better, lost fat, and increased lean muscle mass.

In a second study, researchers in Japan found that athletes who ate the same number of calories a day from either two or six meals lost an average of 11 pounds in 2 weeks. But the ones who ate six meals a day lost 3 pounds more fat and 3 pounds less muscle than the ones who ate only two meals. Snacking keeps you full, keeps your metabolism revving, and keeps you from bingeing at mealtimes. You just need to keep these simple guidelines in mind.

- **Don't snack if you're not hungry.** French researchers found that when people who weren't hungry ate a snack a few hours after lunch, they did not eat fewer calories at dinner—regardless of whether the snack was high in carbohydrates or fat.

- **Go for high-protein, not high-carb.** Another group of French researchers found that high-protein snacks help people feel full longer and eat less at their next meal. Study participants ate 200 calories of protein or carbs or nothing at all. Those who ate high-carbohydrate snacks were hungry again just as quickly as those who ate no snacks.

- **Keep the salt down, especially for your kids.** A study published in an American Heart Association journal found that kids who eat salty snacks get thirstier—duh—but they're also more likely to drink calorie- and sugar-laden sodas to tame their thirst.

According to the USDA, most of the sodium in the American diet comes from packaged and processed foods. Naturally occurring salt accounts for only 13 percent of total intake, while 77 percent is added by food manufacturers.

● **Take the family to the movies.**
A study of popcorn consumers published in the *Journal of the American Dietetic Association* found that popcorn eaters had a 22 percent higher intake of fiber and a 250 percent higher intake of whole grains than noneaters. (But order it without the scary faux-butter topping, to save hundreds of calories.)

● **Go nuts and dark chocolate.**
Purdue University researchers found that snackers who ate peanuts, peanut butter, almonds, chestnuts, or chocolate were significantly less hungry than those who ate rice cakes or pickles.

● **Reward yourself with ice cream.**
British researchers conducted MRI scans and found that a single spoonful of ice cream triggers the pleasure centers in the brain. Plus, just half a cup of vanilla ice cream gives you

18 milligrams of choline, which recent USDA research shows lowers blood levels of homocysteine by 8 percent. That translates into protection from cancer, heart attack, stroke, and dementia. Best pick: Dreyer's Slow Churned Rich & Creamy Light. One serving has at most 3 grams of saturated fat.

● **Think dips.** The average corn chip is hardly a model of nutrition. But you can turn it into something much healthier by pairing it with the right dip. Sour cream and dried onion soup? I don't think so. But mix a little avocado, some lime juice, half a jalapeño, and a few sprinkles of salt and you have instant guacamole—and a delivery system for fiber, vitamins and minerals, and heart-healthy monounsaturated fat. Low-cal, high-in-vitamins salsa and fiber-rich bean dips are also smart choices.

The Science of Serving Vessels

Four countermoves against the forces of fat

1. Downsize your dishes: Unless you're eating off decades-old dishes, you probably have the newer, plus-size plates—the kind that cause your eyes to override your appetite. Give them to Goodwill, and pick up either the 16-piece Santiago set by Dansk (10½-inch dinner plates, 8-inch salad plates, and 7-inch soup bowls, $80) or the 20-piece Platinum Band set by Majestry (10⅝-inch dinner plates, 7¾-inch salad plates, and 7¾-inch soup bowls, $60). Both are sold at bedbathandbeyond.com.

2. Be small-minded about snacks: In a recent experiment at the Cornell University food and brand lab, research-ers gave study partici-pants either a single bag containing 100 Wheat Thins or four smaller bags holding 25 Thins each, waited for the munching to subside, then did a cracker count. The tally: Those given the jumbo bag ate up to 20 percent more. Out-smart your snack habit by sticking with the tiny 100-calorie packs now being used for everything from Doritos to Goldfish.

3. Raise your glasses: Since even experienced bartenders pour more into short, wide glasses than they do into tall, narrow ones, you'll need to be creative when you play mixmaster at home. Start by using highball glasses to replace the squat tumblers you use for scotch and brandy. Next, put away your pint beer glasses and buy the pilsner kind. Finally, if you own balloon wine glasses, switch them with regular wine glasses. Just watch the red: Cornell researchers found that people inadvertently pour more red wine than white into the same-size glass.

4. Divide and dine: Until all restaurants become BYOP (bring your own plate), you'll need to shrink your serving in a different way: When your entrée arrives, dive in and eat half, then wait at least 10 minutes before coming out for round 2. While you chat and sip water, your stomach will have a chance to digest and decide whether you've had enough—no matter what the plate's saying.

For more savvy snacking tips and top supermarket picks, go to eatthis.com

The Pantry Label Decoder

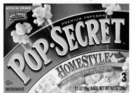

POP-SECRET HOMESTYLE

THE CLAIM: "Made with a sprinkle of salt and a taste of butter"

THE TRUTH: The taste of the butter is actually the taste of partially hydrogenated soybean oil, which imbues on this greasy bag a total of 18 grams of trans fats—more than seven times what you should safely consume in a day, according to the American Heart Association. No area of the supermarket is more riddled with these fats—proven to increase the risk of coronary heart disease—than the snack aisles, so be on high alert.

WHAT YOU REALLY WANT: Unadulterated popcorn. Buy a low-calorie bag like Smart Balance Smart Movie-Style, then flavor it at home with a bit of heart-healthy olive oil, grated Parmesan cheese, and fresh herbs.

INGREDIENTS: WHOLE GRAIN POPCORN, PARTIALLY HYDROGENATED SOYBEAN OIL, SALT, NATURAL AND ARTIFICIAL FLAVOR, COLOR ADDED. FRESHNESS PRESERVED BY PROPYL GALLATE.

DISTRIBUTED B'
GENERAL OFFIC

Carbohydrate C

May be mfg. under U.S. Pat. Nos.
6,333,059; 6,706,296; 5,897,89⁴

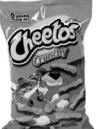

CHEETOS CRUNCHY

THE CLAIM: "Zero grams trans fats"

THE TRUTH: The FDA allows manufacturers to make this claim when their products contain less than 0.5 gram of trans fats per serving. It may seem insignificant, but 0.49 gram of this nefarious fat can add up quickly.

WHAT YOU REALLY WANT: Keep total trans fat intake to no more than 1 percent of total calories—about 2.5 grams per day for most adults. That means reading the ingredients list (especially those that proclaim to be trans-fat free) looking for "partially hydrogenated," "shortening," or "interesterified."

Nutrition Facts

Serving Size 1 oz. (28g/About 21 pieces)
Servings Per Container 9

Amount Per Serving

Calories 160	Calories from Fat 90

	% Daily Value*
Total Fat 10g	**15%**
Saturated Fat 2g	**10%**
Polyunsaturated Fat 5g	
Monounsaturated Fat 2.5g	
Trans Fat 0g	
Cholesterol less than 5mg	**1%**
Sodium 290mg	**12%**
Total Carbohydrate 15g	**5%**

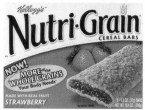

NUTRI-GRAIN STRAW-BERRY CEREAL BAR

THE CLAIM: "Naturally and artificially flavored"

THE TRUTH: While the FDA requires manufacturers to disclose the use of artificial flavoring on the front of the box, the requirements for what is considered "natural" and "real" are not strict: Even trace amounts of the essence or extract of fruit counts as natural. So yes, there is fruit in this bar, but it falls third in the ingredients list, behind HFCS and corn syrup.

INGREDIENTS: FILLING (HIGH FRUCTOSE CORN SYRUP, CORN SYRUP, STRAWBERRY PUREE CONCENTRATE, GLYCERIN, SUGAR, WATER, SODIUM ALGINATE, MODIFIED CORN STARCH, CITRIC ACID, NATURAL AND ARTIFICIAL FLAVOR, SODIUM CITRATE, DICALCIUM PHOSPHATE, METHYLCELLULOSE, CARAMEL COLOR, MALIC ACID, RED #40), WHOLE GRAIN ROLLED OATS, ENRICHED FLOUR (WHEAT FLOUR, NIACIN, REDUCED IRON, THIAMIN MONONITRATE [VITAMIN B₁], RIBOFLAVIN [VITAMIN B₂], FOLIC ACID), WHOLE WHEAT FLOUR, SUNFLOWER AND/OR SOYBEAN OIL WITH TBHQ FOR FRESHNESS, HIGH FRUCTOSE CORN SYRUP, SUGAR, CONTAINS TWO PERCENT OR LESS OF HONEY, DEXTROSE, CALCIUM CARBONATE, SOLUBLE CORN FIBER, NONFAT DRY MILK, WHEAT BRAN, SALT, CELLULOSE, POTASSIUM BICARBONATE (LEAVENING), NATURAL AND ARTIFICIAL FLAVOR, MONO- AND DIGLYCERIDES, PROPYLENE GLYCOL ESTERS OF FATTY ACIDS, SOY LECITHIN, WHEAT GLUTEN, NIACINAMIDE, SODIUM STEAROYL LACTYLATE, VITAMIN A PALMITATE, CARRAGEENAN, ZINC OXIDE, REDUCED IRON, GUAR GUM, PYRIDOXINE HYDROCHLORIDE (VITAMIN B₆), THIAMIN HYDROCHLORIDE (VITAMIN B₁), RIBOFLAVIN (VITAMIN B₂), FOLIC ACID.

CONTAINS WHEAT, MILK AND SOY INGREDIENTS.

WHAT YOU REALLY WANT: An honest snack with nothing to hide. Lärabars, one of our favorite snacks in the aisle, are made with nothing more than dried fruit and nuts.

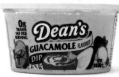

DEAN'S GUACAMOLE

THE CLAIM: "Guacamole"

THE TRUTH: This "guacamole" dip is comprised of less than 2 percent avocado; the rest of the green goo is a cluster of fillers and chemicals, including modified food starch, soybean oils, locust bean gum, and food coloring. Dean's isn't alone in this guacamole caper; most guacs with the word "dip" attached to them suffer from a lack of avocado. This was brought to light when a California woman filed a lawsuit against Dean's after she noticed "it just didn't taste avocadoey." Similarly, a British judge ruled that Pringles are not technically chips, being that they have only 42 percent potato in them.

WHAT YOU REALLY WANT: If you want the heart-healthy fat, you'll need avocado. Wholly Guacamole makes a great guac, or mash up a bowl yourself.

The Snack Matrix

Hundred-calorie snack packs are the hottest thing in the packaged food industry since the hot sauce wars of '87. But while they may provide a decent defense against portion distortion, nearly all of them are total junk. Oreos, Chips Ahoy!, Cheetos—these heavily processed nutritional vortexes do little to stem hunger. Luckily, there are more than a few ways to put a solid snack together. Here, we've created a range of two-piece snack combinations, one part relying on a healthy vehicle like fresh fruit and whole wheat crackers, the other being a tasty topper with real nutritional benefits. Each component adds up to 100 calories, which is ideal since two 200-calorie snacks strategically timed throughout the day are just what your body needs to maximize metabolism and keep you burning calories around the clock. More than anything, you'll see how easy it is to put together a great-tasting combo loaded with the foundations of sound snacking: fiber, lean protein, healthy fat, and a cache of nutrients, or some delicious combination thereof.

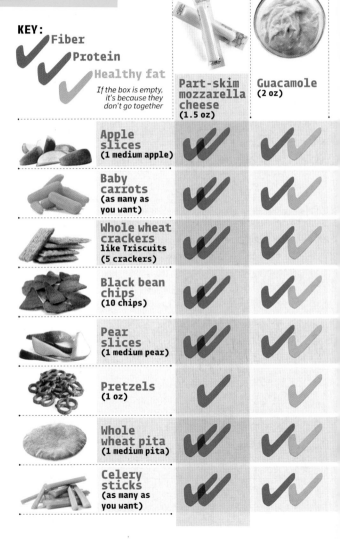

KEY:
Fiber
Protein
Healthy fat
If the box is empty, it's because they don't go together

	Part-skim mozzarella cheese (1.5 oz)	Guacamole (2 oz)
Apple slices (1 medium apple)	Fiber, Protein	Fiber, Healthy fat
Baby carrots (as many as you want)	Fiber, Protein	Fiber, Healthy fat
Whole wheat crackers like Triscuits (5 crackers)	Fiber, Protein	Fiber, Healthy fat
Black bean chips (10 chips)	Fiber, Protein	Fiber, Healthy fat
Pear slices (1 medium pear)	Fiber, Protein	Fiber, Healthy fat
Pretzels (1 oz)	Protein	Healthy fat
Whole wheat pita (1 medium pita)	Fiber, Protein	Fiber, Healthy fat
Celery sticks (as many as you want)	Fiber, Protein	Fiber, Healthy fat

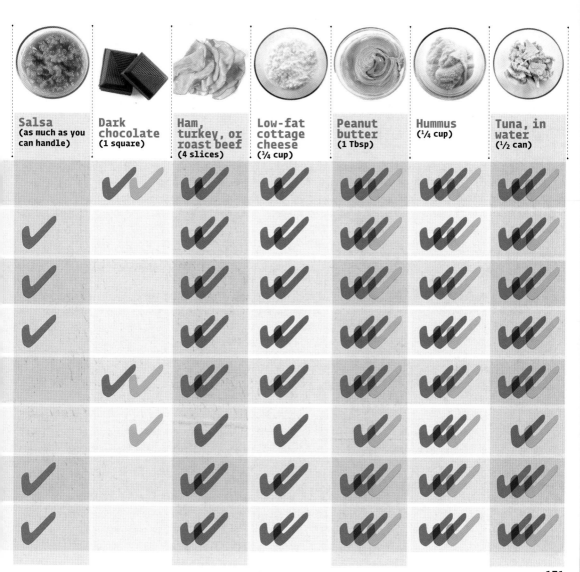

Salsa (as much as you can handle)	Dark chocolate (1 square)	Ham, turkey, or roast beef (4 slices)	Low-fat cottage cheese (¾ cup)	Peanut butter (1 Tbsp)	Hummus (¼ cup)	Tuna, in water (½ can)
	✔✔	✔✔	✔✔	✔✔✔	✔✔✔	✔✔
✔		✔✔	✔✔	✔✔✔	✔✔✔	✔✔
✔		✔✔	✔✔	✔✔✔	✔✔✔	✔✔
✔		✔✔	✔✔	✔✔✔	✔✔✔	✔✔
	✔✔	✔✔	✔✔	✔✔✔	✔✔✔	✔✔
	✔	✔	✔	✔✔✔	✔✔✔	✔
✔		✔✔	✔✔	✔✔✔	✔✔✔	✔✔
✔		✔✔	✔✔	✔✔✔	✔✔✔	✔✔

171

The Trans-Fattiest Foods in the Supermarket

Dangerous trans fat takes many shapes and forms in the supermarket aisles. Here are 10 of the very worst.

COOKIE
10 Pillsbury White Chunk Macadamia Nut Big Deluxe Classics
(1 cookie)

2 g trans fat

180 calories / 13 g sugars
10 g fat (3 g saturated)

Refrigerated you-bake products are a breeding ground for trans fat. Every time you pop one of these cookies into your mouth, you reach the maximum daily amount of trans fat deemed safe by the American Heart Association.

Eat This Instead!
Late July Dark Chocolate Cookies (3 cookies)

150 calories / 9 g sugars
6 g fat (3 g saturated, 0 g trans)

BOXED SIDE
9 Pasta Roni Fettuccine Alfredo
(1 serving, prepared with 2% milk and margarine)

3.5 g trans fat

450 calories / 1140 mg sodium
25 g fat (7 g saturated)

In terms of fat, no sauce compares to the belly-expanding capabilities of Alfredo. So to say that this side is bad even by Alfredo standards does not speak highly of the production standards at Pasta Roni. Lump together the saturated and trans fats, which make up one-fifth of the calories in this box, and you can almost feel your LDL cholesterol building.

Eat This Instead!
Knorr Alfredo Pasta Sides

240 calories / 810 mg sodium
4.5 g fat (2.5 g saturated, 0 g trans)

FROZEN BREAKFAST
8 Jimmy Dean Sausage, Egg, and Cheese Croissant Sandwich (1 sandwich, 128 g)

3.5 g trans fat

430 calories / 740 mg sodium
29 g fat (9 g saturated)

Breakfast breads consistently carry a walloping dose of trans fat. Manufacturers claim it's hard to make biscuits and croissants without trans fat, but we always have the same response: If other companies can do it, then why can't you?

Eat This Instead!
Jimmy Dean D-Lights Muffin made with Whole Grain, Turkey Sausage, Egg White & Cheese
(1 sandwich, 145 g)

260 calories / 840 mg sodium
7 g fat (3.5 g saturated, 0 g trans)

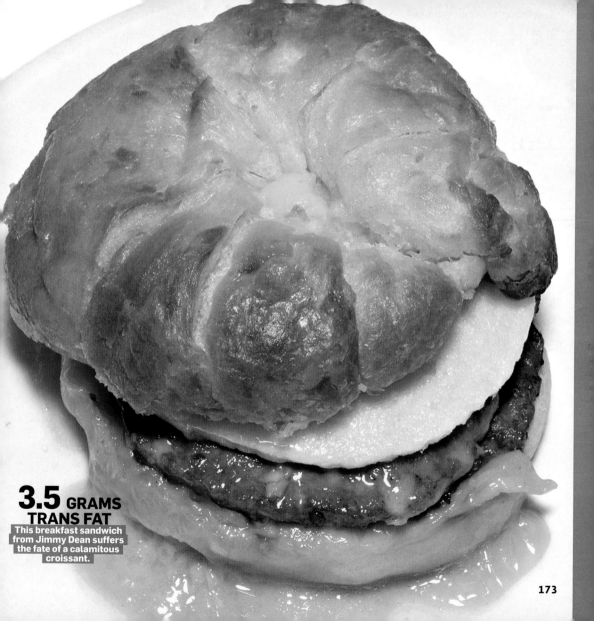

3.5 GRAMS TRANS FAT
This breakfast sandwich from Jimmy Dean suffers the fate of a calamitous croissant.

173

7 Kraft Macaroni & Cheese (1 serving)

4 g trans fat per serving

410 calories / 710 mg sodium
19 g fat (5 g saturated)

Somehow Kraft has determined that it takes a half stick of margarine to get these noodles sufficiently "cheesy." When you follow that advice, the outcome is a pot of noodles with more trans fat than an entire family should eat in a day. If you must succumb to the blue-box allure, please do so responsibly. Replace the margarine with real butter or tub margarine.

Eat This Instead!
Annie's Classic Mac & Cheese (1 serving)

280 calories / 530 mg sodium
4 g fat (2 g saturated, 0 g trans)

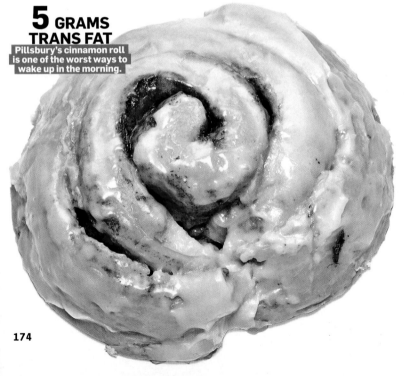

5 GRAMS TRANS FAT
Pillsbury's cinnamon roll is one of the worst ways to wake up in the morning.

6 Pillsbury Perfect Portions Buttermilk Biscuits (1 biscuit)

4 g trans fat

190 calories / 440 mg sodium
9 g fat (2.5 g saturated)

Semi-solid fats like Crisco make biscuits flaky, and most manufacturers refuse to give them up in favor of healthier alternatives. Pillsbury, by no means shy with the trans fat, is the biggest offender of all.

Eat This Instead!
Pillsbury Crusty French Oven Baked Dinner Rolls (1 roll)

90 calories / 190 mg sodium
1 g fat (0 g saturated, 0 g trans)

5 Austin Cheese Crackers with Cheddar Jack Cheese (1 package)

4.5 g trans fat

200 calories / 390 mg sodium
11 g fat (2.5 g saturated)

These classic lunch-box stuffers are contributing more than their share to the obesity epidemic facing this country. Trans fat alone accounts for a fifth of the calories in each cracker.

Eat This Instead!
Kraft Handi-Snacks Mister Salty Pretzels 'n Cheese (1 packet)

90 calories / 380 mg sodium
3.5 g fat (1 g saturated, 0 g trans)

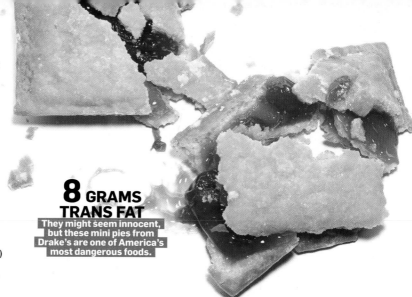

8 GRAMS TRANS FAT
They might seem innocent, but these mini pies from Drake's are one of America's most dangerous foods.

4 Pillsbury Grands! Flaky Supreme Cinnabon Cinnamon Rolls with Icing (1 roll, 99 g)

5 g trans fat

380 calories / 20 g sugars
19 g fat (6 g saturated)

Never start your day with trans fat, especially when it's in a bloated ball of refined carbohydrates and sugar. If this bomb is your breakfast, expect it to be a tough day.

Eat This Instead!
Pepperidge Farm Raisin Cinnamon Swirl Bread (2 slices)

160 calories / 10 g sugars
3 g fat (0 g saturated, 0 g trans)

3 Celeste Original Pizza for One (1 pizza, 158 g)

5 g trans fat

350 calories / 1,090 mg sodium
17 g fat (4 g saturated)

At first glance, Celeste seems to have made a decent pizza. But look closer: That "cheese" is actually imitation cheese, which means water and partially hydrogenated oil. So this pizza is literally covered with a layer of trans fat. Doesn't that sound appetizing?

Eat This Instead!
Lean Cuisine Deluxe French Bread Pizza (1 pizza, 174 g)

340 calories / 760 mg sodium
10 g fat (3.5 g saturated,
0 g trans)

2 Pop-Secret Kettle Corn (1 cup)

6 g trans fat

180 calories / 150 mg sodium
13 g fat (3 g saturated)

How does Pop-Secret manage to turn a healthy snack into this disaster? By using partially hydrogenated oils to pop the kernels. This box has three bags of popcorn, which means every time you buy it, you're bringing 54 grams of dangerous trans fat into your house.

Eat This Instead!
Orville Redenbacher's Smart Pop! Kettle Korn (1 cup)

130 calories / 370 mg sodium
2.5 g fat (0.5 g saturated, 0 g trans)

1 Drake's Cherry Fruit Pie (2 small pies)

8 g trans fat

460 calories / 26 g sugars
27 g fat (7 g saturated)

Individually wrapped snacks are a festering cesspool of partially hydrogenated oils. With these mini pies, you'll gobble down more than 4 days' worth of trans fat! Make sure you have your doctor on speed dial.

Eat This Instead!
Lärabar Cherry Pie Bar

190 calories / 21 g sugars
8 g fat (0.5 g saturated,
0 g trans)

Corn Chips
Eat This

Guiltless® Gourmet All Natural Chili Lime

(~18 chips, 28 g)

120 calories
3 g fat
(0 g saturated)
200 mg sodium

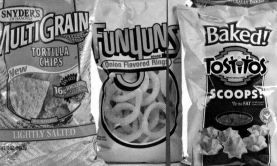

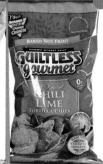

Fewer ingredients, less fat, and double the fiber of Tostitos.

Que Pasa White Corn

(~14 chips, 28 g)

140 calories
7 g fat
(0.5 g saturated)
50 mg sodium

Save across the board with one of the most reliable plain tortilla chips in the supermarket.

Snyder's® of Hanover MultiGrain

(~ 8 chips, 28 g)

130 calories
5 g fat
(0 g saturated)
110 mg sodium

With 3 grams of fiber from whole corn and bran, Snyder's is the king of corn chips.

Funyuns®

(~13 pieces, 28 g)

140 calories
7 g fat
(1 g saturated)
240 mg sodium

The puff of air that fills each Funyun keeps the potential damage to a minimum.

Sun Chips® Original

(~16 chips, 28 g)

140 calories
6 g fat
(1 g saturated)
120 mg sodium

By using only whole grains, Sun Chips keep your blood sugar stable and your belly feeling fed.

Baked! Tostitos Scoops!

(~15 chips, 28 g)

120 calories
3 g fat
(0.5 g saturated)
130 mg sodium

These guys scoop just as well with less than half the fat of Fritos. And if you crack them in half, they're roughly the same size, too.

Baked! Doritos Nacho Cheese

(~15 chips, 28 g)

120 calories
3.5 g fat
(0.5 g saturated)
220 mg sodium

Doritos beat Cheetos any way you bag them, but Baked Doritos also offer 2 grams of fiber.

Not That!

**Tostitos®
Hint of Lime**
(~6 chips, 28 g)

*150 calories
8 g fat
(1 g saturated)
160 mg sodium*

For Tostitos,
a "hint of lime" includes
partially hydrogenated
soybean oil and
artificial coloring.

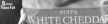

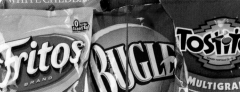

**El Sabroso®
Original
Guacachip®**
(28 g)

*150 calories
9 g fat
(1.5 g saturated)
160 mg sodium*

Unless you like
chemicals and artificial
colorings, spring for
real guac.

**Natural Cheetos®
White Cheddar**
(~32 pieces, 28 g)

*150 calories
9 g fat
(1.5 g saturated)
290 mg sodium*

Don't be fooled by
the term "natural."
It means nothing in
the eyes of the FDA.

**Fritos®
Original**
(~32 chips, 28 g)

*160 calories
10 g fat
(1.5 g saturated)
160 mg sodium*

Great for transporting
bean dip to mouth.
Not so good for keeping
off the belly flat.

**Fritos®
Pinch of Salt™**
(~34 chips, 28 g)

*160 calories
10 g fat
(1.5 g saturated)
75 mg sodium*

They may be light
on sodium, but they
still have 90 calories
from fat.

**Bugles™
Original**
(1⅓ cups, 30 g)

*160 calories
9 g fat
(8 g saturated)
310 mg sodium*

Each horn is nearly
50% saturated
fat by weight!

**Tostitos®
Multigrain**
(~8 chips, 28 g)

*150 calories
8 g fat
(1 g saturated)
135 mg sodium*

Half of the calories
come from vegetable
oil—enough to fill out
each serving with a full
gram of saturated fat.

177

Potato Chips
Eat This

178

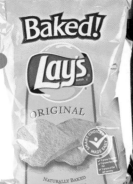
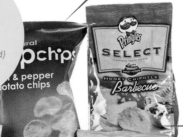
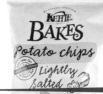
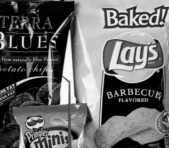
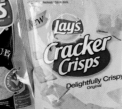

Popchips™ Salt & Pepper
(~20 chips, 28 g)

120 calories
4 g fat
(0 g saturated)
290 mg sodium

Popchips are neither fried nor baked—the potatoes "pop" with heat and pressure. Delicious ingenuity.

Baked! Lay's® Original
(~15 crisps, 28 g)

120 calories
2 g fat (0 g saturated)
180 mg sodium

Pringles® Select Honey Chipotle Barbecue
(~28 crisps, 28 g)

140 calories
8 g fat
(1.5 g saturated)
210 mg sodium

If you're going to eat Pringles, you may as well save calories.

Kettle™ Bakes Lightly Salted
(28 g)

120 calories
3 g fat
(0.5 g saturated)
115 mg sodium

Purest spud in the chip aisle—just russet potatoes lightly salted and baked with oil.

Baked! Lay's has 10 fewer calories per serving than almost any other brand of baked chips.

Pringles® Minis Sour Cream & Onion
(1 bag, 23 g)

130 calories
8 g fat
(2 g saturated)
170 mg sodium

Mini chips equate to more munching for your caloric buck.

Terra Blues®
(~15 chips, 28 g)

130 calories
6 g fat
(1 g saturated)
115 mg sodium

The 3 grams of fiber will ensure that this snack sticks in your stomach for a while.

Baked! Lay's® Barbecue
(~14 chips, 28 g)

120 calories
3 g fat
(0.5 g saturated)
210 mg sodium

Regardless of the flavor, you can never go wrong with Baked! Lay's.

Lay's® Cracker Crisps
(~38 pieces, 28 g)

130 calories
4 g fat
(1 g saturated)
250 mg sodium

Meet the potato chip–wheat cracker hybrid, with more fiber and less than half the fat of a thick-cut potato chip.

Not That!

Boulder™ Canyon Malt Vinegar & Sea Salt
(~14 chips, 28 g)

150 calories
7 g fat
(1 g saturated)
410 mg sodium

Nearly double the sodium of all the other major brands.

Pringles® Original
(~14 crisps, 28 g)

160 calories
11 g fat
(3 g saturated)
170 mg sodium

A British court found that Pringles aren't actually potato chips, since they contain only 42% potato.

Lay's® Light® Original
(~20 chips, 28 g)

75 calories
0 g fat
200 mg sodium

Olestra can cause nutritional deficiencies when carotenoids and other fat-soluble nutrients get flushed out in loose stools.

Ruffles® Original
(~12 chips, 28 g)

160 calories
10 g fat (1 g saturated)
160 mg sodium

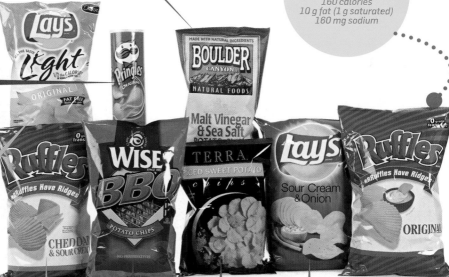

Ruffles Cheddar & Sour Cream
(~11 chips, 28 g)

160 calories
11 g fat
(1.5 g saturated)
230 mg sodium

Thick cut and crinkled means more fried potato is stuffed into each bite.

Wise® BBQ
(15 chips, 28 g)

150 calories
10 g fat
(3 g saturated)
210 mg sodium

Just potatoes cooked in vegetable oil with a bunch of junk added in.

Terra® Spiced Sweet Potato
(~17 chips, 28 g)

160 calories
11 g fat
(1 g saturated)
150 mg sodium

Even a good chip can go bad with too much oil.

Lay's® Sour Cream & Onion
(~17 chips, 28 g)

160 calories
10 g fat
(1 g saturated)
210 mg sodium

These classic chips suffer from a too-long list of ingredients tainted with partially hydrogenated oils.

Why don't we like crinkled chips? If you stretched out the crinkles, you'd have a massive hunk of fried potato.

Dips

Try using guac as a sub for mayo on a turkey sandwich. The monounsaturated fats from the avocado make for a great heart-healthy spread.

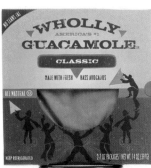

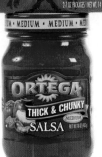

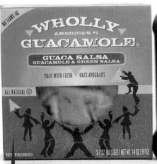

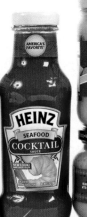

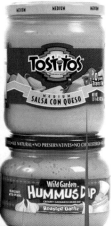

Wholly Guacamole™ Classic
(2 Tbsp, 30 g)
50 calories
4 g fat (0.5 g saturated)
75 mg sodium

Ortega® Thick & Chunky Salsa Medium
(2 Tbsp, 31 g)
10 calories
0 g fat
210 mg sodium
The planet's finest condiment, packed with antioxidants that help prevent cancers and macular degeneration.

Wholly Guacamole™ Guaca Salsa
(2 Tbsp, 30 g)
30 calories
2 g fat
(0 g saturated)
190 mg sodium
Avocados are rich with oleic acid, a healthy fat that helps to lower the bad cholesterol and raise the good.

Heinz Cocktail Sauce
(¼ cup, 60 g)
60 calories
0 g fat
690 mg sodium
Choosing cocktail sauce over tartar is like choosing tomatoes over mayo. It's a no-brainer.

Wild Garden™ Hummus Dip Roasted Garlic
(2 Tbsp, 30 g)
35 calories
2 g fat
(0 g saturated)
70 mg sodium
A fiber- and protein-rich Mediterranean staple perfect for dipping and slathering.

Tostitos® Salsa Con Queso Medium
(2 Tbsp, 34 g)
40 calories
2.5 g fat
(1 g saturated)
280 mg sodium
With the nutritional perks of tomatoes and peppers, salsa con queso beats straight cheese dip every time.

Not That!

Mission® Guacamole Dip
(2 Tbsp, 31 g)

40 calories
3 g fat (0 g saturated)
150 mg sodium

The first 3 ingredients in this "guacamole" are water, oil, and food starch. The only mention of avocadoes comes from "avocado powder."

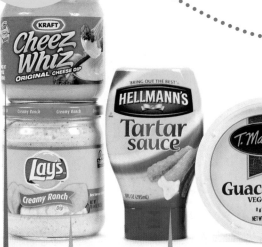
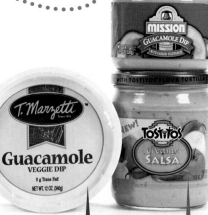

Kraft® Cheez Whiz Original Cheese Dip
(2 Tbsp, 33 g)

90 calories
7 g fat
(1.5 g saturated)
440 mg sodium

This is pure junk. If you have a taste for cheese, save your calories for the real thing.

Lay's™ Creamy Ranch Dip
(2 Tbsp, 33 g)

60 calories
5 g fat
(2.5 g saturated)
240 mg sodium

Make ranch your staple dip and you could be adding hundreds of low-quality calories to your snacking.

Hellmann's® Tartar Sauce
(4 Tbsp, 60 g)

160 calories
14 g fat
(2 g saturated)
660 mg sodium

Tartar is basically glorified mayo, waiting to drown fish's nutritional benefits in a tide of fat.

T. Marzetti™ Guacamole Veggie Dip
(2 Tbsp, 29 g)

130 calories
13 g fat
(2.5 g saturated)
240 mg sodium

Guacamole imposters are hiding in every cooler in the country. This one is mostly oil and sour cream.

Tostitos® Creamy Salsa
(2 Tbsp, 32 g)

35 calories
3 g fat
(0 g saturated)
150 mg sodium

To make it creamy, Tostitos has polluted this good salsa with a dose of oil.

181

Eat This

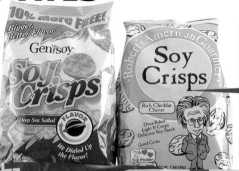

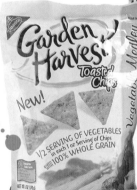

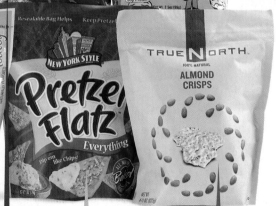

Nabisco Garden Harvest Toasted Vegetable Medley
(~16 chips, 28 g)

120 calories
3.5 g fat (0 g saturated)
240 mg sodium

Robert's American Gourmet Rich Cheddar Cheese Soy Crisps
(28 g)

120 calories
4 g fat
(0.5 g saturated)
210 mg sodium

Soy crisps have as much as 4 times the protein and 3 times the fiber in rice chips.

The first 2 ingredients are whole grain wheat and a vegetable blend. Each serving has 3 grams of fiber.

GeniSoy® Soy Crisps Deep Sea Salted
(17 crisps, 28 g)

100 calories
1.5 g fat
(0 g saturated)
270 mg sodium

It's not the lower calories that make this a good snack—it's the 2 grams of fiber and 8 grams of protein per serving.

New York Style® Pretzel Flatz Everything
(12 Flatz, 28 g)

120 calories
2 g fat
(0 g saturated)
290 mg sodium

The nutritional profile of a pretzel (a good thing) with the dipability of a chip (a great thing).

TrueNorth™ Almond Crisps
(~15 crisps, 28 g)

140 calories
7 g fat
(0.5 g saturated)
240 mg sodium

The base of this chip is almonds, which brings a host of healthy fat and naturally occurring nutrients such as phosphorus, magnesium, and vitamin E.

isps

Not That!

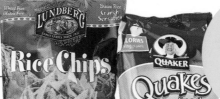

Lundberg Nacho Cheese Rice

(~10 chips, 28 g)

140 calories
7 g fat
(0.5 g saturated)
140 mg sodium

Nobody's bagged rice compares to Lundberg's. Too bad the same can't be said of its chips.

Nabisco Ritz Toasted Sour Cream & Onion

(~14 chips, 28 g)

130 calories
6 g fat (1 g saturated)
270 mg sodium

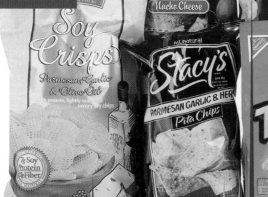

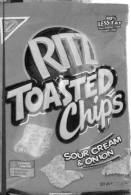

Snyder's® of Hanover EatSmart Soy Crisps Parmesan, Garlic & Olive Oil

(~22 chips, 30 g)

160 calories
9 g fat
(1 g saturated)
290 mg sodium

There are too many tasty, healthy options in this category to fall back on these.

Stacy's® Parmesan Garlic & Herb Pita Chips

(~12 chips, 28 g)

140 calories
5 g fat
(0.5 g saturated)
200 mg sodium

If the goal is low calorie, you can do better than pita chips.

Quaker® Quakes® Rice Snacks Cheddar Cheese

(18 mini cakes, 30 g)

140 calories
5 g fat (2.5 g saturated)
460 mg sodium

Quaker halves the serving size to make Quakes appear healthier. Doesn't matter how many of these things you eat, there's still not more than a speck of fiber.

Without any fiber to slow its movement through your belly, this load of enriched flour will spike your blood sugar to fat-storing heights.

183

Pretzels and Snack Mix

Eat This

Kraft® Handi-Snacks® Mister Salty® Pretzels 'n Cheez

(1 package, 28 g)

90 calories
3.5 g fat
(1 g saturated)
380 mg sodium

Limit your dipping to half the cup and cut 20 calories from your snack.

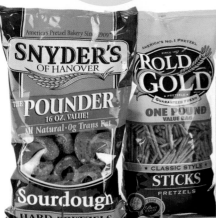
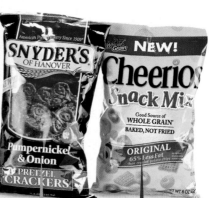

Snyder's® of Hanover Sourdough Hard

(1 pretzel, 28 g)

100 calories
0 g fat
240 mg sodium

Including water, this pretzel has only 5 ingredients—almost half as many as Rold Gold's version of the same pretzel.

Rold Gold Sticks

(~48 pretzels, 28 g)

100 calories
0 g fat
580 mg sodium

Sodium is pretzel's Achilles' heel, and these sticks have plenty. Stick to 24 sticks and you'll have a 50-calorie, fat-free snack.

Cheez-It® Party Mix

(½ cup, 30 g)

120 calories
4.5 g fat
(1 g saturated)
290 mg sodium

This mix has 25% less fat than the Munchies.

Snyder's® of Hanover Pumpernickel & Onion Pretzel

(~11 crackers, 30 g)

130 calories
3 g fat
(1.5 g saturated)
230 mg sodium

Not only do you save on calories and trans fat, but you gain big on fiber.

Cheerios® Snack Mix Original

(⅔ cup)

120 calories
3.5 g fat
(0.5 g saturated)
330 mg sodium

By creating a mix that wins in every nutritional category, Cheerios could replace Chex as the snack mix king.

es

Not That!

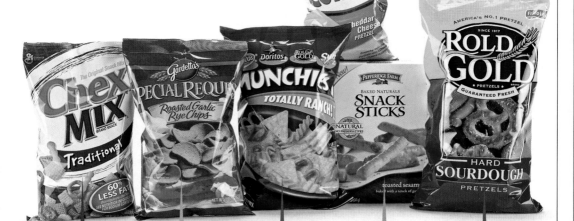

The core of the combo is packed with saturated fats; not even its pretzel armor can protect you.

**Combos®
Cheddar Cheese**
(~1/3 cup, 28 g)

*130 calories
4.5 g fat
(3 g saturated)
440 mg sodium*

**Chex Mix®
Traditional**
(2/3 cup, 30 g)

*130 calories
4 g fat
(0.5 g saturated)
380 mg sodium*

The "original snack mix" is no longer the only player in the game.

**Gardetto's®
Special Request
Roasted Garlic
Rye** (1/2 cup, 30 g)

*160 calories
10 g fat
(2 g saturated,
2.5 g trans)
340 mg sodium*

The gratuitous use of partially hydrogenated oils makes this line one to limit.

**Frito-Lay®
Munchies®
Totally Ranch!™**
(3/4 cup, 28 g)

*140 calories
6 g fat
(1 g saturated)
260 mg sodium*

The snack mix market has exploded in recent years, which means you don't have to settle for lackluster products.

**Pepperidge
Farm® Snack
Sticks Toasted
Sesame**
(12 sticks, 31 g)

*140 calories
5 g fat
(1 g saturated)
330 mg sodium*

Bigger sticks mean more calories. Go small and eat more for less.

**Rold Gold®
Hard Sourdough**
(1 pretzel, 26 g)

*100 calories
0.5 g fat
(0 g saturated)
500 mg sodium*

It's not just the double dose of sodium that has us concerned; it's the superfluous ingredients like corn syrup.

Boxed Crackers
Eat This

Nabisco Triscuit Original
(6 crackers, 29 g)

120 calories
4.5 g fat (1 g saturated)
180 mg sodium

About as unadulterated as wheat gets without chewing on chaff. Your reward: Nearly half a gram of fiber in every cracker.

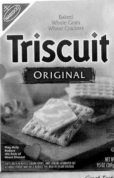

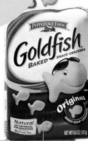

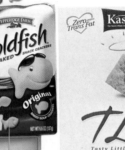

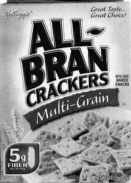

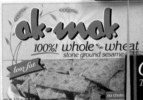

Ak-Mak® 100% Whole of the Wheat
(5 crackers, 28 g)

115 calories
2 g fat
(<0.5 g saturated)
220 mg sodium

Four grams of fiber, 5 grams of protein, and seasoned with sesame seeds and honey instead of oil and sugar.

Pepperidge Farm Goldfish Original
(55 pieces, 30 g)

150 calories
6 g fat
(0.5 g saturated)
230 mg sodium

Each fish sets you back just 2.5 calories. Eat them one at a time and feel the craving vanish.

Carr's® Table Water®
(~5 crackers, 17 g)

70 calories
1.5 g fat
(0.5 g saturated)
100 mg sodium

Each box has a quarter of the fat and 1,220 fewer calories than Ritz.

Kashi™ TLC™ Original 7 Grain
(15 crackers, 30 g)

130 calories
3 g fat
(0 g saturated)
160 mg sodium

Avoid overeating by filling up individual baggies with a single serving of crackers.

Kellogg's® All-Bran® Multi-Grain
(18 crackers, 30 g)

130 calories
6 g fat
(1 g saturated)
270 mg sodium

The 5 grams of fiber in these crackers will slow your digestion to keep your stomach feeling full.

Not That!

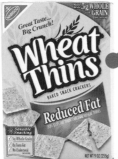

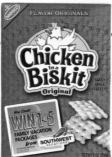

Nabisco Wheat Thins Reduced Fat
(16 crackers, 29 g)

130 calories
4 g fat (0.5 g saturated)
260 mg sodium

Most of the flour is refined, so this "wheat" cracker has 4 times as much sugar (4 grams) as fiber (1 gram).

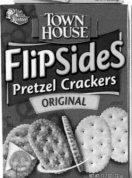

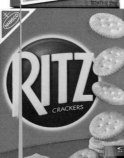

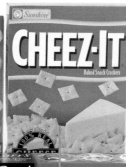

Town House® FlipSides® Pretzel Original
(10 crackers, 30 g)

140 calories
7 g fat
(1 g saturated)
400 mg sodium

The FlipSide doesn't offer much besides empty calories and novelty appeal.

Chicken in a Biskit Original
(12 crackers, 31 g)

160 calories
8 g fat
(1.5 g saturated)
310 mg sodium

Don't eat a cracker that doesn't have 1 full gram of fiber in a serving. Especially when said cracker is 45% pure fat.

Ritz
(10 crackers, 32 g)

160 calories
9 g fat
(2 g saturated)
270 mg sodium

The most famous name in crackers is also an easy way to get fat. Each cracker contains 2 grams of refined carbohydrates and nearly 1 gram of fat.

Cheez-It
(27 crackers, 30 g)

160 calories
8 g fat
(2 g saturated)
250 mg sodium

The "100% real cheese" stamp on the box is a stretch; these crackers contain far more vegetable oil than cheese.

Carr's® Whole Wheat
(4 crackers, 34 g)

160 calories
8 g fat
(3 g saturated)
200 mg sodium

The generous use of vegetable oil provides much more fat than a wheat cracker needs.

187

Individually Packaged
Eat This

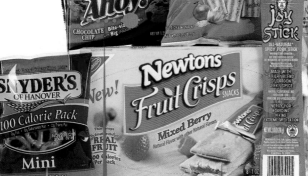
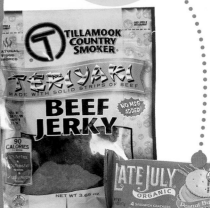

Sun Chips® French Onion
(1 package, 28.3 g)

140 calories
6 g fat
(1 g saturated)
130 mg sodium

Choosing Sun Chips over Ruffles will halve the fat and double the fiber.

Late July® Peanut Butter
(1 package, 37 g)

160 calories
8 g fat (2 g saturated)
2 g sugars

Snyder's® of Hanover Mini Pretzels
(1 bag, 26 g)

100 calories
0 g fat
220 mg sodium

Sub in a bag of Snyder's every day for a year, you'll lose more than 4 pounds of stored fat.

Chips Ahoy! Mini
(1 bag, 35 g)

170 calories
8 g fat
(2.5 g saturated)
10 g sugars

Nutritious? No, but as far as cookies go, the small serving size makes them relatively safe.

Newtons Fruit Crisps Mixed Berry
(2 crisps, 28 g)

100 calories
2 g fat
(0 g saturated)
8 g sugars

A reliably low-calorie way to quell your cravings.

Applegate Farms® Natural Joy Stick Pepperoni
(1 stick, 28 g)

100 calories
7 g fat
(3 g saturated)
700 mg sodium

This stick is nitrate-free, a rare feat for packaged meats.

Tillamook Country Smoker® Teriyaki Beef Jerky (1 oz, 28 g)

90 calories
1 g fat
(0.5 g saturated)
650 mg sodium

A good low-cal dose of protein to beat back midday hunger.

Just the way we like it: light on the sugar and heavy on the peanuts.

Snacks
Not That!

NutterButter Peanut Butter Sandwich
(1 package, 53 g)

250 calories
10 g fat (2.5 g saturated)
15 g sugars

Ruffles® Cheddar & Sour Cream
(~11 chips, 28 g)

160 calories
11 g fat
(1.5 g saturated)
230 mg sodium

There are too many healthier chip options to ever settle for these Ruffles.

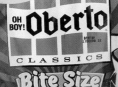

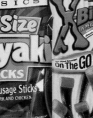

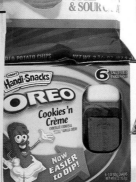

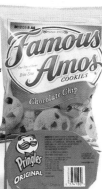

This is not a snack; it's a dessert, and it has only 10 fewer calories than a pack of Reese's Peanut Butter Cups.

Oberto® Bite Size Teriyaki Smoked Sausage Sticks
(5 pieces, 31 g)

140 calories
12 g fat
(3.5 g saturated)
650 mg sodium

This pork/chicken mix is 75% fat.

Jack Link's® X-Bites™ Pepperoni Extra
(½ package, 28 g)

120 calories
10.5 g fat
(4 g saturated)
455 mg sodium

Two sticks per wrapper means double trouble.

Kraft Handi-Snacks Oreo Cookies'n Crème
(1 unit, 28 g)

140 calories
6 g fat
(2.5 g saturated)
13 g sugars

Sugar and fat together make up 75% of the calories.

Famous Amos® Chocolate Chip (1 pack, 56 g)

280 calories
13 g fat
(4 g saturated)
18 g sugars

It's too easy to thoughtlessly wolf down 12% of your daily calories.

Pringles® Original
(1 tub, 23 g)

140 calories
10 g fat
(3 g saturated)
150 mg sodium

The majority of the calories in the tub come from fat.

189

Fruits, Nuts, and Seeds
Eat This

Planters Pistachio Lovers Mix
(~35 pieces, 28 g)
*160 calories
13 g fat (1.5 g saturated)
80 mg sodium*

Ocean Spray® Craisins® Original
(⅓ cup, 40 g)
*130 calories
0 g fat
26 g sugars*

Sugar is used to cut cranberry's natural tartness. Keep it to a handful and still reap the nutritional benefits.

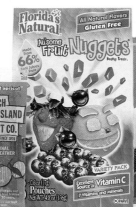
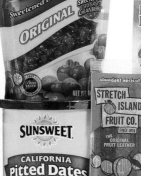
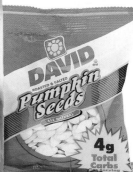
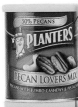
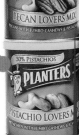

Choosing a nut mix with pistachios instead of macadamias sheds fat and calories while earning 33% more protein and 50% more fiber.

Planters Pecan Lovers Mix
(~24 pieces, 28 g)
*180 calories
17 g fat
(2 g saturated)
70 mg sodium*

The antioxidant powers of pecans with a fraction of the fat.

Sunsweet® California Pitted
(40 g, 5–6 dates)
*120 calories
0 g fat
27 g sugars*

No added sugar makes this a great source of quick energy that won't spin your blood sugar into a wild state of flux.

Stretch Island Fruit Co.® The Original Fruit Leather Abundant Apricot®
(1 strip, 14 g)
*45 calories
0 g fat
8 g sugars*

The best fruit chew at your grocery store.

Florida's Natural® Au'some Fruit Nuggets Strawberry
(1 pouch, 17 g)
*50 calories
0 g fat
10 g sugars*

Made from real fruit concentrates and purees.

David® Pumpkin Seeds Roasted & Salted
(¼ cup, 30 g of kernels)
*160 calories
12 g fat
(2.5 g saturated)
10 mg sodium*

Packed with magnesium and iron.

190

Not That!

**Sun-Maid®
Yogurt
Cranberries
Vanilla**
(30 g)

*120 calories
3.5 g fat
(3 g saturated)
20 g sugars*

Yogurt here equals
sugar and partially
hydrogenated oil.

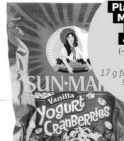

**Planters Select
Macadamias,
Cashews
& Almonds**
(~26 pieces, 28 g)

*180 calories
17 g fat (2.5 g saturated)
95 mg sodium*

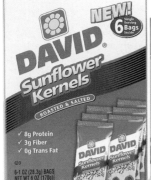

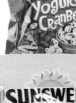

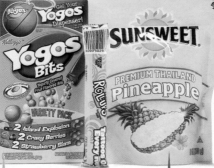

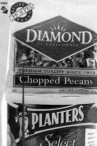

*Macadamias
are the low
nuts on the
nutritional
totem pole.*

**David®
Sunflower
Kernels Roasted
& Salted**
(1 pkg, 28 g)

*180 calories
14 g fat
(1.5 g saturated)
210 mg sodium*

Polluted with partially
hydrogenated oils.

**Yogos® Bits,
Island Explosion®**
(1 pouch, 23 g)

*90 calories
1.5 g fat
(1.5 g saturated)
15 g sugars*

The first ingredient?
Sugar.

**Fruit Roll-ups®
Strawberry**
(1 roll, 14 g)

*50 calories
1 g fat
(0 g saturated)
7 g sugars*

"Fruit snack" means
an amalgamation
of corn syrup, sugar,
oil, and artificial
colors.

**Sunsweet®
Premium
Thailand
Pineapple**
(⅓ cup, 40 g)

*130 calories
0 g fat
31 g sugars*

Added sweeteners
and preservatives
make this a less-
worthy dried fruit.

**Diamond®
Chopped Pecans**
(¼ cup, 30 g)

*210 calories
22 g fat
(2 g saturated)
0 mg sodium*

Pecans can help
lower LDL cholesterol,
but eat them sparingly.

191

Popcorn

Eat This

American's Best Microwave Butter
(2 cups popped)

*40 calories
1 g fat (0 g saturated)
84 mg sodium*

You're unlikely to find a better popcorn—American's Best packs in 4 grams of fiber per serving.

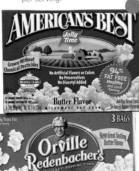

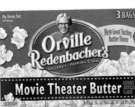

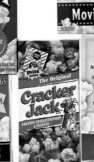

Orville Redenbacher's® Kettle Korn
(2 cups popped)

*70 calories
4 g fat
(2 g saturated)
50 mg sodium*

Sweetened with sucralose to keep the calories down.

Cracker Jack® The Original
(½ cup, 28 g)

*120 calories
2 g fat
(0 g saturated)
70 mg sodium
15 g sugars*

Relatively low in calories with 30% less sodium than Crunch 'n Munch.

Orville Redenbacher's® Movie Theater Butter
(2 cups popped)

*70 calories
5 g fat
(2 g saturated)
110 mg sodium*

The same rich taste as Pop-Secret, without the harmful trans fat.

Orville Redenbacher's® Natural Simply Salted
(2 cups popped)

*70 calories
5 g fat
(2 g saturated)
220 mg sodium*

Never settle for an inferior bag.

Good Health® Half Naked with Olive Oil
(2 cups, 14 g)

*60 calories
1.5 g fat
(0 g saturated)
70 mg sodium*

Save 100 calories and double up on fiber.

Not That!

**Newman's Own®
Pop's Corn
Light Butter**
(2 cups popped)

*70 calories
2.5 g fat (1 g saturated)
100 mg sodium*

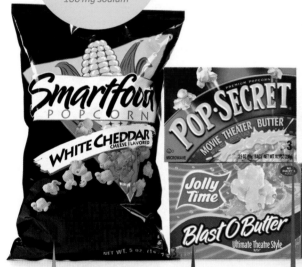

*Newman's Own is one
of the supermarket's
better brands, but that
doesn't make it
infallible.*

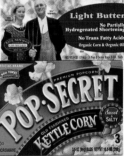

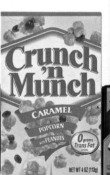

**Smartfood®
White Cheddar
Cheese**
(1¾ cups, 28 g)

*160 calories
10 g fat
(2 g saturated)
290 mg sodium*

A thick oil slick gives
this bag 5 times more
fat than the popcorn
you'd pop at home.

**Jolly Time®
Blast O Butter®**
(2 cups popped)

*90 calories
6 g fat
(2 g saturated,
2 g trans)
170 mg sodium*

The name should make
you worry. If that
doesn't do it, the
nutrition label will.

**Pop-Secret®
Movie Theater
Butter**
(2 cups popped)

*90 calories
6 g fat
(1.5 g saturated,
2.5 g trans)
150 mg sodium*

The only "secret" here is
that the company has no
qualms with trans fat.

**Crunch 'n Munch
Caramel**
(⅔ cup, 31 g)

*150 calories
6 g fat
(2 g saturated)
100 mg sodium
11 g sugars*

One serving is the
caloric equivalent of
10 Milk Duds.

**Pop-Secret®
Old Fashioned
Kettle Corn**
(2 cups popped)

*80 calories
3.5 g fat
(0.5 g saturated,
1.5 g trans)
40 mg sodium*

The calories aren't
too bad, but the trans
fat is atrocious.

193

Granola and Cereal Bars
Eat This

The 9 grams of fiber are sure to annihilate even the most persistent hungers.

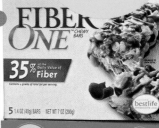

Fiber One™ Oats & Chocolate

(1 bar, 40 g)

140 calories
4 g fat (1.5 g saturated)
10 g sugars
9 g fiber

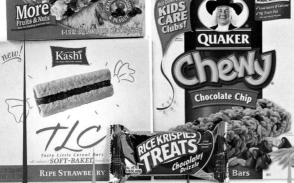

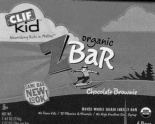

Nutri-Grain® Cranberry, Raisin & Peanut

(1 bar, 32 g)

120 calories
3.5 g fat
(1 g saturated)
11 g sugars
3 g fiber

Don't confuse this with the regular Nutri-Grain bar. It's vastly superior.

Kashi™ TLC® Ripe Strawberry

(1 bar, 35 g)

110 calories
3 g fat
(0 g saturated)
9 g sugars
3 g fiber

More fiber, fewer calories, and less sugar than the Nutri-Grain bar.

Kellogg's® Rice Krispies Treats® Chocolatey Drizzle

(1 bar, 22 g)

100 calories
3 g fat
(1 g saturated)
8 g sugars
0 g fiber

An average snack, but a very safe dessert.

Quaker Chewy® Chocolate Chip

(1 bar, 24 g)

100 calories
3 g fat
(1.5 g saturated)
7 g sugars
1 g fiber

Think of it more as a modest dessert than as a healthy bar.

Clif® Kid™ Organic Z Bar™ Chocolate Brownie

(1 bar, 36 g)

120 calories
3 g fat
(1 g saturated)
12 g sugars
3 g fiber

A candy bar name with 3 grams of fiber. Perfect for a kid.

Not That!

(2 bars, 44 g)

*180 calories
4 g fat (2 g saturated)
18 g sugars
1 g fiber*

Special K shrinks their bar down to half the normal size, but the truth is that it's 40% sugar and doesn't even have 1 gram of fiber. You'll feel twice as hungry half an hour after eating it.

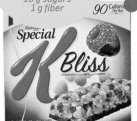

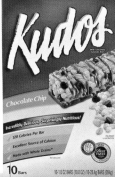

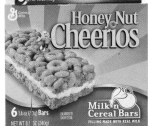

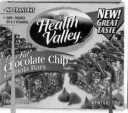

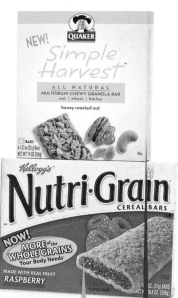

Honey Nut Cheerios® Milk 'n Cereal
(1 bar, 40 g)

*160 calories
4 g fat
(2 g saturated)
14 g sugars
1 g fiber*

You know how Cocoa Puffs are so bad for you? Yeah, well . . .

Kudos® Chocolate Chip
(1 bar, 28 g)

*120 calories
3.5 g fat
(2 g saturated)
11 g sugars
1 g fiber*

A third of the calories are from added sugars, which by our best estimation makes Kudos a candy bar.

Health Valley® Low Fat Chocolate Chip
(1 bar, 42 g)

*160 calories
2.5 g fat
(1 g saturated)
13 g sugars
1 g fiber*

The main ingredient is brown rice syrup—a euphemism for sugar.

Kellogg's® Nutri-Grain® Raspberry
(1 bar, 37 g)

*140 calories
3 g fat
(0.5 g saturated)
13 g sugars
2 g fiber*

Refined flour on the outside, high-fructose corn syrup inside.

Quaker® Simple Harvest™ Honey Roasted Nut
(1 bar, 35 g)

*160 calories
7 g fat
(1 g saturated)
7 g sugars
2 g fiber*

You could do worse, but why not do a bit better?

195

Meal Replacement and

Eat This

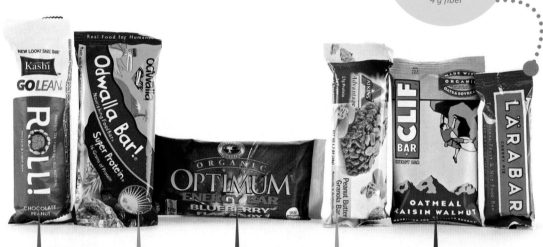

Lärabar® Cherry
(1 bar, 48 g)

190 calories
8 g fat (0.5 g saturated)
4 g protein
21 g sugars
4 g fiber

Made from exactly 3 ingredients: dates, almonds, and cherries. Lärabar is the closest thing to real food in the bar section of the grocery store.

Kashi™ GoLean® Protein & Fiber Chocolate Peanut
(1 bar, 55 g)

190 calories
5 g fat
(1.5 g saturated)
12 g protein
14 g sugars
6 g fiber

High fiber, high protein, low calorie: Perfect.

Odwalla Bar!® Super Protein®
(1 bar, 62 g)

230 calories
4.5 g fat
(1.5 g saturated)
16 g protein
16 g sugars
4 g fiber

Mega protein makes this bar a powerful weapon against hunger.

Nature's Path Optimum® Blueberry Flax & Soy
(1 bar, 56 g)

200 calories
3 g fat
(0 g saturated)
6 g protein
20 g sugars
5 g fiber

Figs and raisins supply the natural sweetness.

Atkins™ Advantage Peanut Butter Granola Bar
(1 bar, 48 g)

200 calories
7 g fat
(1 g saturated)
17 g protein
1 g sugars
6 g fiber

Great postworkout meal.

Clif® Bar Oatmeal Raisin Walnut
(1 bar, 68 g)

240 calories
5 g fat
(1 g saturated)
10 g protein
20 g sugars
5 g fiber

The bonus takeaway is a healthy dose of vitamin A and your day's intake of vitamin E.

Protein Bars
Not That!

PowerBar® Energize Berry Blast Smoothie
(1 bar, 57 g)

210 calories
3.5 g fat (0.5 g saturated)
6 g protein
24 g sugars
<1 g fiber

Besides the fact that it doesn't contain a single gram of fiber, the Energize BerryBlast Smoothie lists evaporated cane juice (aka sugar) as its first ingredient.

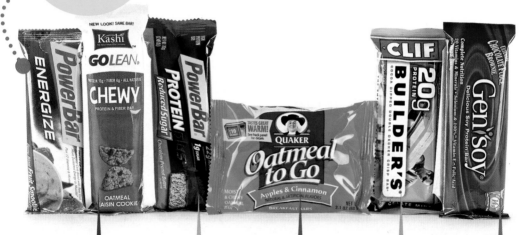

Kashi™ GoLean® Chewy Oatmeal Raisin Cookie
(1 bar, 78 g)

280 calories
5 g fat
(3 g saturated)
13 g protein
33 g sugars
6 g fiber

47% of the bar's calories come from sugars.

PowerBar® Protein Plus Reduced Sugar
(1 bar, 70 g)

270 calories
9 g fat
(4 g saturated)
22 g protein
1 g sugars
2 g fiber

The high protein and low sugar counts almost make up for the calories and fat. Almost.

Quaker® Oatmeal to Go Apples & Cinnamon
(1 bar, 60 g)

220 calories
4 g fat
(1 g saturated)
4 g protein
22 g sugars
5 g fiber

High-fructose corn syrup and margarine pollute this package.

Clif® Builder's Chocolate Mint
(1 bar, 68 g)

270 calories
8 g fat
(5 g saturated)
20 g protein
20 g sugars
4 g fiber

The extra calories, sugar, and fat don't justify the extra 4 grams of protein.

Genisoy® Ultimate Chocolate Fudge Brownie
(1 bar, 62 g)

240 calories
5 g fat
(3 g saturated)
14 g protein
22 g sugars
2 g fiber

197

Cookies

Eat This

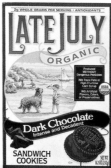

At 60 calories per cookie, this is the least destructive Chips Ahoy! on the shelf.

Chips Ahoy! Chewy
(2 cookies, 27 g)

120 calories
6 g fat (3 g saturated)
10 g sugars

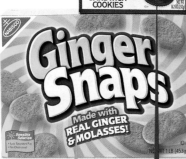

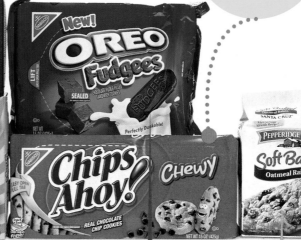

Nabisco Ginger Snaps
(4 cookies, 28 g)

120 calories
2.5 g fat
(0.5 g saturated)
11 g sugars

Ginger Snaps come with the benefit of ginger's natural anti-inflammatory and anticarcinogenic effects.

Late July® Organic Dark Chocolate
(3 cookies, 33 g)

150 calories
6 g fat (3 g saturated)
9 g sugars
2 g fiber

A good, honest cookie short on ingredients and long on satisfying richness. Three cookies should be plenty to satisfy even the sweetest tooth.

Oreo Fudgees
(2 cookies, 31 g)

140 calories
6 g fat
(3 g saturated)
12 g sugars

Although it is by no means a health cookie, the Fudgees have 20 fewer calories per serving than even the original Oreos.

Pepperidge Farm® Soft Baked Oatmeal Raisin
(1 cookie, 31 g)

130 calories
4.5 g fat
(1.5 g saturated)
13 g sugars

Big cookies take a toll, but as an occasional treat, this one's not too bad. Just keep it to one, okay?

Not That!

Oreo
(3 cookies, 34 g)

160 calories
7 g fat (2 g saturated)
14 g sugars

America's most popular cookie unfortunately is not one of its healthiest. The reduced-fat version will only save you 10 calories a cookie.

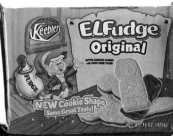

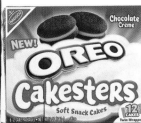

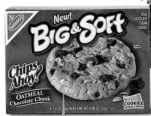

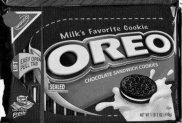

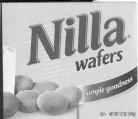

Chips Ahoy! Big & Soft Oatmeal Chocolate Chunk
(1 cookie, 39 g)

180 calories
8 g fat
(3 g saturated)
13 g sugars

The caloric equivalent of an entire cantaloupe, but without the fiber and natural sugars.

E.L. Fudge® Original
(2 cookies, 36 g)

180 calories
7 g fat
(3 g saturated)
12 g sugars

Many E.L. Fudge offerings turn to flab, and at 90 calories apiece, the original cookie is no exception.

Oreo Cakesters Chocolate Creme
(2 cakes, 57 g)

250 calories
12 g fat
(3 g saturated)
23 g sugars

Eat this if you want to try the get-fat-quick diet. Every cake packs another 125 calories into your gut.

Nilla Wafers
(8 wafers, 30 g)

140 calories
6 g fat
(1.5 g saturated)
11 g sugars

If you must have a Nilla Wafer, go for the reduced-fat version. It will save you 30 calories per serving.

199

Pudding
Eat This

Jell-O Sugar Free Dark Chocolate
(1 snack, 106 g)

60 calories
1.5 g fat (0 g saturated)
0 g sugar

Sugar is the biggest concern with yogurts and puddings, so worry less about fat and find one that is minimally sweetened, instead.

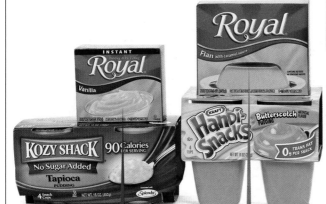

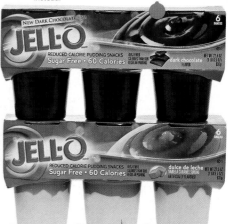

Royal® Instant Vanilla
(½ cup prepared)

80 calories
0 g fat
17 g sugars

The goal with pudding is to find the lowest amount of sugar. You can always use a handful of raisins to sweeten it at home.

Kozy Shack® No Sugar Added Tapioca
(1 snack cup, 113 g)

90 calories
3 g fat
(2 g saturated)
5 g sugars

This pudding is fortified with 4 grams of inulin fiber so that your blood sugar remains stable.

Royal® Flan with Caramel Sauce
(½ cup prepared)

70 calories
0 g fat
18 g sugars

The dry-mix route is often the safest. And if you want to cut an extra 40 calories, go easy on the caramel sauce.

Handi-Snacks® Butterscotch
(1 snack, 99 g)

90 calories
1 g fat
(1 g saturated)
16 g sugars

Make Handi-Snacks your default pudding cup. In flavor-to-flavor matchups, they win over Snack Pack every time.

Jell-O Sugar Free Dulce De Leche
(1 snack, 106 g)

60 calories
1 g fat
(1 g saturated)
0 g sugars

In small amounts, most alternative sweeteners are harmless. Here, they help to cut calories by 60%.

Not That!

Jell-O Fat Free Chocolate
(1 snack, 113 g)

*100 calories
0 g fat
17 g sugars*

Two-thirds of the calories in this cup come from added sugars.

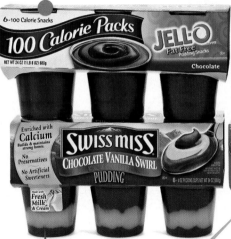

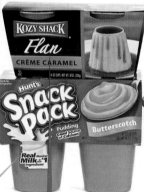

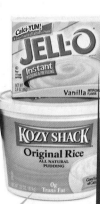

**Swiss Miss®
Chocolate
Vanilla Swirl**

(1 pudding cup, 113 g)

*150 calories
4 g fat
(3 g saturated)
20 g sugars*

There's almost a full teaspoon of sugar in every ounce of this cup.

**Hunt's®
Snack Pack®
Butterscotch**

(1 pudding cup)

*120 calories
3 g fat
(1.5 g saturated)
16 g sugars*

Buying a 4-pack is a commitment to eating an extra 120 unnecessary calories.

**Kozy Shack®
Restaurant Style
Flan Crème
Caramel**

(1 flan, 113 g)

*150 calories
4 g fat
(2 g saturated)
20 g sugars*

Every tablespoon packs nearly 3 grams of sugar and 18 calories.

**Kozy Shack®
Original Rice**

(½ cup, 113 g)

*130 calories
3 g fat
(2 g saturated)
14 g sugars*

These tubs make it far too easy to overindulge, so be careful which one you buy.

**Jell-O Instant
Vanilla**

(½ cup prepared, 25 g)

*150 calories
0 g fat
19 g sugars*

And don't even think about swapping for Jell-O's Sugar-Free, Fat-Free Pudding; it's sweetened with the suspected carcinogen aspartame.

Snack Cakes

Eat This

WARNING:
Nothing on this page has even the slightest hint of real nutritional value. Snack cakes—like candy—will always be a lesser-of-two-evils choice. Since most of these products are made from the same cache of refined flour, oils, and synthetic sweeteners, the key is to limit the serving size. The items on this page do that best.

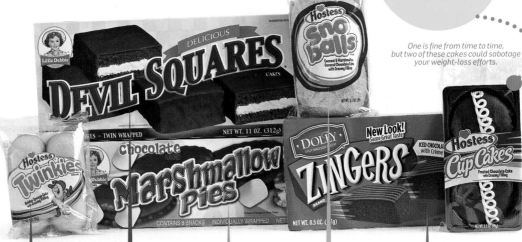

Hostess® Cup Cakes
(1 cake, 50 g)

*180 calories
6 g fat (3 g saturated)
22 g sugars*

One is fine from time to time, but two of these cakes could sabotage your weight-loss efforts.

Hostess® Twinkies®
(1 cake, 43 g)

*150 calories
4.5 g fat
(2.5 g saturated)
19 g sugars*

Surprisingly mild on the fat scale. But as with all starchy, sugary snacks, you must proceed cautiously.

Little Debbie® Devil Squares®
(1 cake, 31 g)

*135 calories
6 g fat
(3 g saturated)
13 g sugars*

That tricky devil has twin-wrapped these cakes, so you better have somebody nearby to pawn one off on.

Little Debbie Marshmallow Pies
(1 cookie, 43 g)

*180 calories
7 g fat
(4 g saturated)
15 g sugars*

Little Debbie has a ton of dubious desserts. This one's surprisingly decent.

Hostess® SnoBalls®
(1 cake, 50 g)

*170 calories
5 g fat
(3.5 g saturated)
23.5 g sugars*

If you don't trust yourself to eat just one, you'd better just leave them on the shelf.

Dolly Madison Zingers® Iced Chocolate
(1 cake, 40 g)

*150 calories
5 g fat
(2.5 g saturated)
18 g sugars*

When possible, opt for individually wrapped snacks.

Not That!

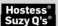

Hostess® Suzy Q's®
(1 cake, 58 g)

*220 calories
8.5 g fat (4.5 g saturated,
0.5 g trans)
28 g sugars*

One Suzy Q's has 60 more calories than a Wendy's Junior Frosty.

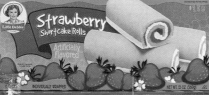
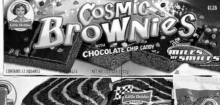
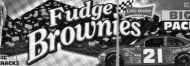

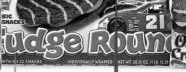

**Little Debbie®
Fudge**
(1 brownie, 66 g)

*310 calories
14 g fat
(4 g saturated)
26 g sugars*

This brick of calories and fat is best left for actors looking to gain weight for a role.

**Little Debbie®
Strawberry
Shortcake**
(1 roll, 61 g)

*240 calories
9 g fat
(3 g saturated)
30 g sugars*

You'd have to eat 60 strawberries to equal the number of calories in this shortcake.

**Little Debbie®
Fudge Rounds**
(1 cookie, 67 g)

*300 calories
11 g fat
(4.5 g saturated)
30 g sugars*

Before you buy the box, think about when you'll find time to burn off the 2,480 calories within.

**Little Debbie®
Cosmic™ with
Chocolate Chip
Candy**
(1 brownie, 62 g)

*280 calories
13 g fat
(3.5 g saturated)
24 g sugars*

More calories than a slice of supreme pizza from Pizza Hut.

**Little Debbie®
Double Decker
Oatmeal
Creme Pie**
(1 cookie, 108 g)

*470 calories
18 g fat
(5 g saturated,
0.5 trans)
39 g sugars*

More calories than 3 Twinkies!

203

Cake Mixes and Frosti

Eat This

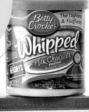

Bob's Red Mill® Gingerbread Cake Mix

(1 slice, 43 g prepared)

220 calories
0.5 g fat (0 g saturated)
13 g sugars

Bob's gingerbread is perhaps the best cake mix on the market. Not only is it made with whole wheat flour, but it's also one of the few mixes with absolutely zero trans fat.

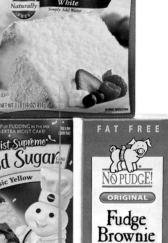

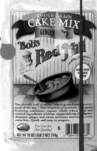

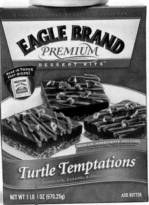

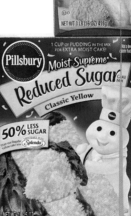

Betty Crocker® Whipped Frosting Milk Chocolate

(2 Tbsp, 24 g)

100 calories
4.5 g fat
(1.5 g saturated, 1 g trans)
12 g sugars

If you must frost, go whipped.

Eagle Brand Turtle Temptations®

(28 g mix, prepared)

130 calories
6 g fat
(2 g saturated)
13 g sugars

Cut bite-size brownies so you don't have to commit to a massive brownie boat.

Pillsbury Moist Supreme® Reduced Sugar Cake Mix Classic Yellow

(43 g mix prepared)

230 calories
3 g fat
(1 g saturated)
10 g sugars

Reduced sugar equates to 15% fewer calories.

Betty Crocker® Angel Food Cake Mix White

(38 g mix prepared)

140 calories
0 g fat
23 g sugars

Angel food keeps the calories low by keeping out the fats.

No Pudge!® Fat Free Original Fudge Brownie Mix

(32 g mix prepared)

120 calories
0 g fat
22 g sugars

The No Pudge! formula replaces oil and eggs with nonfat yogurt.

ngs

Not That!

Krusteaz® Cinnamon Crumb Cake Mix

(33 g mix prepared, with 2 Tbsp cinnamon topping)

230 calories
7 g fat (2 g saturated, 2 g trans)
26 g sugars

You'd have to scrub a floor for more than half an hour to burn off one piece of this cake.

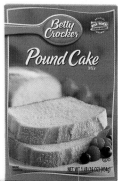

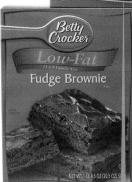

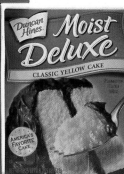

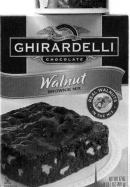

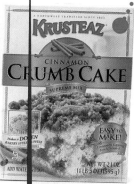

Betty Crocker® Low-Fat Fudge Brownie Mix
(32 g mix prepared)

140 calories
2 g fat
(0.5 g saturated, 0.5 g trans)
20 g sugars

Popular brands get the best shelf space. Look around for better options.

Betty Crocker® Pound Cake Mix
(37 g mix prepared)

170 calories
4.5 g fat
(1.5 g saturated, 1.5 g trans)
17 g sugars

More than half the fats in this pound cake are the kinds you should be avidly avoiding.

Duncan Hines® Moist Deluxe® Cake Mix Classic Yellow
(43 g prepared)

270 calories
12 g fat
(2.5 g saturated)
20 g sugars

"Deluxe" usually means more fat, sugar, and calories.

Ghirardelli® Walnut Brownie Mix (1 2" brownie, 30 g, prepared)

170 calories
5 g fat
(1.5 g saturated, 1 g trans)
16 g sugars

The fourth ingredient is partially hydrogenated oil.

Pillsbury Creamy Supreme® Milk Chocolate Frosting
(2 Tbsp, 35 g)

140 calories
6 g fat
(1.5 g saturated, 2 g trans)
19 g sugars

Nothing but sugar and fat.

Candy

Eat This

Werther's® Original®
(3 pieces, 16 g)

70 calories
1.5 g fat
(1 g saturated)
10 g sugars

Hard candies make for a longer-lasting treat with fewer calories.

Red Hots®
(40 pieces, 34 g)

120 calories
0 g fat
26 g sugars

Half the size of a Hot Tamale, so you get more for less.

Trolli® Sour Brite Crawlers®
(~13 pieces, 39 g)

110 calories
0 g fat
22 g sugars

Pure sugar, yes, but so are nearly all "fruit" candies. Limit yourself to a dozen Crawlers.

Jelly Belly® 30 Flavors
(35 pieces, 40 g)

140 calories
0 g fat
28 g sugars

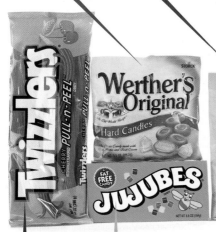
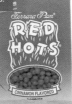
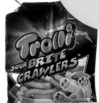

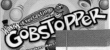

Twizzlers® Pull-n-Peel™ Cherry
(1 piece, 33 g)

100 calories
0 g fat
15 g sugars

Just because a candy is fat-free doesn't mean you can gorge. Show some restraint.

Jujubes®
(52 pieces, 40 g)

110 calories
0 g fat
18 g sugars

At just over 2 calories apiece, you can afford to indulge.

Life Savers Gummies®
(10 pieces, 39 g)

130 calories
0 g fat
23 g sugars

Go for sweets that don't include fattening oils. You lose a little texture, but you also lose body flab.

Jolly Rancher® Gummies
(10 pieces, 39 g)

120 calories
0 g fat
22 g sugars

Like everything else on this page, this is basically pure sugar, just in slightly more restrained quantities.

Wonka® Gobstopper®
(18 pieces, 30 g)

120 calories
0 g fat
28 g sugars

"Everlasting" candies like this are always better bets.

Believe it or not, Jelly Belly contains trace amounts of real fruit puree.

206

Not That!

**Skittles®
Original Fruit**
(~¼ cup, 42 g)
*170 calories
2 g fat (1.5 g saturated)
32 g sugars*

**Wonka® Laffy
Taffy®**
(5 bars, 43 g)
*160 calories
2 g fat
(1.5 g saturated)
27 g sugars*
Taffy sits squarely
at the bottom
of the nutritional
totem pole
for candy.

Hot Tamales®
(20 pieces, 40 g)
*150 calories
0 g fat
23 g sugars*
It takes six
different artificial
colors to make
the perfect Hot
Tamale shade
of red.

**Werther's®
Original®
Chewy
Caramels**
(3 pieces, 19 g)
*85 calories
2.5 g fat
(1.5 g saturated)
7 g sugars*

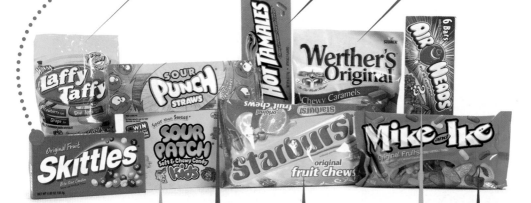

*With 75% sugar,
10% fat, and an
artist's palette
of artificial colors,
Skittles is one
of the worst fruit
candies in
America.*

**Sour Patch
Kids**
(16 pieces, 40 g)
*140 calories
0 g fat
25 g sugars*
You would have
to run a mile just
to burn off a small
handful of these.

**Sour Punch®
Straws**
(~6 pieces, 40 g)
*150 calories
0.5 g fat
(0.5 g saturated)
18 g sugars*
This little treat
has as many
calories as 4 strips
of bacon.

**Starburst®
Fruit Chews**
(8 pieces, 40 g)
*160 calories
3.5 g fat
(3 g saturated)
23 g sugars*
One Starburst
serving per day for
a year will add
21.5 pounds
of body fat.

Airheads®
(2 bars, 31 g)
*120 calories
1.5 g fat
(1 g saturated)
17 g sugars*
Each Airhead
relies on a gob
of partially
hydrogenated oil
to help it stretch.

**Mike and Ike®
Original Fruits**
(~23 pieces, 40 g)
*140 calories
0 g fat
26 g sugars*
Each serving
contains almost
2 tablespoons
sugar.

Chocolate Candy
Eat This

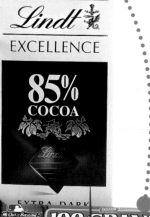

Coming in under 200 calories is a rare feat for an impulse-rack candy bar. And since it comes in 2 pieces, it's perfect for splitting.

Nestlé® 100 Grand®
(2 bars, 43 g)

180 calories
8 g fat (5 g saturated)
21 g sugars

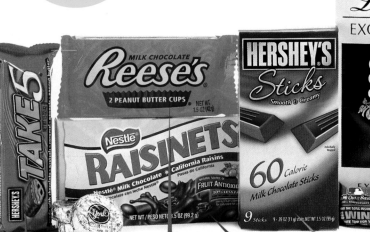

Hershey's® Take 5®
(1 package)

210 calories
11 g fat (5 g saturated)
18 g sugars

Take 5 stays in the nutritional safe zone by replacing the nougat with pretzel.

York® Dark Chocolate Covered Peppermint Patties
(3 patties)

140 calories
3 g fat (1.5 g saturated)
26 g sugars

A safe bet when indulging.

Reese's® Peanut Butter Cups
(1 package)

230 calories
13 g fat (4.5 g saturated)
20 g sugars

The iconic cups take down the sticks in the better peanut butter battle.

Nestlé® Raisinets®
(¼ cup)

190 calories
8 g fat (5 g saturated)
27 g sugars

Raisins are rich with flavanols, so milk-chocolate lovers can still get similar antioxidant benefits.

Hershey's® Sticks Smooth & Creamy
(1 stick)

60 calories
3 g fat (2 g saturated)
6 g sugars

The same pocket-carry appeal with a third less sugar and calories.

Lindt Excellence 85% Cocoa Extra Dark Chocolate
(4 squares)

210 calories
18 g fat (11 g saturated)
5 g sugars

Fat in real chocolate is relatively safe.

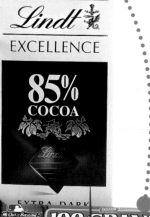

Not That!

One Snickers bar has as much sugar as 3 Krispy Kreme Glazed Doughnuts.

Snickers®
(1 bar, 59 g)

280 calories
14 g fat (5 g saturated)
30 g sugars

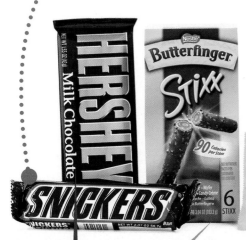
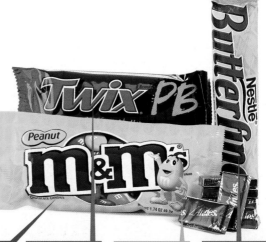

**Hershey's®
Milk
Chocolate**
(1 bar)

*230 calories
13 g fat
(8.5 g saturated)
22 g sugars*

The first ingredient in milk chocolate is sugar.

**Nestlé®
Butterfinger®
Stixx** (1 stick)

*90 calories
4 g fat
(2.5 g saturated)
9 g sugars*

It has only a third as many calories as the original Butterfinger, but there are better sticks to snack on.

**M&M's®
Peanut**
(~¼ cup)

*220 calories
11 g fat
(4.5 g saturated)
22 g sugars*

Unlike Raisinets, M&M's can't claim that any of its sugar is natural.

**Twix® Peanut
Butter**
(2 cookies)

*280 calories
17 g fat
(8 g saturated)
19 g sugars*

One of the fattiest, oil-saturated candy bars on the market.

**Andes® Crème
De Menthe
Thins (8 pieces)**

*200 calories
13 g fat
(11 g saturated)
20 g sugars*

Each serving provides more than half your recommended daily intake of saturated fat.

**Nestlé®
Butterfinger®**
(1 bar)

*270 calories
11 g fat
(6 g saturated)
28 g sugars*

Nobody should lay a finger on this Butterfinger.

209

Chapter 7

THE FREEZER SECTION

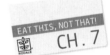

EAT THIS, NOT THAT!
CH. 7

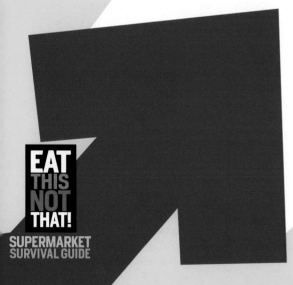

EAT THIS NOT THAT!
SUPERMARKET SURVIVAL GUIDE

The Big Freeze

In 1924, Clarence Birdseye was working on the Peninsula of Labrador in Canada when he noticed something about the way the Eskimos preserved their food: Quickly freezing food prevents the formation of the large ice crystals that damage the cells in fruits and vegetables. Birdseye's brainstorm led us to where we are today: standing outside a row of enormous industrial freezers, contemplating dinner.

There's an old saw that says the best place to meet single men and women is in the frozen food section of your supermarket. The idea, of course, is that only single folks are shopping for frozen dinners. (As comedian Dave Attell once joked: "Hungry-Man Dinners? Why don't we call them what they really are: Lonely-Man Dinners!") So there can be something slightly unnerving about turning your grocery cart into the frozen section. Will people think you're lonely? Or just lazy? Shouldn't you be loitering instead in the crisp produce and meat sections, planning out some Mario Batali—style feast?

Well, forget about the creepy peer pressure. First of all, everyone seeks help in the freezer section: From August 2007 to August 2008, supermarkets sold more than $30 billion of frozen foods—and that doesn't even include all the chilled chow bought at Wal-Mart and other superstores. And here are the facts, Jack: While not everything you find in the supermarket's freezer is the embodiment of nutrition, you might be surprised to learn just how healthy many frozen foods can be. Consider:

● **Fresher doesn't always mean healthier.** Frozen foods can be not only cheaper but healthier—especially when it comes to fruits and vegetables in the winter and spring months. As Birdseye realized, fast freezing means more nutrition: One study found that vegetables such as green beans and spinach lose 75 percent of their vitamin C after being stored in the fridge for a week. And at Arizona State University, an analysis found that ready-to-drink orange juice has less than half the vitamin C of frozen OJ and loses all of its C within 4 weeks of opening the package. So freezing really does help foods retain the vast majority of their nutrients. Additionally, food processors pick "fresh" produce when it's still unripe, and then it sits on trucks and boats during its long journey—sometimes thousands of miles—to your supermarket. But produce intended to be sold frozen is picked at the peak of ripeness—which means it has more time to suck up nutrients from the sun and the soil. So not only are frozen foods higher in nutrition to begin with, but they also don't lose nutrients sitting in trucks and then in the fridge.

- **Frozen foods are better for the environment.** Unlike those "fresh" strawberries you buy in February, which need to be grown in hothouses in tropical climes and shipped all the way to your market, frozen foods can be picked in season and stored—you can find low-impact, organic food

more readily in the frozen section (tip: buy frozen wild blueberries whenever you can find them—they're far more nutritious than the domesticated kind).

- **You can mix and match frozen dinners.** Hey, just because the folks at Swanson thought a tiny piece of beef and some rice made a meal doesn't mean you have to agree. You can bolster the nutritional content of any frozen—or fresh—meal by quickly nuking up some frozen corn, peas, or a vegetable medley.

On Thin Ice
A quick guide to buying smart in the freezer section

1. Watch the salt. Sodium and other preservatives help the freezing process but don't help your health. Read labels carefully to make sure you're not getting more salt than you would with fresh foods—and avoid any ingredients you can't pronounce.

2. Inspect the packages. Look for packages that have been vacuum sealed—extra air means extra moisture, which leaves room for extra frost and, eventually, freezer burn. Also, buy packages that look clean and firm (especially when they're made of paper products). And don't buy packages that are covered in frost—according to the National Frozen and Refrigerated Foods Association (NFRA), these packages may have been handled improperly.

3. Keep it cool. The NFRA suggests making the frozen food department your last stop in the supermarket, grouping frozen foods together in your shopping cart, and unpacking them before you unpack anything else.

- **You can prevent freezer burn.**

  Here's a little science for steak lovers: A water molecule is like a teenage boy—always looking for the coolest place to be. In your freezer, that's down by the cooling coils. So water molecules try to escape from your chicken and steak and drift down to the coils if they can. Once the meat has lost enough of these molecules, you get dried-out steak—the dreaded freezer burn. But this doesn't have to happen: Mammoth flesh found preserved in the ice of Siberia has stayed edible for at least 15,000 years. To keep your steaks tasty forever, remove the fresh meat from its package and wrap it snugly in plastic wrap, then slip it into a freezer bag, squeezing out as much air as possible first.

- **Always keep a full freezer.**

  Would you believe that having a full freezer will not only keep you 60 seconds away from a burrito but also lower your electric bill? Chilling air requires more energy than chilling food, and the more food in your freezer, the less air.

All in all, it seems like old Clarence Birdseye had some pretty good ideas back there. And there's a good reason why Birdseye was inducted in 2005 into the Inventors Hall of Fame, alongside the folks who brought us Valium and the electric guitar. (Hold on a second: Valium, frozen dinners, and the electric guitar? Who was on the voting committee, Keith Richards??)

How Long Can You Keep Meat?

Here are the guidelines, courtesy of the USDA.

MEAT	STORAGE LENGTH
Hot dogs, deli slices	1 to 2 months
Ground meat	3 to 4 months
Pork chops	4 to 6 months
Fish	2 to 3 months
Beef, veal, lamb	6 to 12 months
Poultry	9 months

Freezer Label Decoder

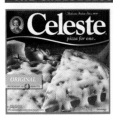

MAMA CELESTE ORIGINAL PIZZA

THE CLAIM: "Original Pizza"

THE TRUTH: Ever had a pizza without cheese? Well, if you eat this one you will have, since Mama Celeste doesn't use a single shred of real cheese in making this problematic pie. What *does* she use? Imitation mozzarella, which is the second ingredient on the list and is composed mostly of partially hydrogenated soybean oil, endowing each serving with 5 grams of nasty trans fats. Also watch out for the attachment of the word "flavored," as in "strawberry-flavored"; it's a surefire sign that the product is utterly fruitless.

WHAT YOU REALLY WANT: Cheese, strawberries, or whatever you think it is you're getting. If the name or flavor in the food's title isn't one of the first few ingredients, find another product.

INGREDIENTS: TOPPING: TOMATO PUREE (WATER, TOMATO PASTE), IMITATION MOZZARELLA CHEESE (WATER, PARTIALLY HYDROGENATED SOYBEAN OIL, CASEIN [MILK], MODIFIED FOOD STARCH, TRISODIUM CITRATE, SODIUM ALUMINUM PHOSPHATE, LACTIC ACID, NATURAL FLAVOR, DISODIUM PHOSPHATE, ARTIFICIAL COLOR, GUAR GUM, SORBIC ACID [TO PRESERVE FRESHNESS], ARTIFICIAL FLAVOR). CONTAINS 2% OR LESS OF: SEASONING BLEND (SALT, SPICES, SUGAR, SOYBEAN OIL, GARLIC POWDER), GREEN BELL PEPPERS, FLAVOR BLEND (MALTODEXTRIN, DEXTROSE, NATURAL SPICE OLEORESINS), MODIFIED FOOD STARCH, CORN OIL, XANTHAN GUM. CRUST: WHEAT FLOUR WITH MALTED BARLEY FLOUR, WATER, VEGETABLE SHORTENING (PARTIALLY HYDROGENATED SOYBEAN AND COTTONSEED OILS, SOY LECITHIN, NATURAL AND ARTIFICIAL FLAVOR, ARTIFICIAL COLOR, CITRIC ACID [PRESERVATIVE], SOYBEAN OIL, YEAST, HIGH FRUCTOSE CORN SYRUP, SALT, PRESERVATIVES (CALCIUM PROPIONATE), DOUGH CONDITIONER (L-CYSTEINE MONOHYDROCHLORIDE). CONTAINS: MILK, SOY, WHEAT

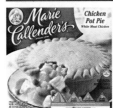

MARIE CALLENDER'S CHICKEN POT PIE

THE CLAIM: "Serving size: 1 cup"

THE TRUTH: Beware of the misleading serving size. Have you ever split a small pot pie between two people? Companies who peddle individually packaged products routinely play games with the serving size, hoping to trick less-observant label readers into believing they're getting only a fraction of the calories and fat. Other offenders include 20-ounce soft drinks, frozen pizzas, and candy bars, among others.

WHAT YOU REALLY WANT: Conservative portions. When purchasing individually packaged products, check the total weight. Drinks should be 12 ounces or less, snacks should be in the 1.5-ounce range, and dinners like this shouldn't exceed 275 grams.

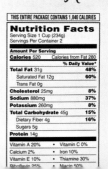

Food from the heart... prepared with love and care. *Love, Marie*

THIS ENTIRE PACKAGE CONTAINS 1,040 CALORIES

Nutrition Facts

Serving Size 1 Cup (234g)
Servings Per Container 2

Amount Per Serving

Calories 520	Calories from Fat 280

	% Daily Value*
Total Fat 31g	48%
Saturated Fat 12g	60%
Trans Fat 0g	
Cholesterol 25mg	8%
Sodium 880mg	37%
Potassium 260mg	8%
Total Carbohydrate 45g	15%
Dietary Fiber 4g	16%
Sugars 5g	
Protein 14g	

Vitamin A 20%	•	Vitamin C 0%
Calcium 2%	•	Iron 10%
Vitamin E 10%	•	Thiamine 30%
Riboflavin 25%	•	Niacin 50%

215

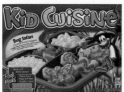

KID CUISINE ALL STAR CHICKEN NUGGETS

THE CLAIM: "Made with real chicken"; "made with real cheese"

THE TRUTH: Yes, there is actual chicken in these "nugget-shaped patties," but it shares space with 17 other ingredients, including textured soy protein and modified food starch. The mac with "real cheese" does have cheddar, but it also has 34 other ingredients, including the cheap carb filler maltodextrin. Rule of thumb: If a product makes claims about its realness on the package, be skeptical.

WHAT YOU REALLY WANT: To eat more food and fewer science experiments. While it's tricky with our industrialized food complex, stick to items with as few ingredients as possible. If they're chicken nuggets, that means chicken, bread crumbs, and oil. Foster Farms Breast Nuggets fit the bill.

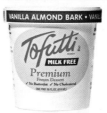

TOFUTTI VANILLA ALMOND BARK

THE CLAIM: "No butterfat"; "no cholesterol"

THE TRUTH: Though both of these claims are technically true, they paint a false sense of security in the person looking for a healthy indulgence. Ignore front label claims (Tofutti is not made with dairy, so by definition it can't have butterfat or cholesterol) and flip the package for the straight scoop; here you'll see that this ice cream substitute still has 15 grams of fat and 16 grams of sugar per serving—as high as most full-fledged ice creams.

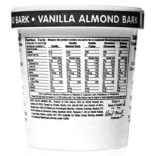

WHAT YOU REALLY WANT: If you're lactose intolerant, both Soy Delicious and Soy Dream make reliably low-cal nondairy creams. If you're just looking for a healthy ice cream fix, try Breyers Double Churn.

INGREDIENTS: BREADED FUN-SHAPED CHICKEN PATTIES: CHICKEN BREAST WITH RIB MEAT, WATER, BREADER (WHEAT FLOUR, SALT, DEXTROSE, SOYBEAN OIL, WHEY, COLORED WITH OLEORESIN PAPRIKA), TEXTURED SOY PROTEIN (SOY PROTEIN AND SOY CARBOHYDRATE), WHEAT FLOUR, RICE FLOUR, MODIFIED FOOD STARCH, SALT, SPICES, FLAVORING, BLACK PEPPER (DEXTROSE, SPICE EXTRACTIVES), FRIED IN VEGETABLE OIL WITH TBT. MACARONI AND CHEESE: ELBOW MACARONI (DURUM SEMOLINA ENRICHED WITH NIACIN, FERROUS SULFATE [IRON], THIAMINE MONONITRATE, RIBOFLAVIN, FOLIC ACID), EGG WHITES], WATER, CONTAINS 2% OR LESS OF EACH OF THE FOLLOWING: CHEDDAR CLUB CHEESE (PASTEURIZED CULTURED MILK, SALT, ENZYMES, ANNATTO [COLOR]), BLEND SWEET WHEY, SOYBEAN OIL, MODIFIED FOOD STARCH, DRIED SWEET CREAM (SWEET CREAM, NONFAT MILK, SODIUM CASEINATE), CITRIC ACID, LACTIC ACID, YELLOW #5 AND #6), BUTTER (SWEET CREAM, SALT), WHEY PROTEIN CONCENTRATE, ACETIC ACID (STEPS OF WORK) AND DIGLYCERIDES WITH MALTODEXTRIN, POTASSIUM CHLORIDE, SODIUM PHOSPHATE, SALT, FLAVORING (MALTODEXTRIN, NATURAL FLAVOR), CITRIC ACID, BETA CAROTENE (COLOR OIL, BETA CAROTENE). BOXED SNACKS PACKETS: CORN SYRUP, SUCROSE, GELATIN, MODIFIED FOOD STARCH, APPLE JUICE CONCENTRATE, PECTIN, CITRIC ACID, MALIC ACID, SODIUM CITRATE, COCONUT OIL, CARNAUBA WAX, NATURAL AND ARTIFICIAL FLAVOR, COLOR ADDED, RED #40, YELLOW #5, AND BLUE #1, KETCHUP SAUCE PACKET: WATER, TOMATO PASTE, SUGAR, DISTILLED VINEGAR, SALT, MODIFIED FOOD STARCH, SOYBEAN OIL, SODIUM BENZOATE AND POTASSIUM SORBATE (PRESERVATIVES), DEXTROSE, XANTHAN GUM, ONION POWDER, GUAR GUM, SPICE, NATURAL FLAVOR. CONTAINS: WHEAT, SOY, MILK, EGGS.

ConAgra Foods, Inc.
P.O. Box 3768, Dept. KC
Omaha, NE 68103-0768 U.S.A.

THE "HEALTH FOOD" THAT ISN'T

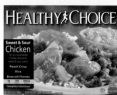

HEALTHY CHOICE SWEET & SOUR CHICKEN

THE CLAIM: "Healthy Choice"

THE TRUTH: A company can call itself whatever it wants, but that doesn't give credence to the name. Healthy Choice even provides a handful of nutritional stats—430 calories, 9 grams fat, 600 milligrams sodium—to back up the name, but they neglect to mention the 29 grams of added sugars used in this dish. The six different forms of sweeteners in the ingredient list combine to give this less-than-healthy choice almost the same amount of sugar as a Snickers bar. Many Healthy Choice selections are reliably nutritious; this is not one of them.

WHAT YOU REALLY WANT: Dinner that doesn't taste like a bowl of ice cream. While fat and calories are important considerations in everything you eat, be sure to read the fine print. Companies with healthy label claims often pull the bait and switch, going low in fat but then elevating the sugar or sodium to up the flavor quotient.

Need to upgrade your frozen fare? Learn more about the supermarket's worst freezer burns and the healthy foods you should be stocking in the ice box instead at **eatthis.com**

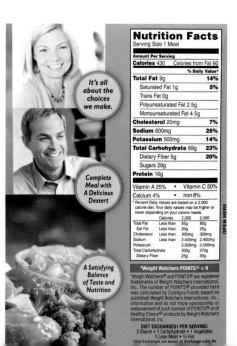

It's all about the choices we make.

Complete Meal with A Delicious Dessert

A Satisfying Balance of Taste and Nutrition

Nutrition Facts
Serving Size 1 Meal

Amount Per Serving		
Calories 430	Calories from Fat 90	
		% Daily Value*
Total Fat 9g		14%
Saturated Fat 1g		5%
Trans Fat 0g		
Polyunsaturated Fat 2.5g		
Monounsaturated Fat 4.5g		
Cholesterol 20mg		7%
Sodium 600mg		25%
Potassium 500mg		14%
Total Carbohydrate 69g		23%
Dietary Fiber 5g		20%
Sugars 29g		
Protein 16g		
Vitamin A 25%	•	Vitamin C 50%
Calcium 4%	•	Iron 8%

* Percent Daily Values are based on a 2,000 calorie diet. Your daily values may be higher or lower depending on your calorie needs.

	Calories	2,000	2,500
Total Fat	Less than	65g	80g
Sat Fat	Less than	20g	25g
Cholesterol	Less than	300mg	300mg
Sodium	Less than	2,400mg	2,400mg
Potassium		3,500mg	3,500mg
Total Carbohydrate		300g	375g
Dietary Fiber		25g	30g

OPEN HERE

*Weight Watchers® POINTS® = 9

*Weight Watchers® and POINTS® are registered trademarks of Weight Watchers International, Inc. The number of POINTS® provided here was calculated by ConAgra Foods based on published Weight Watchers International, Inc., information and do not imply sponsorship or endorsement of such number of POINTS® or of Healthy Choice® products by Weight Watchers International, Inc.

DIET EXCHANGES† PER SERVING:
3 Starch • 1 Carbohydrate • 1 Vegetable
1 Lean Meat • ½ Fat
†Diet Exchanges are based on Exchange Lists for

The Perfect Freezer

SHRIMP

3 OUNCES: *90 calories, 1 g fat (0 g saturated), 17 g protein*
Just defrost and give salads, stir-fries, and pasta a virtually fat-free boatload of appetite-quelling protein, bone-strengthening vitamin D, and the antioxidant selenium, which researchers believe can protect against prostate cancer.
POWER PLAY: Stir-fry shrimp, zucchini, onions, peanuts, and a scoop of chili-garlic sauce.

NATURE'S PATH HEMP PLUS WAFFLES

2 WAFFLES: *210 calories, 9 g fat (1 g saturated), 6 g protein, 28 g carbs, 5 g fiber*
Hemp seeds give these whole-grain waffles a shot of heart-healthy omega-3 fats. Plus, there's more protein and fiber than most on the market.
POWER PLAY: Swap out syrup for nutritious apple or almond butters.

KASHI SOUTHWEST STYLE CHICKEN FROZEN DINNER

1 SERVING: *240 calories, 5 g fat (0 g saturated), 16 g protein, 32 g carbs, 6 g fiber*
Fast and simple, Kashi's big-flavored entrées use whole grains and pony up plenty of protein and fiber without the harmful fats.
POWER PLAY: Make any frozen meal taste a little more homemade by adding fresh herbs such as parsley and rosemary after it's done cooking.

WILD BLUEBERRIES

1 CUP: *79 calories, 1 g protein, 19 g carbs, 4 g fiber*
Nutritional stars plump with brain-boosting phytochemicals called anthocyanins and pterostilbene—a compound that lowers cholesterol. Frozen blueberries cost about a third the price of fresh and are available year-round.

BIRDS EYE FROZEN BROCCOLI, CAULIFLOWER, AND CARROTS

¾ CUP: *30 calories, 0 g fat, 1 g protein, 5 g carbs, 2 g fiber*
An array of good-for-you phytochemicals in a no-fuss medium. Keep two on hand.
POWER PLAY: Steam; boiling vegetables can pillage their nutritional treasures. A bit of olive oil helps your body absorb the fat-soluble nutrients.

BIRDS EYE FROZEN BABY SWEET PEAS

⅔ CUP: *70 calories, 0 g fat, 4 g protein, 4 g fiber*
Shelling pricey fresh peas is a time-consuming, wallet-emptying process. Luckily, studies show frozen vegetables maintain their nutrients as well as fresh—sometimes better. That's because peas are picked at the height of season and frozen and packaged on the spot.
POWER PLAY: Stir peas straight from the bag into rice or pasta dishes.

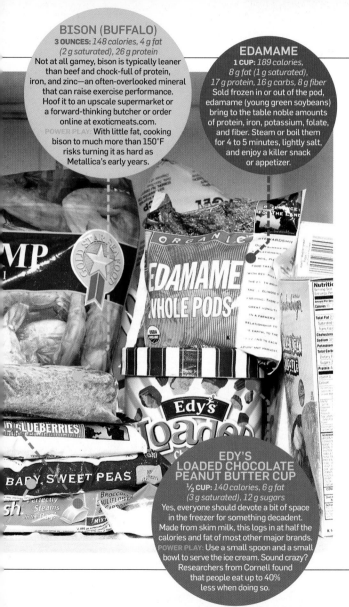

BISON (BUFFALO)

3 OUNCES: *148 calories, 4 g fat (2 g saturated), 26 g protein*

Not at all gamey, bison is typically leaner than beef and chock-full of protein, iron, and zinc—an often-overlooked mineral that can raise exercise performance. Hoof it to an upscale supermarket or a forward-thinking butcher or order online at exoticmeats.com. **POWER PLAY:** With little fat, cooking bison to much more than 150°F risks turning it as hard as Metallica's early years.

EDAMAME

1 CUP: *189 calories, 8 g fat (1 g saturated), 17 g protein, 16 g carbs, 8 g fiber*

Sold frozen in or out of the pod, edamame (young green soybeans) bring to the table noble amounts of protein, iron, potassium, folate, and fiber. Steam or boil them for 4 to 5 minutes, lightly salt, and enjoy a killer snack or appetizer.

EDY'S LOADED CHOCOLATE PEANUT BUTTER CUP

½ CUP: *140 calories, 6 g fat (3 g saturated), 12 g sugars*

Yes, everyone should devote a bit of space in the freezer for something decadent. Made from skim milk, this logs in at half the calories and fat of most other major brands. **POWER PLAY:** Use a small spoon and a small bowl to serve the ice cream. Sound crazy? Researchers from Cornell found that people eat up to 40% less when doing so.

In or Out?

Fresh Fish: Out

If you're going to pay serious green-backs for a good cut of wild salmon or mahimahi, don't ruin its texture and flavor by coming home and sending it to cryo-heaven.

WHERE IT BELONGS: The fridge and, in a day or two, down your gullet.

Overripe Bananas: In

Any way you slice it, going back for seconds and likely thirds of butter-smothered banana bread is a fast track to pudge town. Instead, place your brown monkey food in the freezer and—when it comes time to whirl up a protein shake—simply run it under hot water for a minute or so, peel, and then add the potassium superstar to the blender.

Coffee: Out

Freezing breaks down the oils that give your java its distinct flavor. Being porous, coffee also absorbs flavors and moisture from the freezer (remember that catfish sale a few weeks back?).

WHERE IT BELONGS: In an airtight container placed in a dark cupboard.

Ice Cream

Eat This

Edy's Slow Churned creates one of the safest ice creams at the supermarket. For an extra health boost, go for a flavor like Rocky Road, which contains real nuts.

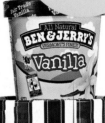

Edy's™ Slow Churned® Rocky Road
(½ cup)
120 calories
4 g fat (2 g saturated)
12 g sugars

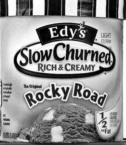

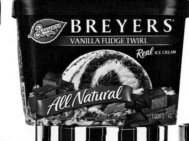

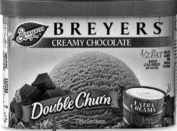

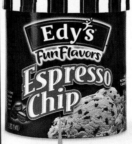

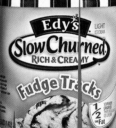

Breyers® Double Churn™ Creamy Chocolate (½ cup)

100 calories
3.5 g fat
(2 g saturated)
13 g sugars

We couldn't find a lighter ice cream. Keep this in your freezer and you'll drastically blunt the damage of any potential sugar binge.

Breyers® All Natural Vanilla Fudge Twirl (½ cup)

130 calories
6 g fat
(3.5 g saturated)
15 g sugars

Try replacing chocolate ribbons with an ice cream that blends flavors.

Edy's Fun Flavors Espresso Chip (½ cup, 65 g)

130 calories
5 g fat
(3.5 g saturated)
15 g sugars

Edy's and Breyers have cornered the market on low-calorie ice cream. This is just another great example.

Edy's® Slow Churned® Fudge Tracks (½ cup)

120 calories
4.5 g fat
(2.5 g saturated)
13 g sugars

Marshmallows carry far fewer calories than fudge, cookie dough, or chocolate ribbons.

Ben & Jerry's® Vanilla (½ cup)

230 calories
14 g fat
(9 g saturated)
19 g sugars

Not exactly light ice cream, but it's the lesser evil among indulgences. And because B&J's vanilla is Fair Trade Certified, it's soothing to conscience and palate.

Not That!

**Häagen-Dazs®
Chocolate Peanut
Butter**
(½ cup)

*360 calories
24 g fat (11 g saturated)
24 g sugars*

*One of the most
calorie-packed scoops
in the supermarket.
This carton weighs in
with a whopping 1,440
calories per pint.*

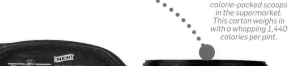

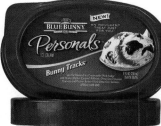

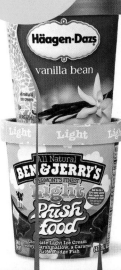

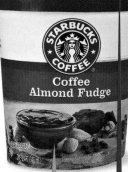

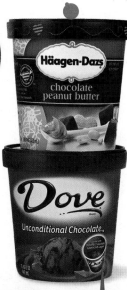

**Häagen-Dazs®
Vanilla Bean**
(½ cup)

*290 calories
18 g fat
(11 g saturated,
0.5 g trans)
26 g sugars*

Häagen-Dazs shows
restraint with ingredients
(6, in this case), but they
still make some of the
fattiest ice creams.

**Ben & Jerry's®
Light Phish Food®**
(½ cup)

*210 calories
6 g fat
(4.5 g saturated)
23 g sugars*

Despite having 22%
fewer calories than the
full-flavor version, Phish
Food Light still suffers
from a gratuitous
dose of sugar.

**Starbucks®
Coffee® Coffee
Almond Fudge**
(½ cup)

*250 calories
13 g fat
(7 g saturated)
26 g sugars*

The "chocolaty coated
almonds" are coated
with sugar and partially
hydrogenated oil.

**Blue Bunny®
Bunny Tracks**
(½ cup)

*190 calories
11 g fat
(6 g saturated)
19 g sugars*

Choose your chunks and
swirls wisely. Many are
just blends of sugars and
fats, often partially
hydrogenated.

**Dove®
Unconditional
Chocolate™ (½ cup)**

*290 calories
17 g fat
(11 g saturated)
27 g sugars*

Dove doesn't make
one ice cream with
fewer than 240
calories. Move this
brand into the rare-to-
never category.

221

Frozen Yogurt and Sor

Eat This

Ben & Jerry's blueberry, blackberry, and lemon swirled sorbet beats Häagen-Dazs by using a third less sugar.

**Ben & Jerry's®
Sorbet
Berried Treasure™**
(½ cup)
110 calories
0 g fat
24 g sugars

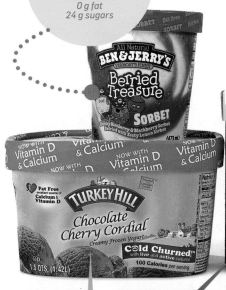

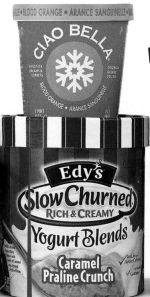

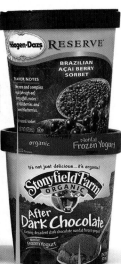

**Turkey Hill®
Creamy Frozen
Yogurt Chocolate
Cherry Cordial**
(½ cup)
100 calories
0 g fat
17 g sugars
Turkey Hill uses real cherries and fudge to make this light yogurt a genuinely rich treat.

**Edy's Slow
Churned® Yogurt
Blends Caramel
Praline Crunch**
(½ cup)
120 calories
3.5 g fat
(2 g saturated)
16 g sugars
Try Edy's Fat Free Vanilla Yogurt—each serving has only 90 calories.

**Ciao Bella®
Blood Orange
Sorbetto**
(½ cup)
98 calories
0 g fat
23 g sugars
Only 5 ingredients, starting with blood orange juice, orange juice, and sugar.

**Häagen-Dazs®
Reserve® Sorbet
Brazilian Acai
Berry** (½ cup)
120 calories
2 g fat
(0 g saturated)
20 g sugars
The Amazonian acai fruit is one of nature's most antioxidant-dense foods.

**Stonyfield Farm®
Nonfat Frozen
Yogurt After
Dark Chocolate**
(½ cup)
100 calories
0 g fat
18 g sugars
Believe it or not, many of Stonyfield's dessert yogurts are better than their breakfast yogurts.

bet

Not That!

At least a third of the sugar comes from real fruit, but no matter how you scoop it, 36 grams is a massive sugar load.

Häagen-Dazs® Fat Free Sorbet Mango
(½ cup)

*150 calories
0 g fat
36 g sugars*

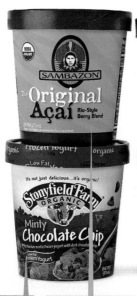

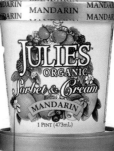

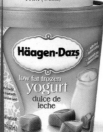

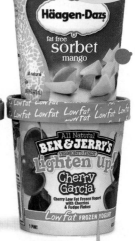

Stonyfield Farm Low Fat Frozen Yogurt Minty Chocolate Chip
(½ cup)

*140 calories
3 g fat
(1.5 g saturated)
21 g sugars*

Not bad but there are plenty of healthier scoops.

Sambazon® The Original Rio-Style Berry Blend Acai
(½ cup)

*150 calories
8 g fat
(2 g saturated)
13 g sugars*

Sombazon's acai blend is nearly 50% fat.

Julie's™ Organic Sorbet & Cream Mandarin
(½ cup)

*160 calories
6 g fat
(3.5 g saturated)
24 g sugars*

This "sorbet" is actually sugar, cream, and eggs. Sounds like ice cream.

Häagen-Dazs® Low Fat Frozen Yogurt Dulce de Leche
(½ cup)

*180 calories
2.5 g fat
(1.5 g saturated)
26 g sugars*

This has 3 fewer grams of sugar than a pack of Rolos.

Ben & Jerry's Lighten Up!® Frozen Yogurt Cherry Garcia
(½ cup)

*160 calories
3 g fat
(2 g saturated)
20 g sugars*

One of Ben & Jerry's best-selling flavors, unfortunately.

223

Nondairy Creams
Eat This

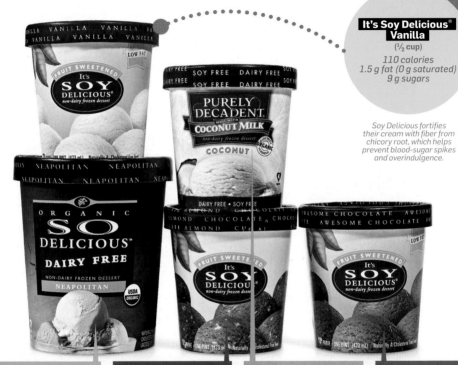

It's Soy Delicious® Vanilla
(½ cup)

110 calories
1.5 g fat (0 g saturated)
9 g sugars

Soy Delicious fortifies their cream with fiber from chicory root, which helps prevent blood-sugar spikes and overindulgence.

SO Delicious™ Neapolitan
(½ cup)

120 calories
3.5 fat (0.5 g saturated)
13 g sugars

The USDA Organic stamp ensures that this ice cream is free from pesticides, herbicides, and genetically modified soybeans.

It's Soy Delicious® Chocolate Almond
(½ cup)

140 calories
4.5 g fat (0.5 g saturated)
12 g sugars

Each serving has 8% of your daily fiber, a rare feat for a frozen treat and one which slows the rate of digestion and protects your body from extreme fat-storage mode.

Purely Decadent® Coconut made with Coconut Milk (½ cup)

170 calories
10 g fat (9 g saturated)
11 g sugars

The saturated fat found in coconut milk might actually reduce bad cholesterol levels. Lauric acid, the primary source of the saturated fat, has been shown to have immune-boosting antiviral and antibacterial properties.

It's Soy Delicious® Awesome Chocolate
(½ cup)

115 calories
1.5 g fat (0 g saturated)
12 g sugars

It's Soy Delicious proves to be an incredibly reliable brand for vegans, people who are lactose-intolerant, or someone looking to shave off a few calories from their ice cream habit.

224

Not That!

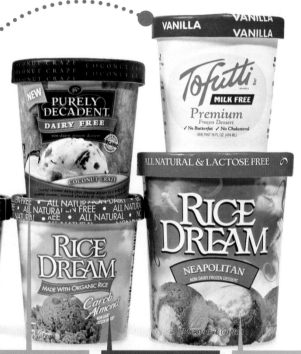

Tofutti® Vanilla
(½ cup)

210 calories
13 g fat (2 g saturated)
16 g sugars

Tofutti's vanilla has 10 grams more fat than any of Ben & Jerry's frozen yogurts, most of which comes from corn oil.

Purely Decadent® Mint Chocolate Chip
(½ cup)

190 calories
8 g fat (2 g saturated)
21 g sugars

Purely Decadent lives up to its name with this one, offering up a heavy helping of fat and sugars.

Purely Decadent® Coconut Craze (½ cup)

240 calories
12 g fat (4.5 g saturated)
24 g sugars

The Coconut Craze earns 85% of its calories from sugar and fat alone.

Rice Dream® Carob Almond
(½ cup)

190 calories
9 g fat (0 g saturated)
12 g sugars

Carob might be a healthy alternative to chocolate, but not when it's adrift in a sea of sugars and fats.

Rice Dream Neapolitan
(½ cup)

150 calories
6 g fat (0.5 g saturated)
18 g sugars

Rice Dream is consistently worse than the other nondairy alternatives.

225

Ice Cream Bars and San

Eat This

In the world of frozen decadence, an ice cream sandwich is one of the few reasonable indulgences.

Turkey Hill Vanilla Bean Ice Cream Sandwich
(1 sandwich, 70 g)

*160 calories
2.5 g fat (1.5 g saturated)
16 g sugars*

SO Delicious™ Creamy Fudge
(1 bar, 63 g)

*90 calories
2 g fat
(0 g saturated)
9 g sugars*

Dairy-free or not, this is one of the lightest fudge bars at the supermarket.

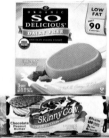

The Skinny Cow® Skinny Dippers
(1 bar, 38 g)

*80 calories
6 g fat
(2 g saturated)
7 g sugars*

Nary an ice cream bar can so much as compare with Skinny Cow's low-cal recipes.

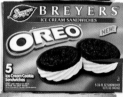
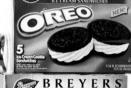

Breyers® Oreo® Ice Cream Sandwiches
(1 sandwich, 55 g)

*170 calories
6 g fat
(2.5 g saturated)
13 g sugars*

This swap will save you more than 50 calories of pure fat and sugar.

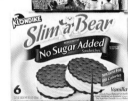

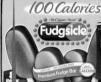

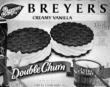

Good Humor® Chocolate Eclair (1 bar, 59 g)

*160 calories
8 g fat
(3.5 g saturated)
11 g sugars*

Too big for a daily dessert, but with 200 fewer calories than the Drumstick, it makes a pretty decent treat.

Klondike® Slim a Bear® No Sugar Added Ice Cream Sandwiches
(1 sandwich, 49 g)

*100 calories
2 g fat
(1 g saturated)
3 g sugars*

The Skinny Cow® Chocolate Peanut Butter Ice Cream Sandwiches
(1 sandwich, 71 g)

*150 calories
2 g fat
(1 g saturated)
15 g sugars*

Fudgsicle® Fudge Bar
(1 bar, 64 g)

*100 calories
2.5 g fat
(2 g saturated)
13 g sugars*

Replace a daily Carb Smart bar with an old-fashioned Fudgsicle and you'll lose half a pound of body fat in 3 weeks.

So Delicious™ Big Buddy
(1 sandwich, 89 g)

*240 calories
8 g fat
(1.5 g saturated)
19 g sugars*

If you insist on a massive ice cream sandwich, at least choose one short on saturated fat and ingredients.

Breyers® Double Churn™ Creamy Vanilla Ice Cream Sandwiches
(1 sandwich, 61 g)

*130 calories
1.5 g fat
(0.5 g saturated)
13 g sugars*

Not That!

What would you do for a Klondike bar? Inject your bloodstream with nearly a pound of hamburger's worth of saturated fat? No? Oh, okay.

Tofutti® Marry Me™ Dessert Bars (1 bar, 70 g)

168 calories
8 g fat
(3 g saturated)
18 g sugars

The name "Tofutti" implies something healthy, but this brand leaves much to be desired.

Weight Watchers® English Toffee Crunch Ice Cream Bars (1 bar, 80 g)

110 calories
6 g fat
(5 g saturated)
10 g sugars

25% of your day's saturated fat.

M&M's® Cookie Ice Cream Sandwiches (1 sandwich, 66 g)

220 calories
10 g fat
(5 g saturated)
20 g sugars

This is the small version. Tack on an extra 40 calories if you buy it individually packaged.

Klondike® The Original (1 sandwich, 81 g)

250 calories
17 g fat (13 g saturated)
18 g sugars

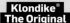
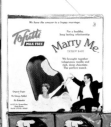
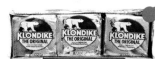
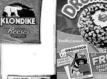
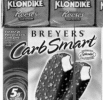
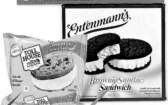
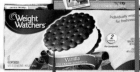

Nestlé® Toll House® Chocolate Chip Cookie Sandwich (1 sandwich, 142 g)

499 calories
23 g fat
(12 g saturated)
39 g sugars

Want to gain weight fast? Eat this.

Entenmann's Brownie Sundae Sandwich (1 sandwich, 89 g)

320 calories
14 g fat
(7 g saturated)
29 g sugars

More calories than a Burger King cheeseburger.

Breyers® Carb Smart™ Almond Bar (1 bar, 56 g)

180 calories
15 g fat
(10 g saturated)
5 g sugars

"Carb smart" means it's sweetened with Splenda and sugar alcohols. It's still loaded up with fat.

Klondike® Reese's® (1 bar, 76 g)

260 calories
16 g fat
(10 g saturated)
21 g sugars

If the original bar is so fattening, it makes sense that blending it with a candy bar is not the solution.

Weight Watchers® Vanilla Ice Cream Sandwiches (1 sandwich, 75 g)

140 calories
2 g fat
(0.5 g saturated)
12 g sugars

Heavy on the sugar for a weight loss treat.

Nestlé® Classic Drumstick Vanilla Caramel (1 drumstick, 100 g)

360 calories
22 g fat
(11 g saturated)
29 g sugars

It weighs as much as a McDonald's hamburger with 110 more calories.

227

Fruit Bars and Frozen

Eat This

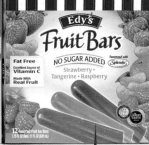

Edy's™ Smoothie Strawberry Banana

(1 bar, 69 g)

100 calories
2 g fat (1 g saturated)
13 g sugars

This bar contains real strawberries and 3 grams of fiber.

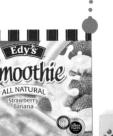

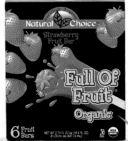

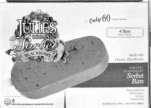

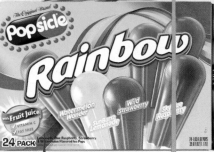

Julie's® Organic Sorbet Blackberry

(1 bar, 54 g)

60 calories
0 g fat
14 g sugars

Blackberries are pureed into this bar, and they are loaded with a flavonoid called anthocyanidin that helps improve communication among your neural cells.

Popsicle® Rainbow

(1 bar, 53 g)

40 calories
0 g fat
7 g sugars

It's a classic for a reason. One of the most innocent indulgences you'll find in the supermarket.

Natural Choice™ Full of Fruit® Organic Strawberry

(1 bar, 78 g)

60 calories
0 g fat
13 g sugars

The organic strawberries and strawberry puree in this bar contribute a heaping load of possible cancer-preventing antioxidants.

Edy's™ No Sugar Added Strawberry, Tangerine, Raspberry

(1 bar, 69 g)

30 calories
0 g fat
1 g sugars

All three flavors are made with real fruit.

Treats
Not That!

Blue Bunny® Sundae Crunch Strawberry
(1 bar, 62 g)

170 calories
9 g fat (3.5 g saturated)
14 g sugars

The "cake crunch" that covers this bar is sugar and wheat flour held together with partially hydrogenated vegetable oils.

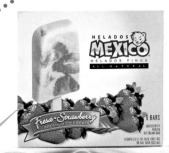

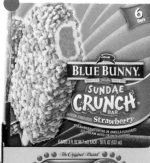

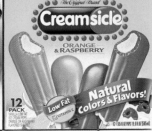

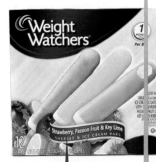

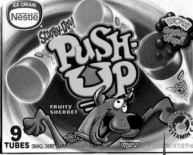

Weight Watchers® Strawberry, Passion Fruit & Key Lime
(1 bar, 45 g)

60 calories
0.5 g fat (0 g saturated)
10 g sugars

The concentrated juice in the sherbet coating is as close as these bars come to real fruit, and it's listed after both sugar and high-fructose corn syrup.

Helados Mexico® All Natural Strawberry
(1 bar, 88 g)

150 calories
7 g fat (4.5 g saturated)
14 g sugars

This bar is essentially heavy cream and sugar blended with strawberries and corn syrup.

Nestlé® Push-Up Fruity Sherbet
(1 piece, 62 g)

80 calories
1 g fat (0.5 g saturated)
16 g sugars

Push-Ups beat most ice cream bars, but will always lose to popsicles.

Creamsicle® Orange & Raspberry
(1 pop, 43 g)

70 calories
1 g fat (0.5 g saturated)
8 g sugars

Don't mistake the sherbet-coated bars for fruit bars. They're nothing more than ice cream with fruit-flavored coating.

Frozen Pies

Eat This

Smart Ones key lime beats Edwards by more than a full calorie for every gram of pie.

Smart Ones® Key Lime Pie
(1 slice, 79 g)

190 calories
4.5 g fat (2 g saturated)
25 g sugars

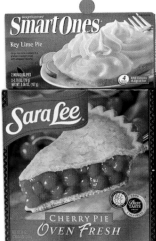

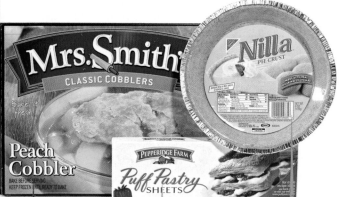

Sara Lee® Cherry Pie
(⅙ pie, 131 g)

340 calories
16 g fat
(7 g saturated)
14 g sugars

Your first goal is to find a pie free of trans fat. Next, try to keep calories, sugar, and saturated fat low.

Mrs. Smith's® Peach Cobbler
(1/16 cobbler, 126 g)

250 calories
9 g fat
(4 g saturated)
20 g sugars

For the size of the cobbler, Mrs. Smith's isn't too bad. Split it with friends and you've got a low-cal dessert.

Pepperidge Farm® Puff Pastry Sheets
(⅙ sheet, 41 g)

170 calories
11 g fat
(6 g saturated)
1 g sugars

For a healthy dessert, warm and mash some frozen berries, pour them over the baked pastry. Dollop on some light whipped cream.

Nilla Pie Crust
(⅛ crust, 21 g)

110 calories
6 g fat
(2.5 g saturated)
8 g sugars

You won't find this one in the cooler section. Look near the baking goods to find a decent pie crust.

Not That!

Edwards® Singles Key Lime Pie

(1 slice, 92 g)

*330 calories
16 g fat (10 g saturated,
2 g trans)
33 g sugars*

More than a third of the fat in this pie is either saturated or trans, helping to push the caloric load to 3.6 calories per gram.

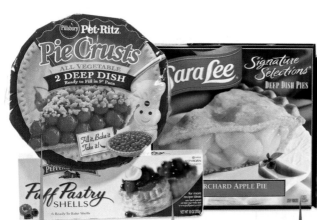
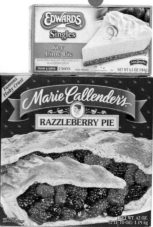

Pillsbury Pet-Ritz All Vegetable Deep Dish Pie Crusts

(1/8 shell, 28 g)

*90 calories
5 g fat (3 g saturated,
1.5 g trans)
1 g sugars*

It's worth taking on a few extra calories if it means cutting out the trans fat from your diet.

Pepperidge Farm® Puff Pastry Shells

(1 shell, 47 g)

*190 calories
13 g fat
(3.5 g saturated,
5 g trans)
2 g sugars*

How do the food scientists at Pepperidge Farm decide when to ladle in gobs of trans fats? We don't know, but they'll likely stop when we stop buying.

Sara Lee® Signature Selections® Orchard Apple Pie (1/10 pie, 133 g)

*390 calories
23 g fat
(10 g saturated)
21 g sugars*

Each slice has half of your day's saturated fat and about a fifth of your total energy intake.

Marie Callender's® Razzleberry Pie

(1/10 pie, 119 g)

*350 calories
19 g fat
(4.5 g saturated,
5 g trans)
18 g sugars*

Not exactly made with love, now is it? Unless, that is, you consider love to be a big helping of trans fat.

231

Frozen Pizza

Eat This

Margherita pizza relies on traditional Italian ingredients such as tomatoes, cheese, basil, and olive oil, all of which are nutritionally superior to America's popular topping, pepperoni.

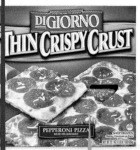

Palermo's® Primo Thin™ Margherita
(⅓ pizza, 140 g)

*260 calories
12 g fat (5 g saturated)
520 mg sodium*

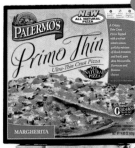

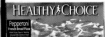

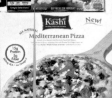

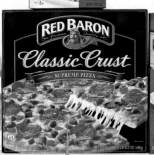

Amy's® Mushroom & Olive
(⅓ pizza, 123 g)

*250 calories
9 g fat
(3 g saturated)
560 mg sodium*

Not all of Amy's pizzas are so easy on the gut, but Mushroom & Olive is one of the best.

Healthy Choice® French Bread Pizza Pepperoni
(1 pizza, 170 g)

*350 calories
4.5 g fat
(1.5 g saturated)
600 mg sodium*

You can eat two Healthy Choice pizzas and still save 70 calories over the DiGiorno.

Kashi™ Mediterranean
(⅓ pizza, 120 g)

*290 calories
9 g fat
(4 g saturated)
640 mg sodium*

One of the healthiest pies in the market, complete with 5 grams of fiber thanks to the flaxseed.

Red Baron® Classic Crust Supreme
(⅕ pizza, 137 g)

*330 calories
15 g fat
(7 g saturated)
630 mg sodium*

If you insist on pepperoni and sausage, at least balance it out with a few veggies.

Lean Pockets® Pepperoni
(1 piece, 127 g)

*290 calories
8 g fat
(4 g saturated)
680 mg sodium*

Pizza for one? A lean pocket is better than any single-serving pizza in the cooler.

DiGiorno Thin Crispy Crust Pepperoni
(⅕ pizza, 125 g)

*320 calories
15 g fat
(7 g saturated,
0.5 g trans)
790 mg sodium*

If you go pepperoni, go thin crust—it cuts the fat by nearly half.

Not That!

**Wolfgang Puck®
Four Cheese,
Tomato, and Pesto**
(⅓ pizza, 116 g)

*330 calories
17 g fat (7 g saturated)
690 mg sodium*

*Wolfgang could have
a healthy pizza if he'd only
lighten up on the oil,
honey, and salt.*

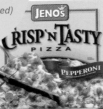
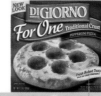
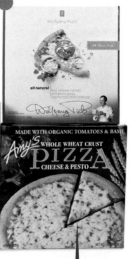
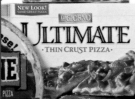
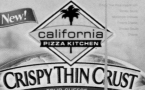

**Tombstone
Original
Pepperoni**
(¼ pizza, 153 g)

*390 calories
20 g fat
(8 g saturated)
880 mg sodium*

The thick layer of
cheese and pepperoni
shoots their slices
up to nearly 20% of
your daily calories
per serving.

**Jeno's® Crisp
'N Tasty®
Pepperoni**
(1 pizza, 192 g)

*490 calories
25 g fat
(6 g saturated,
4.5 g trans)
1,180 mg sodium*

This represents
40% of your daily fat,
half your daily
sodium, and 2 days
of trans fat.

**DiGiorno
Ultimate Four
Meat Thin
Crust**
(⅕ pizza, 142 g)

*390 calories
20 g fat
(8 g saturated)
1,010 mg sodium*

Four meats =
serious saturated
fat influx.

**California
Pizza Kitchen®
Crispy Thin
Crust Four
Cheese**
(⅓ pizza, 127 g)

*330 calories
16 g fat
(8 g saturated,
1 g trans)
690 mg sodium*

It's best to avoid
most CPK pizzas.

**DiGiorno For
One Traditional
Crust
Pepperoni**
(1 pizza, 263 g)

*770 calories
35 g fat
(14 g saturated,
3 g trans)
1,430 mg sodium*

This pizza has
as many calories
as 17 Chicken
McNuggets.

**Amy's®
Whole Wheat
Crust Cheese
& Pesto**
(⅓ pizza, 132 g)

*360 calories
18 g fat
(4 g saturated)
680 mg sodium*

It sounds perfectly
healthy, but the oily
pesto pushes the
calories way up.

233

Frozen Pastas
Eat This

Choosing the right skillet meal can save you 390 calories and 27 grams of fat.

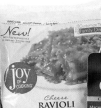

**Bertolli®
Shrimp & Penne
Primavera**

(½ package, 340 g)

*320 calories
15 g fat (1.5 g saturated)
890 mg sodium*

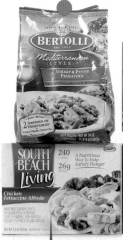

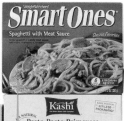

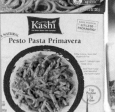

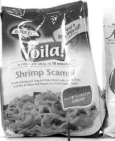

South Beach Living™ Chicken Fettuccine Alfredo

(1 package, 263 g)

*240 calories
7 g fat
(3.5 g saturated)
690 mg sodium*

South Beach keeps the cream and cheese in check in this normally disastrous dish.

Smart Ones® Spaghetti with Meat Sauce

(1 package, 326 g)

*310 calories
6 g fat
(2 g saturated)
580 mg sodium*

The first 4 ingredients: noodles, water, tomatoes, and beef crumbles—exactly as it should be.

Kashi™ Pesto Pasta Primavera

(1 package, 283 g)

*290 calories
11 g fat
(2 g saturated)
750 mg sodium*

Kashi keeps the calories down by using pesto as it should be used—as a seasoning instead of a blanket.

Birds Eye Voila!® Shrimp Scampi

(1¾ cups, 222 g)

*190 calories
2.5 g fat
(1 g saturated)
540 mg sodium*

This dish earns a quarter of your daily vitamin C through a massive portion of bell peppers.

Joy of Cooking Cheese Ravioli Pomodoro with Basil-Marinara Sauce (1 cup, 220 g)

*250 calories
7 g fat
(3.5 g saturated)
710 mg sodium*

The tomato-based sauce makes for a healthy partner to the ricotta- and Parmesan-stuffed ravioli.

Michelina's® Budget Gourmet® Macaroni & Cheese with Cheddar and Romano

(1 package, 227 g)

*260 calories
7 g fat
(2.5 g saturated)
550 mg sodium*

Single servings combat portion distortion.

Not That!

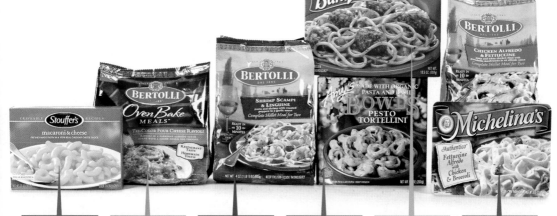

**Bertolli®
Chicken Alfredo &
Fettuccine**
(½ package, 340 g)

*710 calories
42 g fat (22 g saturated)
1,370 mg sodium*

*The wrong skillet meal
can mean a world
of difference to your belt.
This one has more
saturated fat
in 1 serving than you
should eat in an
entire day.*

Stouffer's® Macaroni & Cheese (½ package, 225 g)	**Bertolli® Oven Bake Meals™ Tri-Color Four Cheese Ravioli** (⅓ package, 227 g)	**Bertolli® Shrimp Scampi & Linguine** (⅓ bag, 227 g)	**Amy's® Bowls Pesto Tortellini** (1 package, 269 g)	**Banquet® Spaghetti and Meatballs** (1 package, 297 g)	**Michelina's® Fettuccine Alfredo with Chicken & Broccoli** (1 package, 241 g)
350 calories 17 g fat (7 g saturated) 920 mg sodium	*420 calories 22 g fat (13.5 g saturated) 793 mg sodium*	*353 calories 17 g fat (7 g saturated) 793 mg sodium*	*430 calories 19 g fat (8 g saturated) 640 mg sodium*	*400 calories 17 g fat (7 g saturated, 0.5 g trans) 940 mg sodium*	*310 calories 11 g fat (6 g saturated) 680 mg sodium*
Even if you actually split this package 2 ways, you still get 35% of your day's worth of saturated fat.	Bertolli's ravioli achieves two-thirds of your saturated fat by saucing its 4-cheese ravioli with a 2-cheese cream sauce.	A cream-sauce overload provides this with more than 6 times the saturated fat as the same dish by Voila!	We love pesto, but even love has boundaries. In this case, the boundary is a bowl with nearly half a day's worth of saturated fat.	These meatballs are actually beef and pork blended with bread crumbs and soy flour.	Compared with the South Beach Alfredo, Michelina's has 42% less protein and 71% less fiber.

Frozen Fish

Eat This

Albertson's® Cooked Shrimp
(~8 shrimp, 57g)

30 calories
0 g fat
230 mg sodium

Gorton's® Grilled Fillets Lemon Pepper
(1 fillet, 108 g)

100 calories
3 g fat
(0.5 g saturated)
290 mg sodium

One of the healthiest staples you can keep on hand in your freezer. Pair it with brown rice and grilled vegetables for an exceptional dinner.

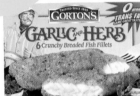

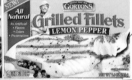

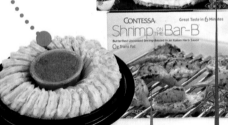

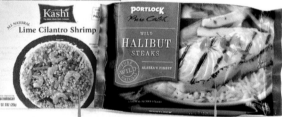

Most supermarkets provide a simple steamed shrimp pack, an excellent choice. Shrimp is an incredibly lean source of protein loaded with the amino acid tryptophan, which boosts serotonin in the brain to help regulate mood.

Contessa® Shrimp on the Bar-B
(~4 pieces with sauce, 140 g)

150 calories
7 g fat
(1 g saturated)
960 mg sodium

Each shrimp delivers 4.25 grams of protein lightly sweetened with half a gram of sugar.

Gorton's® Garlic and Herb Crunchy Breaded Fish Fillets
(2 fillets, 104 g)

230 calories
12 g fat
(3 g saturated)
770 mg sodium

Not the best option in the freezer, but you get the crunch of fried fish with less of the oily effects of the deep fryer.

Kashi™ Lime Cilantro Shrimp
(1 package, 283 g)

250 calories
8 g fat
(2 g saturated)
690 mg sodium

This meal delivers 120% of your daily vitamin A, which boosts your immune system and helps maintain smooth skin.

Pure Catch® Wild Halibut Steaks
(6 oz, 170 g)

180 calories
4 g fat
(0 g saturated)
90 mg sodium

One of the best sources of selenium, which works with vitamins E and C to help protect the body's cells from oxidative stress.

Not That!

Gorton's®
Premium Fillets
Flounder

(1 fillet, 98 g)

230 calories
14 g fat
(3.5 g saturated)
400 mg sodium

More than twice the
calories and nearly
5 times the fat of its
grilled counterpart.

Sea Pak® Crispy
Light Shrimp with
Pineapple Cayenne
Dipping Sauce

(~8 shrimp, 85 g, and 28 g sauce)

235 calories
10 g fat (1.5 g saturated)
925 mg sodium

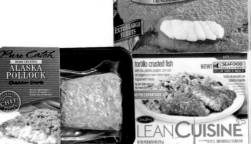

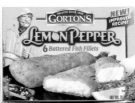

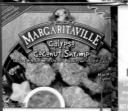

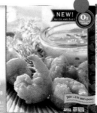

Pure Catch® Herb
Crusted Alaska
Pollock

(1 piece, 170 g)

260 calories
10 g fat
(2 g saturated)
560 mg sodium

Bread crumbs are best
at one thing: soaking up
fat. And between the
soybean oil, butter, and
vegetable shortening,
there's plenty here.

Lean Cuisine®
Tortilla Crusted
Fish

(1 package, 226 g)

330 calories
9 g fat
(2.5 g saturated)
540 mg sodium

The tortilla-chip
crusted fish has only
half the fiber of
Kashi's shrimp meal.

Gorton's®
Lemon Pepper
Battered Fish
Fillets

(2 fillets, 104 g)

270 calories
18 g fat
(4.5 g saturated)
580 mg sodium

Gorton's Lemon Pepper
batter has 50% more
fat than their garlic
and herb breading.

Margaritaville®
Calypso Coconut
Shrimp with
Mango Chutney
Dippin' Sauce

(~5 shrimp and sauce, 150 g)

360 calories
17 g fat
(9 g saturated)
645 mg sodium

Each serving has
13 grams of sugar, too.

*Sea Pak's Crispy Light Shrimp
actually has more calories than
their regular popcorn shrimp.
The solution?
Stick to nonfried shrimp.*

Frozen Chicken Entrées
Eat This

Swanson® Classics Boneless Fried Chicken with Mashed Potatoes and Corn

(1 package, 213 g)

*330 calories
17 g fat (3.5 g saturated)
610 mg sodium*

Swapping in the Swanson will slash almost half the fat and calories from your fried chicken.

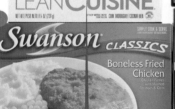

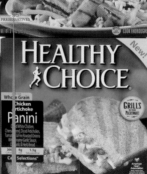

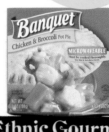

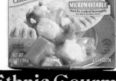

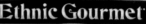

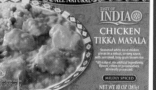

Lean Cuisine® Chicken Marsala with Green Beans and Carrots

(1 package, 230 g)

*140 calories
4 g fat (1.5 g saturated)
620 mg sodium*

It earns hunger-crunching cred with 14 grams of protein and 3 of fiber.

Stouffer's® Grilled Chicken Teriyaki

(1 package, 265 g)

*300 calories
3.5 g fat
(1 g saturated)
880 mg sodium*

The other nutritional boons: 90% of your vitamin A and 21 grams of protein.

Healthy Choice® Chicken Artichoke Panini

(1 package, 170 g)

*300 calories
4 g fat
(1.5 g saturated)
600 mg sodium*

A hundred of these calories come from protein, and another 25 from fiber.

Ethnic Gourmet® Chicken Tikka Masala (1 package, 283 g)

*260 calories
6 g fat
(2 g saturated)
680 mg sodium*

Tikka masala is a blend of spices, tomato, and yogurt served over all-white chicken meat.

Banquet® Chicken & Broccoli Pot Pie (1 pie, 198 g)

*350 calories
20 g fat
(9 g saturated)
800 mg sodium*

No potpie, no matter how carefully constructed, will ever be truly healthy. But this one is about as good as it gets.

Not That!

Banquet Select Recipes™ Classic Fried Chicken Thigh with Mashed Potatoes and Corn

(1 package, 228 g)

690 calories
29 g fat (7 g saturated, 1.5 g trans)
950 mg sodium

There's nothing redeeming about this meal: not the calorie count, not the sodium level, and certainly not the trans fats.

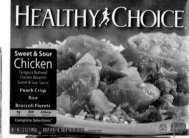
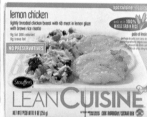
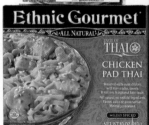
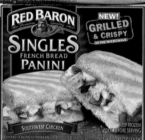
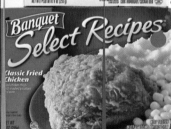

Marie Callender's® Chicken Pot Pie	Ethnic Gourmet® Chicken Pad Thai	Red Baron® Singles French Bread Panini Southwest Chicken	Healthy Choice® Sweet & Sour Chicken	Lean Cuisine® Lemon Chicken
(1 pie, 284 g)	**(1 package, 283 g)**	**(1 panini, 167 g)**	**(1 package, 308 g)**	**(1 package, 255 g)**
640 calories	*410 calories*	*360 calories*	*430 calories*	*300 calories*
38 g fat	*7 g fat*	*12 g fat*	*9 g fat*	*9 g fat*
(14 g saturated)	*(1 g saturated)*	*(5 g saturated)*	*(1 g saturated)*	*(1.5 g saturated)*
1,000 mg sodium	*830 mg sodium*	*790 mg sodium*	*600 mg sodium*	*570 mg sodium*
Potpie crust, made from flour and shortening, is one of the least-healthy foods on the planet.	The "peanut sauce" that covers these noodles adds 22 grams of sugar.	Laced with partially hydrogenated oils.	Trust us: Deep-fried chicken slicked with 29 grams of sugar is not a "healthy choice."	Sometimes you're better off opting for the regular line of products and skipping the "light" one.

Frozen Beef Entrées

Eat This

Meat loaf conquers meatballs, and the mashed potatoes contribute healthier carbohydrates than those from the white noodles.

Stouffer's® Meatloaf
(1 package, 279 g)

*340 calories
19 g fat (8 g saturated,
1 g trans)
780 mg sodium*

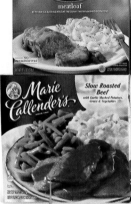

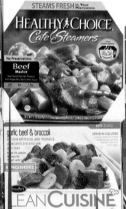

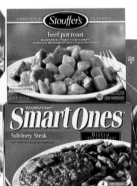

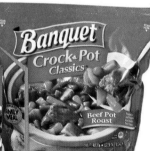

Marie Callender's® Slow Roasted Beef (1 package, 411 g)	**Healthy Choice® Cafe Steamers™ Beef Merlot** (1 package, 284 g)	**Lean Cuisine® Café Classics Garlic Beef & Broccoli** (1 package, 255 g)	**Smart Ones® Salisbury Steak** (1 package, 255 g)	**Stouffer's® Beef Pot Roast** (1 package, 251 g)	**Banquet® Crock-Pot Classics® Beef Pot Roast** (1 cup, 228 g)
340 calories 11 g fat (4 g saturated) 1,360 mg sodium	*220 calories 6 g fat (1.5 g saturated) 600 mg sodium*	*170 calories 6 g fat (2 g saturated) 520 mg sodium*	*200 calories 7 g fat (2.5 g saturated) 660 mg sodium*	*240 calories 8 g fat (2.5 g saturated) 980 mg sodium*	*225 calories 5.5 g fat (3 g saturated) 990 mg sodium*
Lots of food for few calories. The one caveat: Watch the sodium for the rest of the day.	Merlot beats bourbon, and whole potatoes beat mashed and smothered spuds.	Lean Cuisine cuts the fat and calories by more than half.	Asparagus is packed with folate, which helps oxygen travel freely through your blood.	Rich with fresh vegetables and lean meat, pot roast is one of the few nutritious comfort foods.	Teeming with healthy red potatoes, carrots, green beans, and onions.

Not That!

Stouffer's®
Swedish Meatballs
(1 package, 326 g)

*560 calories
27 g fat (12 g saturated,
1 g trans)
1,250 mg sodium*

These mammoth meatballs are loaded with fillers, oils, and food starches.

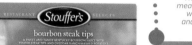
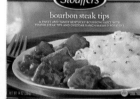
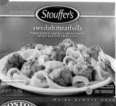
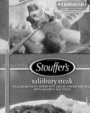
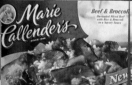
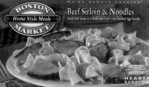
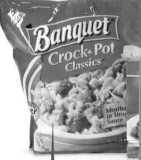

Banquet® Crock-Pot Classics® Meatballs in Stroganoff Sauce (1 cup, 212 g)	Banquet® Beef Pot Pie (1 pie, 198 g)	Stouffer's® Salisbury Steak (1 package, 272 g)	Marie Callender's® Beef & Broccoli (1 package, 369 g)	Stouffer's® Bourbon Steak Tips (1 package, 396 g)	Boston Market® Beef Sirloin & Noodles (1 package, 396 g)
450 calories 21 g fat (7.5 g saturated, 1 g trans) 1,200 mg sodium	*450 calories 27 g fat (11 g saturated, 0.5 g trans) 730 mg sodium*	*410 calories 22 g fat (10 g saturated, 1 g trans) 1,090 mg sodium*	*400 calories 14 g fat (4.5 g saturated) 1,200 mg sodium*	*570 calories 24 g fat (6 g saturated, 0.5 g trans) 1,120 mg sodium*	*470 calories 12 g fat (4 g saturated, 0.5 g trans) 1,310 mg sodium*
	This is the smallest pot pie we could find, and it's still swimming in fat.	The mac and cheese side sinks this dish in saturated fat.	Watch the sodium—this one has more than half of your day's limit.	The word "oil" shows up 3 times on this ingredient list.	Most of the calories come from the refined carbs.

Frozen Meatless Entré

Eat This

Shepherd's pie slashes the fat and calories by covering its veggies with mashed potatoes instead of fat-flecked flour, and with 5 grams of fiber, this is the ultimate high-octane belly filler.

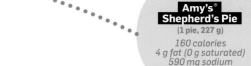

Amy's® Shepherd's Pie
(1 pie, 227 g)

160 calories
4 g fat (0 g saturated)
590 mg sodium

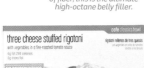

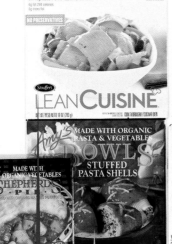

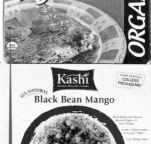

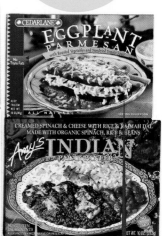

Lean Cuisine® Three Cheese Stuffed Rigatoni
(1 package, 283 g)

240 calories
6 g fat
(3 g saturated)
660 mg sodium

Offers a host of A-list vegetables like zucchini and peppers.

Amy's® Bowls Stuffed Pasta Shells
(1 package, 283 g)

310 calories
13 g fat
(7 g saturated)
740 mg sodium

Amy's shells squeeze in twice the amount of vitamin A and 40% more vitamin C.

Celentano® Vegetarian Lasagne Primavera
(1 tray, 284 g)

290 calories
8 g fat
(1 g saturated)
590 mg sodium

The veggie load boosts the fiber count up to 7 grams.

Kashi™ Black Bean Mango
(1 package, 283 g)

340 calories
8 g fat
(1 g saturated)
430 mg sodium

Loaded with protein, fiber, and antioxidants, black beans should be a staple in everyone's diet.

Amy's Indian Palak Paneer
(1 package, 283 g)

270 calories
9 g fat
(2.5 g saturated)
680 mg sodium

Traditional Indian dishes are long on vegetables and antioxidant-rich spices.

Cedarlane™ Eggplant Parmesan
(1 package, 282 g)

320 calories
16 g fat
(6 g saturated)
780 mg sodium

The first 4 ingredients are eggplant, tomatoes, tomato puree, and onions.

es

Not That!

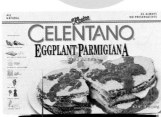

Amy's® Vegetable Pot Pie

(1 pie, 213 g)

420 calories
19 g fat (12 g saturated)
590 mg sodium

Not even a meatless pot pie can successfully hurdle the pitfall of high calories. If you ever get stuck with one of these, save a couple hundred calories by skipping the doughy skin.

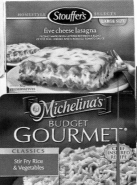

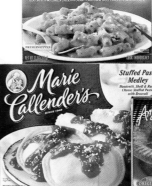

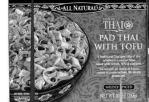

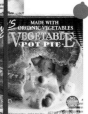

Celentano® Eggplant Parmigiana	**Ethnic Gourmet® Pad Thai with Tofu**	**Michelina's® Budget Gourmet® Stir Fry Rice & Vegetables**	**Stouffer's® Five Cheese Lasagna**	**Marie Callender's® Stuffed Pasta Medley**	**Stouffer's® Cheesy Tomato Rigatoni**
(1 package, 396 g)	(1 package, 283 g)	(1 package, 227 g)	(1 cup, 237 g)	(1 meal, 369 g)	(1 package, 311 g)
660 calories	*420 calories*	*450 calories*	*330 calories*	*420 calories*	*430 calories*
44 g fat	*8 g fat*	*20 g fat*	*14 g fat*	*13 g fat*	*19 g fat*
(10 g saturated)	*(1.5 g saturated)*	*(4 g saturated)*	*(8 g saturated)*	*(6 g saturated)*	*(7 g saturated)*
960 mg sodium	*720 mg sodium*	*700 mg sodium*	*870 mg sodium*	*1,040 mg sodium*	*880 mg sodium*
Even if you saw this meal in half, you're still left with 22 grams of fat.	More sugar (22 g) than 11 Hershey's Kisses.	Vegetables laced with chicken fat.	The idea is to replace the meat with vegetables, not more cheese.	Marie's doles out massive portions. Try splitting them.	Too cheesy to be taken seriously.

Meat Substitutes

Eat This

Lightlife Smart Dogs® Veggie Protein Links

(1 link, 42 g)

45 calories
0 g fat
290 mg sodium

Boca® Meatless Breakfast Links

(2 links, 45 g)

70 calories
3 g fat
(1 g saturated)
330 mg sodium

Boca's formula is twice as lean as Tofurky's.

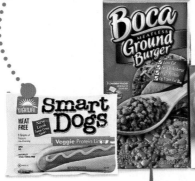
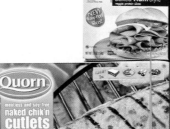
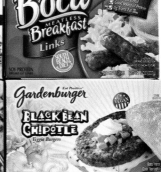

This frank has fewer calories than 5 Ruffles potato chips.

Boca® Meatless Ground Burger

(½ cup, 57 g)

60 calories
0.5 g fat
(0 g saturated)
270 mg sodium

Boca's regular soy blend is the best you can find. By calories, it's nearly 90% pure protein.

Quorn™ Naked Chik 'n Cutlets

(1 cutlet, 69 g)

80 calories
2.5 g fat
(0.5 g saturated)
420 mg sodium

Throw one of these versatile soy-free cutlets on the grill and paint with barbecue sauce for a stand-alone dinner or for a sandwich or salad topping.

Lightlife Smart Deli™ Baked Ham Style

(4 slices, 52 g)

70 calories
1 g fat
(0 g saturated)
390 mg sodium

Another benefit of faux meats: You don't have to deal with dangerous nitrate preservatives.

Gardenburger® Black Bean Chipotle

(1 pattie, 71 g)

90 calories
2.5 g fat
(0 g saturated)
370 mg sodium

Gardenburger's lightest beef-patty substitute is a superlative mix of black beans, brown rice, corn, chiles, and bell peppers.

Not That!

Tofurky® Breakfast Links
(1 link, 45 g)

*130 calories
6 g fat
(0 g saturated)
330 mg sodium*

Canola oil is a healthy source of fat, but when it's the third ingredient on the list, you're probably getting more than you need.

Tofurky® Franks
(1 frank, 45 g)

*80 calories
2 g fat (0 g saturated)
370 mg sodium*

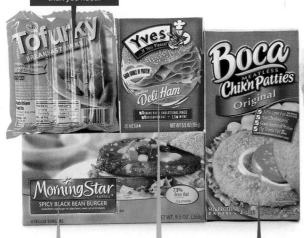
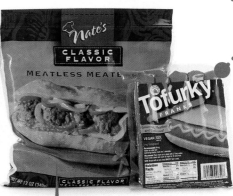

MorningStar Farms® Spicy Black Bean Burger
(1 burger, 67 g)

*120 calories
4 g fat
(0.5 g saturated)
350 mg sodium*

Has 33% more calories than the Gardenburger version.

Yves® Meatless Deli Ham
(4 slices, 62 g)

*100 calories
2 g fat
(0 g saturated)
480 mg sodium*

This meat substitute has more calories and sodium than the real thing.

Boca® Meatless Chik'n Patties Original **(1 patty, 71 g)**

*160 calories
6 g fat
(1 g saturated)
430 mg sodium*

Boca's Chik'n Pattie has about as much protein as real chicken and even manages to cut a few calories, but it still can't compete with Quorn's super-protein formula.

Nate's™ Classic Flavor Meatless Meatballs
(3 meatballs, 43 g)

*90 calories
4.5 g fat
(0 g saturated)
270 mg sodium*

Compared to Boca, Nate's has more calories and less fiber and protein.

For 80 calories, you could switch over to Smart Dogs' jumbo-size dog and get more protein for your caloric buck.

245

Frozen Breakfast

Eat This

Aunt Jemima® Ham & Egg Scramble

(1 package, 193 g)

260 calories
13 g fat (3.5 g saturated)
920 mg sodium

By swapping in ham for bacon and leaving the trans fat out of the potatoes, Aunt Jemima makes a nearly identical breakfast with half the calories.

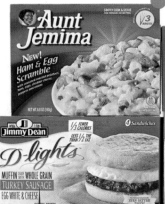

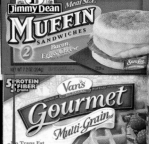

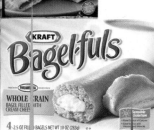

Jimmy Dean® D-Lights™ Muffins made with Whole Grain, Turkey Sausage, Egg White & Cheese

(1 sandwich, 145 g)

260 calories
7 g fat
(3.5 g saturated)
840 mg sodium

Jimmy Dean® Muffin Sandwich Bacon, Egg & Cheese

(1 sandwich, 102 g)

230 calories
9 g fat
(3.5 g saturated)
670 mg sodium

The choice between a croissant and an English muffin is a no-brainer.

Van's® Gourmet Multi-Grain Waffles

(2 waffles, 76 g)

190 calories
6 g fat
(0.5 g saturated)
306 mg sodium

Nearly identical to the Eggo waffle but in one key area: This waffle has 3 times the fiber.

Amy's® Toaster Pops Strawberry

(1 toaster pop, 55 g)

150 calories
3.5 g fat
(0 g saturated)
110 mg sodium

Amy's Toaster Pops are stuffed with real fruit puree.

Kraft Bagel-fuls Whole Grain

(1 filled bagel, 71 g)

180 calories
6 g fat
(3.5 g saturated)
200 mg sodium

This quick breakfast is surprisingly wholesome despite its novelty. It pads your belly with 3 grams of fiber and 7 grams of protein.

Not That!

**Jimmy Dean®
Breakfast Bowls
Bacon**

(1 bowl, 227 g)

*520 calories
33 g fat (13 g saturated,
1.5 g trans)
1,490 mg sodium*

*If the extreme amount of
saturated fat doesn't get you,
the trans fat surely will.*

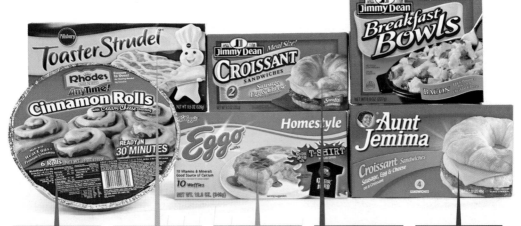

**Rhodes®
Cinnamon Rolls
with Cream
Cheese Frosting**

(1 roll with
frosting, 82 g)

*310 calories
9.5 g fat
(2.5 g saturated)
420 mg sodium*

Lots of refined flour,
plus 21 grams of sugar.

**Pillsbury
Toaster Strudel®
Strawberry**

(1 pastry, 54 g)

*190 calories
9 g fat
(3.5 g saturated,
1 g trans)
190 mg sodium*

Strawberries account
for only 10% of the
filling.

**Kellogg's
Homestyle Eggo®
Waffles**

(2 waffles, 70 grams)

*190 calories
7 g fat
(2 g saturated)
430 mg sodium*

L'Eggo the Eggo: This
popular breakfast offers
only trace amounts of
fiber and protein.

**Jimmy Dean®
Croissant
Sausage, Egg
& Cheese**

(1 sandwich, 128 g)

*430 calories
29 g fat
(9 g saturated,
3.5 g trans)
740 mg sodium*

60% of the calories
come from fat.

**Aunt Jemima®
Croissant
Sausage,
Egg & Cheese**

(1 sandwich, 116 g)

*350 calories
23 g fat
(7 g saturated,
1.5 g trans)
680 mg sodium*

Frozen Quick Bites and

Eat This

This might be the one T.G.I.Friday's appetizer worth eating. Each spud skin packs a gram of fiber, so your idle munching won't leave you hungrier than when you started.

T.G.I. Friday's™ Cheddar & Bacon Potato Skins

(3 pieces, 96 g)

210 calories
12 g fat (4 g saturated)
480 mg sodium

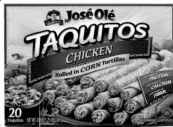

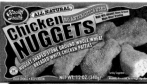

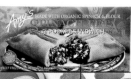

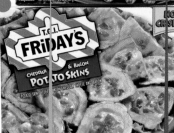

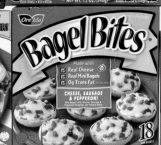

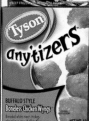

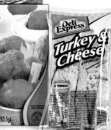

José Olé® Chicken Taquitos

(3 pieces, 85 g)

190 calories
8 g fat
(1 g saturated)
390 mg sodium

The taquitos win by virtue of the corn tortilla, which is better for you than its floury cousin.

Health Is Wealth® Chicken Nuggets

(¼ package, 84 g)

130 calories
4 g fat
(1 g saturated)
230 mg sodium

The best chicken nuggets you'll find in the freezer.

Ore Ida™ Bagel Bites® Cheese, Sausage & Pepperoni

(4 pieces, 88 g)

210 calories
7 g fat
(3 g saturated)
410 mg sodium

Surprisingly decent at just over 50 calories apiece.

Tyson® Any'tizers™ Buffalo Style Chicken Wyngs

(4 pieces, 84 g)

150 calories
7 g fat
(1.5 g saturated)
680 mg sodium

Boneless wings will always prevail.

Amy's® Spinach Feta in a Pocket Sandwich

(1 pocket, 128 g)

260 calories
9 g fat
(4.5 g saturated)
590 mg sodium

A pure product: dough, spinach, and cheese.

Deli Express® Turkey & Cheese Sandwich

(1 sandwich, 119 g)

240 calories
7 g fat
(2.5 g saturated)
970 mg sodium

The whole wheat bread adds 2 grams of fiber to the equation.

Appetizers
Not That!

It's never a good idea to wrap cheese in breading and drop it in a deep fryer. The result here is 100 calories and 6 grams of fat per stick.

T.G.I. Friday's™ Mozzarella Sticks
(3 pieces, 96 g)
300 calories
18 g fat (6 g saturated)
840 mg sodium

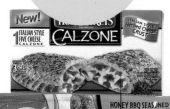
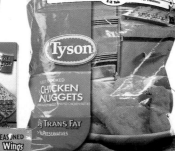
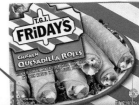
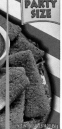
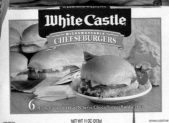
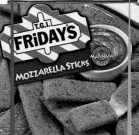

PARTY SIZE

Cedarlane™ "Veggie" Ham & Cheese Veggie Wraps
(1 wrap, 170 g)
350 calories
10 g fat
(4 g saturated)
660 mg sodium
Somehow this "whole wheat" tortilla has just a single gram of fiber.

Hot Pockets® Calzone Italian Style Five Cheese
(½ calzone, 120 g)
280 calories
10 g fat
(4.5 g saturated)
730 mg sodium
The half-calzone serving size is a recipe for disaster.

Tyson™ Any'tizers™ Honey BBQ Seasoned Wings
(4 pieces, 96g)
307 calories
19 g fat
(5 g saturated)
627 mg sodium
Each wing has almost 5 grams of fat.

White Castle® Cheeseburgers
(2 sandwiches, 104 g)
310 calories
17 g fat
(8 g saturated, 1 g trans)
600 mg sodium
The bun is made of partially hydrogenated oil and HFCS.

Tyson® Chicken Nuggets
(4 nuggets, 90 g)
230 calories
16 g fat
(4 g saturated)
360 mg sodium
Compared with the average nugget, Tyson's are on the low side for protein and high side for fat.

T.G.I. Friday's® Chicken Quesadilla Rolls
(2 pieces, 83 g)
230 calories
10 g fat
(3 g saturated, 1 g trans)
470 mg sodium
Frozen flour tortillas are trans-fat vehicles.

249

Frozen Sides
Eat This

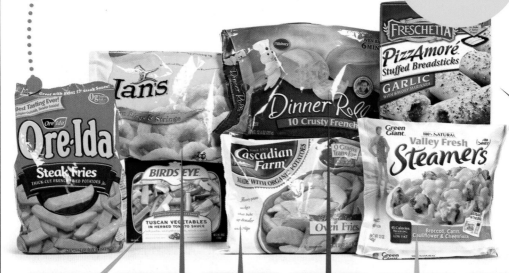

Ore-Ida's Steak Fries have less than a quarter of the fat of the Crispers! And unlike the Crispers!, none of those fats are from partially hydrogenated oils.

Ore-Ida® Steak Fries
(~7 pieces, 84 g)

*110 calories
3 g fat (1.5 g saturated)
300 mg sodium*

Birds Eye® Tuscan Vegetables in Herbed Tomato Sauce
(1 cup, 107 g)

*50 calories
2 g fat
(0 g saturated)
180 mg sodium*

Each serving provides 2 grams of fiber.

Ian's® Onion Rings & Strings
(~6 rings, 70 g)

*152 calories
7 g fat
(1 g saturated)
180 mg sodium*

Ian's smaller rings have less surface area to spackle with fried breading.

Cascadian Farm® Wedge Cut Oven Fries
(~8 pieces, 85 g)

*100 calories
2.5 g fat
(0 g saturated)
10 mg sodium*

Light on oil, these fries rely on apple juice concentrate to help them brown.

Pillsbury Dinner Rolls Crusty French
(1 roll, 35 g)

*80 calories
1 g fat
(0 g saturated)
160 mg sodium*

Rolls are made with flour and water, biscuits with flour and lard. Any questions?

Green Giant® Valley Fresh Steamers™ Broccoli, Carrots, Cauliflower & Cheese Sauce
(1 cup, 109 g)

*45 calories
1 g fat
(0 g saturated)
290 mg sodium*

Freschetta™ PizzAmoré Stuffed Breadsticks Garlic with Savory Marinara
(1 bread stick, 51 g)

*110 calories
3 g fat
(1.5 g saturated)
320 mg sodium*

Not That!

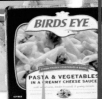
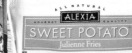

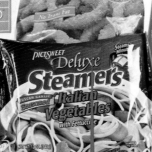
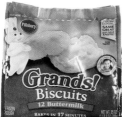
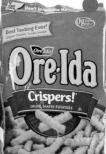

**Ore-Ida®
Crispers!®**
(~20 pieces, 84 g)

*220 calories
13 g fat (2.5 g saturated)
390 mg sodium*

*Crispy means an extra-long
bath in hot oil.*

**New York® The
Original Garlic
Bread Sticks**
(1 bread stick, 50 g)

*170 calories
6 g fat
(1.5 g saturated)
300 mg sodium*

Most breadsticks
are never as
innocuous as they
seem.

**Birds Eye®
Pasta &
Vegetables in
a Creamy
Cheese Sauce**
(1 cup, 130 g)

*160 calories
3.5 g fat
(1.5 g saturated)
590 mg sodium*

**Pillsbury
Grands!®
Biscuits
Buttermilk**
(1 biscuit, 59 g)

*180 calories
9 g fat
(2 g saturated,
3.5 g trans)
560 mg sodium*

**Alexia
Sweet Potato®
Julienne Fries**
(~12 pieces, 85 g)

*150 calories
6 g fat
(0.5 g saturated)
140 mg sodium*

Better than some fry
options, but not the
sweet potato's best
performance.

**Alexia
Onion Rings®**
(~6 rings, 85 g)

*230 calories
12 g fat
(1 g saturated)
230 mg sodium*

As if frying is not
enough, these rings
are sweetened
with sugar.

**PictSweet®
Steamers®
Tuscan Garlic
Seasoned
Italian
Vegetables
with
Fettuccine**
(1 cup, 102 g)

*95 calories
0 g fat
280 mg sodium*

251

Chapter 8
DRINK THIS, NOT THAT!

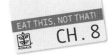

EAT THIS, NOT THAT!
CH. 8

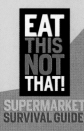

EAT THIS NOT THAT!
SUPERMARKET SURVIVAL GUIDE

Think Before You Drink

If this book has done its job, then I've reinforced the important message that the more you think in advance about what you buy and eat, the more control you'll have over your weight, your health, and your life. And if I've gotten you reading food labels religiously, negotiating your way around the multiple bad ingredients, and making a beeline for the vitamins, minerals, fiber, and other nutrients that are the building blocks of great nutrition, then I'm thrilled.

But there's one important lard-loading culprit out there that most people never think about: beverages. We talk a lot about "watching what we eat," but if you never gave a thought to what you ate and instead watched only what you drank, you could probably cut 450 calories *a day* out of your life.

That's what a study at the University of North Carolina found. Americans today drink about 192 gallons of liquid a year—or about 2 liters a day. But we drink nearly twice as many calories as we did 30 years ago.

Indeed, if you limited yourself to water, seltzer, and unsweetened coffee or tea just *one day a week*, you'd still save enough calories to lose more than 6½ pounds a year. Two days a week and now you're down 13 pounds! And that's without changing your food at all!

Obviously, "drink responsibly" means a lot more than just making sure you have a designated driver. It means taking a hard look at what you sip, as well as what you sup. Twenty-eight percent of all beverages we drink are carbonated soft drinks. And

The Ultimate Fighter's Drinking Plan

Hélio Gracie, the 95-year-old founder of Brazilian jiu-jitsu and the man who started Ultimate Fighting, created a complete regimen for his sons, all of whom went on to become successful fighters. And the first thing every Gracie must do when he awakes in the morning: Drink a glass of water.

Here's why: The Gracie code says that every Gracie must be prepared to fight any opponent at any time. Hélio believes that water throughout the day, especially upon waking, is the key to staying in top fighting shape at all times. (And old Hélio is onto something: Our muscles are 75 percent water.)

among children in fourth through sixth grades, sweetened beverages make up an unreal 51 percent of all fluid intake! (Research shows that students who drink the most sweetened beverages take in an extra 337 calories a day, on average, and less than half the amount of real fruit than their less sugar saturated peers.) And there's a rub-off effect: A Minnesota study found that children were almost three times more likely to drink soda five or more times a week when their parents regularly drank soda.

As I've said throughout this book, you should look at food and drink as weight-control weapons and the supermarket as your armory. Drinking the bad stuff is bad—but not drinking the good stuff is bad, too. The best way to hydrate is to be religious about keeping only low-calorie, high-nutrient beverages in your shopping cart—and to make water and seltzer water regular attendees at all meals. In fact, water was pretty much all our ancestors ever drank for the first 200,000 years humans have been in existence. (Tea—boiled water and leaves—

The Truth about Diet Soda

When confronted with the growing tide of calories from sweetened beverages, the first response is, "Why not just drink diet soda?" Well, for a few reasons:

● **Just because diet soda is low in calories doesn't mean it can't lead to weight gain.** It may have only 5 or fewer calories per serving, but emerging research suggests that consuming sugary-tasting beverages—even if they're artificially sweetened—may lead to a high preference for sweetness overall. That means sweeter (and more caloric) cereal, bread, dessert—everything.

● **Guzzling these drinks all day long forces out the healthy beverages you need.** Diet soda is 100 percent nutrition free, and again, it's just as important to actively drink the good stuff as it is to avoid that bad stuff. So one diet soda a day is fine, but if you're downing five or six cans, that means you're limiting your intake of healthful beverages, particularly water and tea.

● **There remain some concerns over aspartame, the low-calorie chemical used to give diet sodas their flavor.** Aspartame is 180 times sweeter than sugar, and some researchers claim to have linked it to brain tumors and lymphoma. The FDA maintains that the sweetener is safe, but reported side effects include dizziness, headaches, diarrhea, memory loss, and mood changes. Bottom line: Diet soda does you no good, and it might just be doing you wrong.

wasn't even discovered until 3,000 years ago.) As a result, "Our evolution over hundreds of thousands of years didn't prepare us to process liquid calories," says Barry Popkin, PhD, a distinguished professor of nutrition at the University of North Carolina. "High-sugar drinks didn't even exist until 150 years ago, and they weren't consumed in significant amounts until the past 50 years. This is just a blip on our evolutionary timeline."

What about really healthy fare, like fruit juice? Unfortunately, most of what we consider to be "fruit juice" really isn't. You don't believe me? Well, just check out the Label Decoder on the pages to come and you'll see how little fruit is actually in our juice supply.

So we don't really drink as much juice as we think we do. In fact, a study using the national Continuing Survey of Food Intakes by Individuals found that consumption of real fruit juice is higher than other beverages only for very young children. By age 5, fruit drinks, ades, and sodas surpassed that of real fruit juice. (By the time they're 14, children are drinking only one-fifth as much real fruit juice as they are sweetened beverages.)

And even if you do enjoy real fruit juice, the fact is you'd be much better off having a piece of fruit and a glass of water. Consider: A medium orange

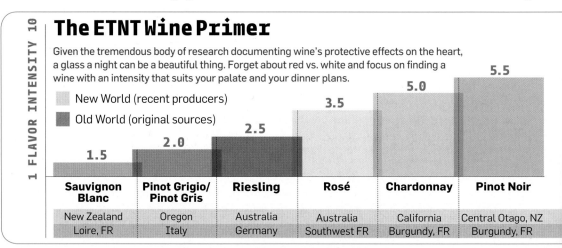

The ETNT Wine Primer

Given the tremendous body of research documenting wine's protective effects on the heart, a glass a night can be a beautiful thing. Forget about red vs. white and focus on finding a wine with an intensity that suits your palate and your dinner plans.

New World (recent producers)
Old World (original sources)

1 FLAVOR INTENSITY 10

	Sauvignon Blanc	Pinot Grigio/ Pinot Gris	Riesling	Rosé	Chardonnay	Pinot Noir
Intensity	1.5	2.0	2.5	3.5	5.0	5.5
New World	New Zealand	Oregon	Australia	Australia	California	Central Otago, NZ
Old World	Loire, FR	Italy	Germany	Southwest FR	Burgundy, FR	Burgundy, FR

contains just 62 calories, 12 grams of sugar, and 3 grams of belly-filling fiber. An 8-ounce glass of Minute Maid orange juice has 110 calories, 24 grams of sugar, and zero fiber.

So what should we be drinking more of?

● **Water.** First and foremost. Keep cold, filtered water in a pitcher in your fridge. You might even want to keep some cut-up limes, oranges, lemons, or cucumber on hand for a quick flavor boost.

● **Tea.** Not only does it contain antioxidants that may help protect against heart disease and cancer, it's also calorie free, as long as you opt for the unsweetened kind.

● **Coffee.** But not the sweet, syrupy specialty drinks that sponge up your paycheck at Starbucks. Gourmet coffee drinkers consume 206 more calories on average than folks who drink regular joe.

● **Milk.** About 73 percent of the calcium in the American food supply comes from dairy foods—critical for growing kids and for adults looking to maintain bone and muscle density.

● **Wine.** Calm down oenophiles, I don't mean you should down a bottle a night. But wine is loaded with heart-healthy resveratrol (pinot noir above all), so trading in beer and booze for a glass or two of vino is a swap worth making.

Tempranillo	Merlot	Zinfandel	Syrah	Cabernet Sauvignon
6.5	6.5	7.5	8.5	9.0
California Spain	Argentina Pomerol, FR	California Italy	California Rhône, FR	California Bordeaux, FR

The Beverage Label Decoder

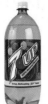

7UP

THE CLAIM: "All Natural Flavors"
THE TRUTH: The FDA doesn't have a definition for this claim. Case in point: 7UP now boasts that it's made with 100 percent natural ingredients. That's because they've switched from carbonated water to filtered water, from citric acid to natural citric acid, and from calcium disodium EDT to natural potassium citrate. Got it? Here's the kicker: The soft drink is still sweetened with high-fructose corn syrup, which can't be made without the help of a centrifuge.
WHAT YOU REALLY WANT: A healthy choice, like lemon and seltzer.
7UP's tactic is employed primarily by companies making junk food (see also: Natural Cheetos). Considering that the calorie counts are nearly always identical with their "unnatural" brethren (in the case of 7UP, calories and sugar counts are the exact same), concentrate on the bigger issues and find reliably healthy drinks and snacks.

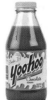

YOO-HOO

THE CLAIM: "Chocolate drink"
THE TRUTH: Ever notice the conspicuous absence of milk in the title of this popular drink? The first ingredient in this kid-favorite is water, the second high-fructose corn syrup; in fact, nonfat dry milk does not appear until the ninth ingredient, three slots below partially hydrogenated soybean oil. As a result, Yoo-Hoo offers less than half the calcium and vitamin D provided by the real thing.
WHAT YOU REALLY WANT: Yoo-hoo is fine for the occasional indulgence, but for a kid in need of nutrition, real milk will always be the better choice. Organic Valley's Chocolate Lowfat Milk comes in 8-ounce cartons for automatic portion control.

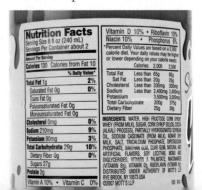

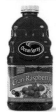

OCEAN SPRAY CRAN-RASPBERRY

THE CLAIM: "Juice drink"
THE TRUTH: Words like "juice drink" and "juice cocktail" are industry euphemisms for a huge dose of sugar water. In this case, the product is also adorned with a cluster of other claims that attempt to hide this simple fact. (Most of Ocean Spray's juice products suffer from a serious lack of juice; this particular one, with just 18 percent juice, is one of the worst offenders.) Ocean Spray, to be sure, is not the only juice purveyor guilty of this sleight of hand: Dozens of manufacturers, including Welch's, Minute Maid, and SunnyD, perpetrate similar nutritional injustices.
WHAT YOU REALLY WANT: Every juice that hits your lips should be 100 percent juice. Period.

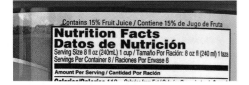

Contains 15% Fruit Juice / Contiene 15% de Jugo de Fruta
Nutrition Facts
Datos de Nutrición
Serving Size 8 fl oz (240mL) 1 cup / Tamaño Por Ración: 8 oz fl (240 ml) 1 taza
Servings Per Container 8 / Raciones Por Envase 8

Amount Per Serving / Cantidad Por Ración

TROPICANA PURE 100% JUICE POMEGRANATE BLUEBERRY

THE CLAIM: "100% juice pomegranate blueberry"
THE TRUTH: Drinks may be labeled 100 percent pure juice, but that doesn't mean they're made exclusively with the advertised juice. Pomegranate and blueberry get top billing here, even though the ingredient list reveals that pear, apple, and grape juices are among the first four ingredients. These juices are used because they're cheap to produce and because they're very sweet— likely to keep you coming back for more. Labels loaded with of-the-moment superfoods like acai and pomegranate are especially susceptible to this type of trickery.
WHAT YOU REALLY WANT: To avoid the huge sugar surge, pick single-fruit juices. POM and R.W. Knudsen both make some reliably pure products.

259

The Worst Beverages in the Supermarket

Americans have a drinking problem. The one we're talking about, though, has nothing to do with alcohol and everything to do with another dangerous substance: sugar. Collectively, we're taking in 66 pounds of added sugar a year, and many of those are waiting for you in your coffee, your juice, and your soft drinks. No matter how harmless they may seem—Vitamin-Packed Water! 100% Juice!—these beverages are at the heart of our national weight issue. We've compiled a list of the worst to be found in the supermarket aisles, and just to give you an idea of how bad they really are, we've paired each with a sugar equivalent and a blueprint for what you'd have to do to work off the liquid calories.

WORST FUNCTIONAL BEVERAGE
Snapple Agave Melon Antioxidant Water (20-ounce bottle)
150 calories
33 g sugars

SUGAR EQUIVALENT:
3 bowls of Honey Comb cereal

PUNISHMENT:
20 minutes
shoveling snow

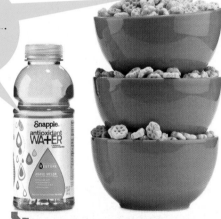

150 calories

33 g sugars

DRINK THIS INSTEAD
Dasani Plus Orange Tangerine Vitamin Enhanced Water (20-ounce bottle)
0 calories
0 g sugars

WORST ICED TEA
**Snapple Lemon Iced Tea
(20-ounce bottle)**
250 calories
58 g sugars

SUGAR EQUIVALENT:
6 Original Fudgsicle Bars

PUNISHMENT:
55 minutes pulling weeds in the garden

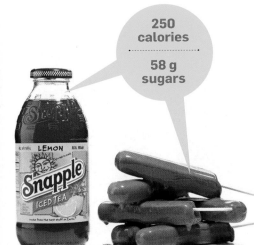

250
calories

58 g
sugars

DRINK THIS INSTEAD
**Honest Tea's Lori's Lemon Tea
(16-ounce bottle)**
60 calories
16 g sugars

WORST COFFEE DRINK
**Starbucks Coffee Frappuccino
(13.7-ounce bottle)**
290 calories
4.5 g fat (2.5 g saturated)
46 g sugars

SUGAR EQUIVALENT:
3½ scoops of Dreyer's Double Fudge
Brownie Ice Cream

PUNISHMENT:
2.75 hours working on a computer

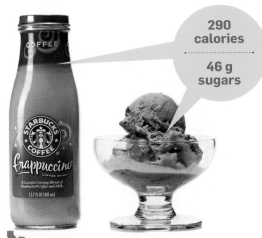

290
calories

46 g
sugars

DRINK THIS INSTEAD
**Starbucks Italian Roast Iced
Coffee (11-ounce can)**
100 calories
22 g sugars

SunnyD Smooth Style (16-ounce bottle)

260 calories
60 g sugars

SUGAR EQUIVALENT:
8 Eggo Choco-'Nilla Flip Flop Waffles

PUNISHMENT:
60 minutes of playing tag

Minute Maid Lemonade (20-ounce bottle)

250 calories
67 g sugars

SUGAR EQUIVALENT:
5 Good Humor Vanilla Ice Cream Sandwiches

PUNISHMENT:
60 minutes of vigorous housecleaning

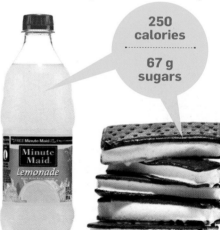

260 calories

60 g sugars

250 calories

67 g sugars

DRINK THIS INSTEAD

Capri Sun Tropical Fruit Roarin' Waters (6.8-ounce pouch)

35 calories
9 g sugars

DRINK THIS INSTEAD

Crystal Light Pink Lemonade Hydration (16-ounce bottle)

10 calories
0 g sugars

WORST ENERGY DRINK
Rockstar Original
(16-ounce can)
280 calories
62 g sugars

- -

SUGAR EQUIVALENT:
7½ Chocolate Drizzle Rice Krispies

- -

PUNISHMENT:
Dance the Macarena
17 times

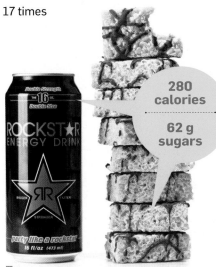

280
calories

62 g
sugars

DRINK THIS INSTEAD
Monster Lo-Ball Java Monster
Coffee + Energy (16-ounce can)
100 calories
8 g sugars

WORST BOTTLED BEVERAGE
Sobe Lizard Lava
(20-ounce bottle)
310 calories
75 g sugars

- -

SUGAR EQUIVALENT:
11 Rainbow Popsicles

- -

PUNISHMENT:
Nearly 2 hours of yoga

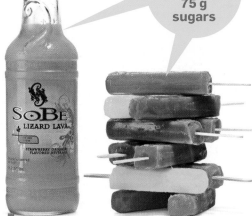

310
calories

75 g
sugars

DRINK THIS INSTEAD
Sobe Lean Blackberry Currant
(20-ounce bottle)
15 calories
2 g sugars

263

Sunkist (20-ounce bottle)
325 calories
88 g sugars

SUGAR EQUIVALENT:
17 Chewy Chips Ahoy! cookies

PUNISHMENT:
Ride your bike 7 miles

Arizona Kiwi Strawberry (23.5-ounce can)
360 calories
84 g sugars

SUGAR EQUIVALENT:
7 bowls of Froot Loops

PUNISHMENT:
Run 13 laps around a high school track

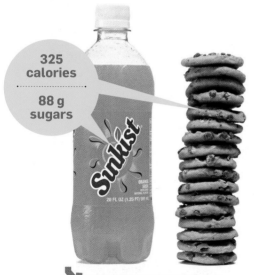

325 calories
88 g sugars

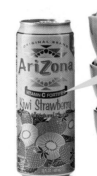

360 calories
84 g sugars

DRINK THIS INSTEAD
Honest Ade Orange Mango (16.9-ounce bottle)
100 calories
24 g sugars

DRINK THIS INSTEAD
Fuze Slenderize Strawberry Melon (18.5-ounce bottle)
23 calories
0 g sugars

Nesquik (16-ounce bottle)

400 calories
10 g fat (6 g saturated)
60 g sugars

SUGAR EQUIVALENT:
4 Little Debbie Oatmeal Cream Pies

PUNISHMENT:
Make beds for 190 minutes straight

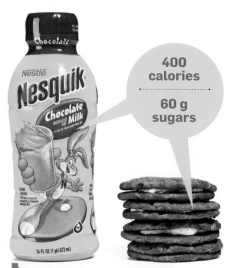

400 calories

60 g sugars

DRINK THIS INSTEAD

Organic Valley Lowfat Chocolate Milk (8-ounce carton)
160 calories / 2.5 g fat (1.5 g saturated)
25 g sugars

WORST "HEALTHY" DRINK

Naked Protein Zone Banana Chocolate (15.2-ounce bottle)

480 calories
3 g fat (1 g saturated)
32 g protein
70 g sugars

SUGAR EQUIVALENT:
5 Breyers Oreo Ice Cream Sandwiches

PUNISHMENT:
135 minutes lifting weights

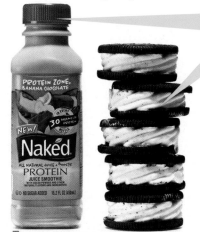

480 calories

70 g sugars

DRINK THIS INSTEAD

Bolthouse Farms Perfect Protein Vanilla Chai (16-ounce bottle)
320 calories
42 g sugars

Juice

Drink This

There's no gimmick in the V-Fusion line, just tasty concoctions of real fruit and vegetable juices.

V8® V-Fusion™ Light Peach Mango
(8 fl oz)

50 calories
0 g fat
10 g sugars

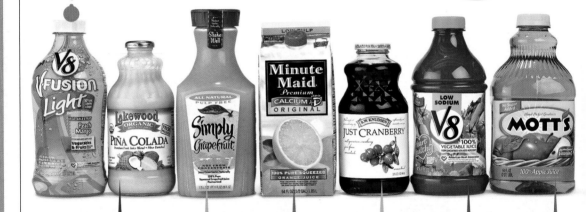

Lakewood Organic Piña Colada
(8 fl oz)

120 calories
1.5 g fat
(0 g saturated)
21 g sugars

Not just a reliable 100% juice, but also considerably better than most piña colada mixers out there.

Simply Grapefruit 100% Pure Squeezed Grapefruit
(8 fl oz)

90 calories
0 g fat
18 g sugars

100% unadulterated juice from a low-sugar, nutrient-dense fruit.

Minute Maid® Original Calcium+D Orange (8 fl oz)

110 calories
0 g fat
24 g sugars

This fortified OJ from Minute Maid contains a quarter of your day's vitamin D, 35% of your calcium, and 120% of your vitamin C.

R.W. Knudsen™ Just Cranberry™
(8 fl oz)

70 calories
0 g fat
9 g sugars

There are no sweeteners or fillers of any sort in this bottle.

V8® Low Sodium 100% Vegetable
(8 fl oz)

50 calories
0 g fat
8 g sugars
140 mg sodium

This is the best of the vegetable-juice lot. The 2 grams of fiber make it feel more like food than drink.

Mott's® 100% Apple
(8 fl oz)

120 calories
0 g fat
28 g sugars

A really simple way to cut back on calories and sugar. Every little bit helps.

Not That!

V8 Splash® Mango Peach
(8 oz)

80 calories
0 g fat
18 g sugars

This juice is closer to Capri Sun punch than regular V8. The first two ingredients are water and high-fructose corn syrup, and it contains only 10% juice.

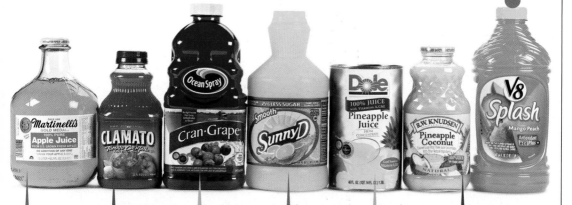

Martinelli's Gold Medal® 100% Apple
(8 fl oz)

140 calories
0 g fat
31 g sugars

Next to grape juice, apple is the sweetest sippable in the aisle.

Clamato® Tomato Cocktail (8 fl oz)

60 calories
0 g fat
8 g sugars
880 mg sodium

Sodium is a major problem with most tomato juices. This one has more than a third of your daily allotment in a single serving.

Ocean Spray® Cran-Grape®
(8 fl oz)

120 calories
0 g fat
31 g sugars

Most of Ocean Spray's cranberry juices are less than 20% actual juice, which means they're filled with sweeteners and colors.

Sunny D® 25% Less Sugar
(8 fl oz)

90 calories
0 g fat
20 g sugars

Actual juice makes up only 5% of this bottle. The rest is diluted high-fructose corn syrup and artificial sweeteners.

Dole® 100% Pineapple
(8 fl oz)

160 calories
0 g fat
32 g sugars

Pineapple juice has nearly twice as many naturally occurring sugars as grapefruit juice.

R.W. Knudsen™ 100% Pineapple Coconut (8 fl oz)

170 calories
1 g fat
(0.5 g saturated)
37 g sugars

A heavy hand with the creamed coconut and the sugar gives this juice a sugar profile akin to a milk shake.

Single-Serving Juices
Drink This

268

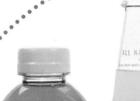

This lighter version of cranberry juice is packed with energizing B vitamins and green tea extracts.

Ocean Spray® Cranergy™ Raspberry Cranberry Lift
(12 fl oz)

50 calories
0 g fat
13 g sugars

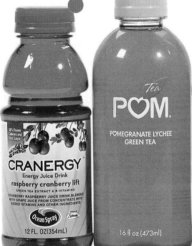

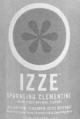

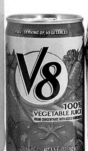

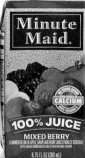

Pom® Pomegranate Lychee Green Tea
(16 fl oz)

140 calories
0 g fat
32 g sugars

Green tea blended with pomegranate juice and fused with extra pomegranate extract antioxidants makes this drink a vacuum cleaner for the free radicals in your bloodstream.

Izze® Sparkling Clementine
(12 fl oz)

120 calories
0 g fat
27 g sugars

Izze fortified drinks consist of 70% fruit juice married with carbonated sparkling water. Replace soft drinks in your fridge with this and you'll be in much better shape.

**V8®
100% Vegetable**
(1 can, 5.5 fl oz)

30 calories
0 g fat
6 g sugars
330 mg sodium

V8 is much more than tomato juice—it also contains spinach, celery, beets, and watercress, helping it earn 4 times as much vitamin A as Campbell's.

Minute Maid® 100% Mixed Berry
(1 box, 6.75 fl oz)

100 calories
0 g fat
23 g sugars

This mutt of juices contains apple, grape, blackberry, and raspberry, but at least it's 100% fruit.

Not That!

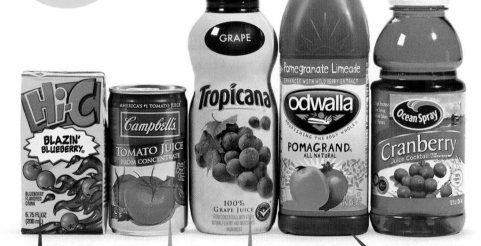

**Ocean Spray®
Cranberry Juice
Cocktail**
(12 fl oz)

*180 calories
0 g fat
45 g sugars*

*Beware of the word
"cocktail" on the label;
here it means there's
only 27% juice inside.*

**Hi-C®
Blazin' Blueberry®**
(1 box, 6.75 fl oz)

*100 calories
0 g fat
26 g sugars*

Hi-C is about as much
a juice as French fries
are a vegetable.

**Campbell's®
Tomato**
(1 can, 5.5 fl oz)

*30 calories
0 g fat
5 g sugars
470 mg sodium*

Each can has 20% of your
daily sodium.

**Tropicana®
100% Grape Juice**
(12 fl oz)

*230 calories
0 g fat
53 g sugars*

This beverage has more
than 10% of your day's calories
and as much sugar as
2 chocolate soft serve cones
from Dairy Queen.

**Odwalla®
Pomagrand
Pomegranate
Limeade**
(15.2 fl oz)

*240 calories
0 g fat
54 g sugars*

Odwalla has a number of great
products, but too often they
pollute their juices with an
abundance of added sugars.

269

Smoothies and Shakes
Drink This

Odwalla® Super Protein® Chocolate Protein
(15.2 fl oz)

340 calories
7 g fat (1 g saturated)
40 g sugars
20 g protein

Another perk of Odwalla's protein shakes is the massive dose of minerals and B vitamins.

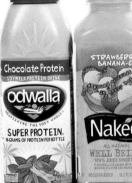

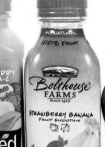

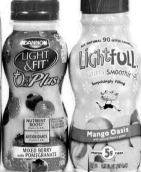

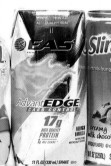

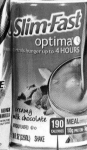

Naked® Strawberry Banana-C
(15.2 fl oz)

240 calories
0 g fat
46 g sugars

Not the insane amount of vitamin C that you get from the Odwalla, but more important, it's lighter on sugar and calories.

Bolthouse® Farms Smoothie Strawberry Banana (8 fl oz)

120 calories
0 g fat
27 g sugars

The smaller serving size keeps the calorie intake in check.

Dannon™ Light & Fit® Mixed Berry with Pomegranate
(7 fl oz)

70 calories
0 g fat
12 g sugars

Nonfat yogurt flavored with berries and fortified with vitamins D, E, and B.

Lightfull™ Satiety Smoothie Mango Oasis
(8.5 fl oz)

90 calories
0 g fat
9 g sugars

It's called a Satiety Smoothie because it has 5 grams of belly-filling fiber.

EAS AdventEdge® Carb Control Ready-to-Drink French Vanilla (11 fl oz)

110 calories
3 g fat
(0 g saturated)
0 g sugars

Packs 15 grams of protein.

Slim-Fast Optima Creamy Milk Chocolate
(11 fl oz)

190 calories
6 g fat
(2.5 g saturated)
18 g sugars

Optima delivers more fiber and vitamins, too.

Not That!

Naked® Protein Zone Banana Chocolate
(15.2 fl oz)

480 calories
3 g fat (1 g saturated)
70 g sugars
32 g protein

Even after adjusting for the extra protein, Naked's protein shakes are consistently more caloric than Odwalla's. This whole bottle has nearly a quarter of your day's calories and as much sugar as a McDonald's Triple Thick Chocolate Shake.

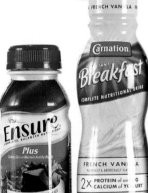
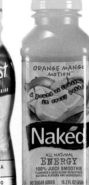
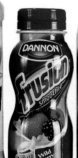
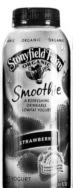
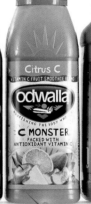
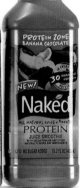

Ensure® Plus Creamy Milk Chocolate
(8 fl oz)
350 calories
11 g fat (1.5 g saturated)
22 g sugars
The excessive fat comes from extra sloshes of corn and canola oils.

Carnation Instant Breakfast French Vanilla
(11 fl oz)
250 calories
5 g fat (1.5 g saturated)
31 g sugars

Naked® Orange Mango Motion™
(8 fl oz)
130 calories
0 g fat
27 g sugars
Not a bad option, but there are better picks in the supermarket mango category.

Dannon™ Frusion® Wild Berry Blend
(7 fl oz)
180 calories
2.5 g fat (1.5 g saturated)
33 g sugars
This mini bottle is packed with more sugar than a Snicker's bar.

Stonyfield Farm® Organic Smoothie Strawberry
(10 fl oz)
230 calories
3 g fat (2 g saturated)
38 g sugars
Sugar alone accounts for 152 calories in this bottle.

Odwalla® C Monster® Citrus C
(15.2 fl oz)
300 calories
0 g fat
54 g sugars
Do you really need 10 times the recommended daily intake of vitamin C? Probably not.

Tea and Fortified Dri

Drink This

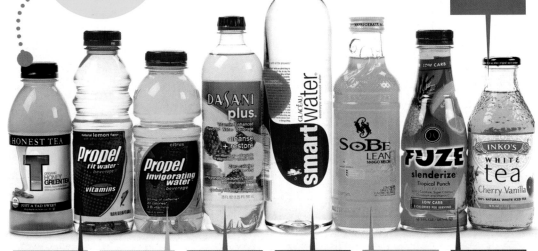

A Men's Health analysis of popular bottled green teas found this one to have a higher concentration of disease-fighting catechins than any other tea analyzed.

Honest Tea® Organic Green Tea Honey

(16.9 fl oz)

74 calories
0 g fat
18 g sugars

Inko's White Tea Cherry Vanilla

(16 fl oz)

56 calories
0 g fat
14 g sugars

Inko is quietly churning out an entire line of teas with modest sugar levels and natural flavors.

Propel Fit Water™ Lemon

(16.9 fl oz)

25 calories
0 g fat
4 g sugars

Propel uses sucralose to keep the calories down. Not great, but better than sugar and an easy way to keep calories down.

Propel Invigorating Water™ Citrus

(20 fl oz)

50 calories
0 g fat
10 g sugars

This drink gives a small energy boost with a few B vitamins and 50 mg of caffeine.

Dasani Plus™ Pomegranate Blackberry

(20 fl oz)

0 calories
0 g fat
0 g sugars

The 2.5 grams of fiber give this product an edge in the crowded functional water category.

Glacéau SmartWater®

(33.8 fl oz)

0 calories
0 g fat
0 g sugars

Loaded up with electrolytes and zero caloric impact.

Sobe Lean Mango Melon

(20 fl oz)

12.5 calories
0 g fat
0 g sugars

Sobe's bottles look similar, but the Lean line replaces the sugar with a blend of sucralose and acesulfame-k.

Fuze® Slenderize® Tropical Punch

(18.5 fl oz)

10 calories
0 g fat
0 g sugars

Provides 40 mg of L-carnitine, an aminoacid that helps the body break down fats for energy.

Not That!

Snapple® White Tea Raspberry
(17.5 fl oz)

120 calories
0 g fat
30 g sugars

Snapple packs in enough sugar to turn an innocent tea into a decadent dessert.

With little evidence to support cancer-causing claims made by those who oppose aspartame and its ilk, and a supermarket's worth of research clearly documenting the ill effects of sugar, we see no clear reason to cut out artificial sweeteners entirely, if it means decreasing sugar and calories in your diet. Still, moderation is key, as is recognizing that some artificial sweeteners are better than others. For more on specific sweeteners, check out the food additive glossary in this book, or log on to eatthis.com

Compared to Honest Tea, Lipton's has a load more calories and only a fraction of the antioxidant levels.

Lipton® PureLeaf™ Green Tea Honey
(16 fl oz)

120 calories
0 g fat
32 g sugars

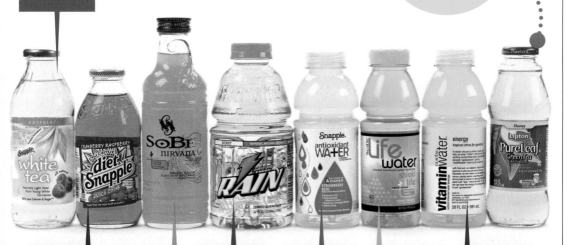

Snapple® Diet Cranberry Raspberry
(16 fl oz)

20 calories
0 g fat
4 g sugars

This bottle contains only 5% juice and is sweetened with aspartame.

Sobe Nirvana Mango Melon
(20 fl oz)

300 calories
0 g fat
72 g sugars

Sobe's drinks have ethereal names like Nirvana, but more accurate names might be Flab, Chubby, and Diabetes.

Gatorade Rain™ Berry
(32 fl oz)

200 calories
0 g fat
56 g sugars

This bottle has nearly 4 tablespoons of sugar, more than a king size Butterfinger. If it's electrolytes you seek, switch to SmartWater and save 200 calories.

Snapple® Antioxidant Water Strawberry Acai
(20 fl oz)

125 calories
0 g fat
19.5 g sugars

Acai is renowned for its antioxidant activity, but you won't find it on this ingredient list. No strawberry, either.

Sobe® Life Water® Orange Tangerine
(16 fl oz)

80 calories
0 g fat
20 g sugars

Don't be wrangled into drinking high-calorie drinks just to get a few easily attainable calories.

Glacéau Vitamin Water Energy Tropical Citrus
(20 fl oz)

125 calories
0 g fat
19.5 g sugars

While it offers some nutritional benefits over plain H$_2$O, they just don't offset the hefty caloric price tag.

Caffeinated and Ener

Drink This

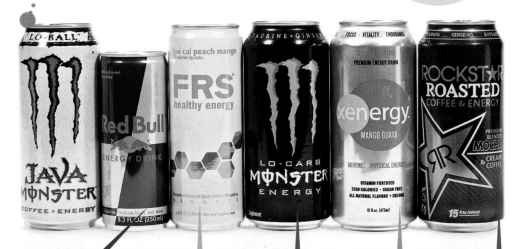

Java Monster™ Lo-Ball Coffee + Energy
(15 fl oz)

100 calories
3 g fat (2 g saturated)
8 g sugars

This is the best of the coffee drinks. It's heavy on the ginseng extract and the B vitamins, and it's light on the sugar.

Red Bull® (8.3 fl oz)

110 calories
0 g fat
27 g sugars

Not that Red Bull's really any better than the competition, but at least they haven't abandoned their moderate-size can. You still get a boost of B vitamins and taurine, but you do it in half the calories.

FRS® Healthy Energy Lo Cal Peach Mango
(11.5 fl oz)

25 calories
0 g fat
5 g sugars

A decent way to stretch your energy reserves without stretching your waistline.

Monster Energy® Lo-Carb
(16 fl oz)

20 calories
0 g fat
6 g sugars

Liquid calories are the easiest to take in, and the easiest to cut off. Start with a few simple swaps.

Xenergy™ Mango Guava
(16 fl oz)

0 calories
0 g fat
0 g sugars

Not only does it taste surprisingly good for a zero-calorie drink, but it has a solid supplemental vitamin package to boot.

Rockstar Roasted Coffee & Energy Premium Blended Mocha
(8 fl oz)

100 calories
1 g fat
(0.5 g saturated)
17 g sugars

Not a health drink, but it does boast coffee's antioxidant profile.

gy Drinks
Not That!

**Starbucks Coffee®
Frappuccino® Coffee**
(9.5 fl oz)

*200 calories
3 g fat (2 g saturated)
32 g sugars*

*Each ounce of this syrupy drink
contains nearly 3.5 grams of sugar.*

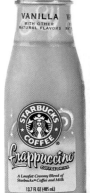
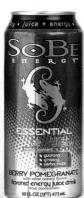
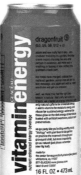
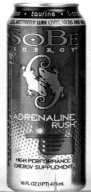
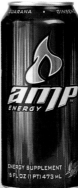
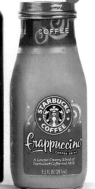

**Starbucks
Coffee®
Frappuccino®
Vanilla** (8 fl oz)

*170 calories
2.5 g fat
(1.5 g saturated)
26 g sugars*

Starbucks is one of
the worst offenders for
sugar-laden drinks.

**Sobe Energy™
Essential Berry
Pomegranate**
(16 fl oz)

*240 calories
0 g fat
56 g sugars*

Add one of these
drinks to your daily
routine and you'll
add a pound of flab
in 2 weeks.

**Glacéau
Vitamin Energy
Dragonfruit**
(16 fl oz)

*200 calories
0 g fat
50 g sugars*

In the same boat as
Glacéau's vitamin
waters, which is to say,
nice on the nutrients,
but why so high
on the sugar?

**Sobe®
Energy™
Adrenaline
Rush®**
(16 fl oz)

*260 calories
0 g fat
66 g sugars*

If it's energy you seek,
then why take in all the
sugar? It will only set
you up for a big crash.

**Amp
Energy™**
(16 fl oz)

*220 calories
0 g fat
58 g sugars*

11% of your
day's calories and
more sugar than 4
scoops of Edy's Loaded
Peanut Butter Cup
ice cream.

Chocolate Milk and Mi

Drink This

This fermented dairy product from the Middle East tastes like drinkable yogurt and has been shown to lower cholesterol, enhance the immune system, and provide important gut-friendly bacteria.

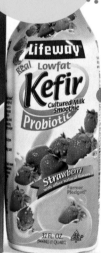

Lifeway® Lowfat Kefir Strawberry
(8 fl oz)

162 calories
2 g fat (1.5 g saturated)
21 g sugars

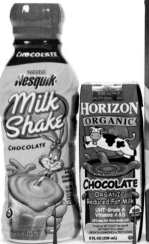

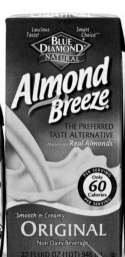

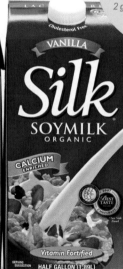

Nesquik® Milk Shake Chocolate
(8 fl oz)

180 calories
5 g fat (3 g saturated)
24 g sugars

With a name like chocolate milk shake, you'd expect this to be a full-on sugar nightmare, but with 20 percent less sugar than Nesquik's Chocolate Milk, it's actually quite manageable.

Horizon Organic® Reduced Fat Chocolate
(8 fl oz)

180 calories
5 g fat (3 g saturated)
27 g sugars

Organic milk completely free from unnatural pesticides, hormones, and chemicals.

Almond Breeze® Original
(8 fl oz)

60 calories
2.5 g fat (0 g saturated)
7 g sugars

Almond Breeze is the best of the milk substitutes, and it's fortified with vitamins A, E, and D.

Silk® Soymilk Vanilla
(8 fl oz)

100 calories
3.5 g fat (0.5 g saturated)
7 g sugars

Another benefit of Silk is that it's fortified with vitamin B_{12}, an essential vitamin that vegetarians struggle to get enough of as its only natural source is meat.

1k Substitutes
Not That!

Half this bottle has 10 percent
of your daily calories.

**Nesquik®
Strawberry Milk**
(8 fl oz)

*200 calories
5 g fat (3.5 g saturated)
29 g sugars*

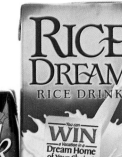

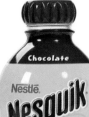

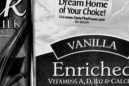

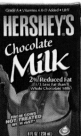

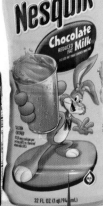

**Silk®
Soymilk
Chocolate**
(8.25 fl oz)

*150 calories
3.5 g fat (0 g saturated)
21 g sugars*

Is having chocolate over
vanilla worth taking in
three times the sugar?

**Rice Dream™
Vanilla**
(8 fl oz)

*130 calories
2.5 g fat (0 g saturated)
12 g sugars*

Rice Dream has almost
twice as much sugar
as Almond Breeze.

**Hershey's®
2% Reduced Fat
Chocolate**
(8 fl oz)

*200 calories
5 g fat (3 g saturated)
29 g sugars*

As a daily habit, the extra
20 calories amounts to a little
more than half a pound of
body fat every 3 months.

**Nesquik® Reduced
Fat Chocolate**
(8 fl oz)

*200 calories
5 g fat (3 g saturated)
29 g sugars*

Watch out: Many flavored-milk
products come in extra-large
servings, which means you need
to double or quadruple the
calorie and sugar counts to fully
assess the impact.

Beer

Drink This

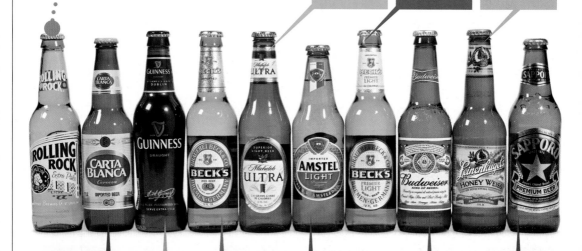

Rolling Rock® Extra Pale
(12 fl oz)
120 calories
10 g carbs
4.5% alcohol

Michelob Ultra™
(12 fl oz)
95 calories
2.6 g carbs
4.2% alcohol

Beck's® Premier Light
(12 fl oz)
64 calories
4 g carbs
3.8% alcohol

Leinenkugel's® Honey Weiss
(12 fl oz)
149 calories
12 g carbs
4.9% alcohol

Carta Blanca (12 fl oz)
128 calories
11 g carbs
4.0% alcohol

Guinness® Draught
(11.2 fl oz)
125 calories
10 g carbs
4% alcohol

Beck's®
(12 fl oz)
143 calories
10 g carbs
5% alcohol

Amstel® Light
(12 fl oz)
95 calories
5.5 g carbs
3.5% alcohol

Budweiser®
(12 fl oz)
143 calories
10.6 g carbs
5% alcohol

Sapporo
(12 fl oz)
140 calories
10.3 g carbs
5.2% alcohol

Not That!

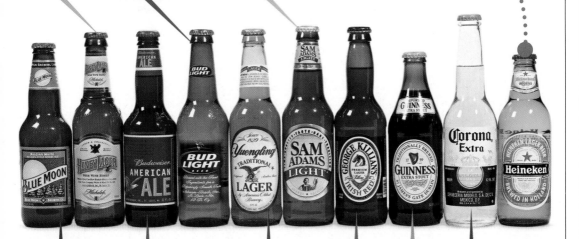

**Michelob®
Honey Lager**
(12 fl oz)

178 calories
19.2 g carbs
4.9% alcohol

Bud Light
(12 fl oz)

110 calories
6.6 g carbs
4.2% alcohol

**Sam Adams
Light®**
(12 fl oz)

119 calories
9.6 g carbs
4% alcohol

Heineken®
(12 fl oz)

166 calories
9.8 g carbs
5.4% alcohol

Blue Moon™
(12 fl oz)

171 calories
12.9 g carbs
5.4% alcohol

**Budweiser®
American Ale**
(12 fl oz)

182 calories
18.1 g carbs
5.3% alcohol

**Yuengling®
Lager**
(12 fl oz)

135 calories
12 g carbs
4.4% alcohol

**George
Killian's®
Irish Red**
(12 fl oz)

163 calories
13.8 g carbs
4.9% alcohol

**Guinness®
Extra Stoudt**
(12 fl oz)

176 calories
12 g carbs
7.5% alcohol

**Corona®
Extra** (12 fl oz)

148 calories
14 g carbs
4.6% alcohol

Mixers

Drink This

The goal with mixers is to keep the sugar count as low as possible. While you'd be better off making margaritas with fresh lime, this will work in a pinch.

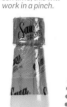
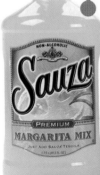
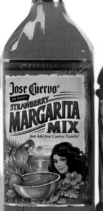
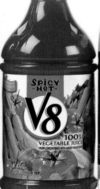
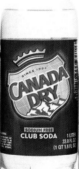
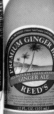
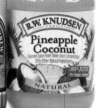

Sauza® Margarita Mix
(4 fl oz)

93 calories
0 g fat
24 g sugars

Jose Cuervo® Strawberry Margarita Mix
(4 fl oz)

100 calories
0 g fat
24 g sugars

Add rum and you've just turned it into a daiquiri, and you've saved a load of sugar calories in the process.

V8® Spicy Hot
(4 fl oz)

25 calories
0 g fat
4 g sugars
310 mg sodium

Low in sugar and high in nutrients, a Bloody Mary is one of the world's healthiest cocktails. By using V8, you'll cut down on the only real drawback—the salt.

Canada Dry® Club Soda
(8 fl oz)

0 calories
0 g fat
0 g sugars

Club soda and its cousin seltzer water are nothing more than carbonated water, which makes them the safest mixers at the party.

Reed's Premium Ginger Brew
(8 fl oz)

100 calories
0 g fat
22 g sugars

Ginger has many known health benefits; just don't fall for the imitation ales that include no actual ginger on their ingredient list, unlike this one.

R.W. Knudsen™ Pineapple Coconut 100% Juice (4 fl oz)

85 calories
0.5 g fat
(0 g saturated)
18.5 g sugars

This is the best piña-colada stand-in you'll find. It's 100% juice and contains no added sweeteners.

280

Not That!

1800™
The Ultimate™
Margarita Mix
(4 fl oz)

170 calories
0 g fat
38 g sugars

Ounce for ounce,
this mix is 3 times
sweeter than most
soda. An 8-ounce
margarita made with
this will top
400 calories.

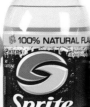

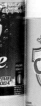

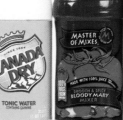

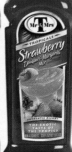

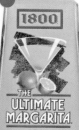

Master of Mixes®
Piña Colada
Mixer (4 fl oz)

210 calories
1.5 g fat
(0 g saturated)
50 g sugars

This typical piña colada
mix contains only 24%
actual juice. The rest
of the calories are
from high-fructose
corn syrup and sugar.

Sprite®
Lemon-Lime
Soda (8 fl oz)

100 calories
0 g fat
26 g sugars

Don't succumb to
the misconception that
Sprite is a "healthier"
soda. It has just as
many calories as nearly
every major type
of soda.

Canada Dry®
Tonic Water
(8 fl oz)

90 calories
0 g fat
23 g sugars

This tonic water is
made from carbonated
water, high-fructose
corn syrup, and
flavoring—basically a
glorified soft drink.

Master of Mixes®
Bloody Mary
Mixer Smooth
& Spicy
(4 fl oz)

50 calories
0 g fat
11 g sugars
910 mg sodium

This mix has as much
sodium as 2 full cups
of salted peanuts.

Mr & Mrs T®
Strawberry
Daiquiri-
Margarita Mix
(4 fl oz)

180 calories
0 g fat
44 g sugars

There's no nutrition
in all these calories,
just a lot of high-
fructose corn syrup.

Chapter 9

YOUR SAVE-MONEY SHOPPING GUIDE

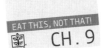

EAT THIS, NOT THAT!
CH. 9

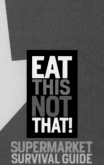

EAT THIS NOT THAT!

SUPERMARKET SURVIVAL GUIDE

Your Save-Money Shopping Guide

It used to be that certain culinary experiences were simply too expensive to contemplate: Taking a whirlwind tour of French wine country. Throwing a dinner party at the Russian Tea Room. Feasting on caviar while floating in a bathtub full of Cristal. Add to those impossible dreams another ridiculously expensive food-related endeavor: Shopping at your local supermarket.

In just the last 2 years, world prices for such staples as corn, wheat, and vegetable oil have risen a shocking 51 percent. And the foods made with, or fed by, these staples—everything from cookies and doughnuts to beef and chicken—have risen right along with them. A combination of high oil prices, bad weather, and a growing world population has turned up the heat on the competition for food.

Well, let me clarify: They've made the competition for healthy food heat up. The cost of vegetables, meat, fruit, and other high-nutrition, low-calorie foods has increased by an average of 19.5 percent over the last 2 years. But junk foods? Their prices have actually decreased slightly, by 1.8 percent. So our economic outlook is not only making it harder to make ends meet—it's making it harder to make the two ends of our belts meet. In fact, researchers recently estimated the cost of a diet based on high-calorie foods versus one based on healthy, low-calorie foods. The high-calorie diet you could eat for $3.52 a day. The low-cal diet? A whopping $36.32 per diem.

Now, that sounds pretty bad. But remember, people in the United States spend a smaller percentage of their incomes on food than almost any other people on Earth. In fact, today you're likely to spend just under 10 percent of what you earn on food. When your great-grandparents were trying to make ends meet in the late 1920s, they were spending a terrifying 24 percent of their income on food!

So all is not bleak, friend. Simply shopping at the supermarket saves you money over eating out. (That cup of latte you like in the morning? Brew your own joe each day and you'll save more than $800 a year!) And there is a lot that we can do to get in and out of the supermarket with as much nutrition—and as little financial damage—as possible.

● **Avoid quickies.** A study published by the Marketing Science Institute found that shoppers who made "quick trips" to the store purchased an average of 54 percent more merchan-dise than they planned. Instead, be thoughtful in your planning—keep a magnet-based notepad on your fridge and make notes throughout the week about what you need. (And avoiding extra trips will cut down on your gasoline costs as well.)

● **Bulk up.** Discount clubs are a great cost-saving alternative, even if you have to pay a fee to join. Not every-thing makes sense to buy in bulk, of course. (Nobody needs a 2-gallon drum of capers.) But focus on items

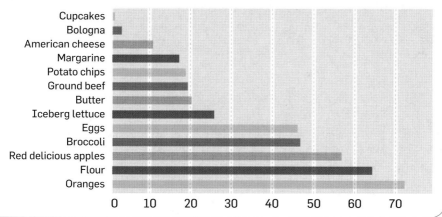

The Real Inflation Problem
Price increases are hitting you in places other than your wallet

Percent Increase for Common Food in Last 5 Years

Food	
Cupcakes	
Bologna	
American cheese	
Margarine	
Potato chips	
Ground beef	
Butter	
Iceberg lettuce	
Eggs	
Broccoli	
Red delicious apples	
Flour	
Oranges	

0   10   20   30   40   50   60   70

you use a lot of and that won't spoil, like paper products and frozen foods. Some shopping clubs also offer discounted gas. Cha-ching!

● **Watch your weight.** Okay, so one brand of crackers costs $4 and the other $4.50. But before you assume which is cheaper, take a closer look at the net weight. You'll often find the more expensive box contains more actual food—and as such, the food is really cheaper. Net weight is also a great way of making sure you're not paying for a lot of packaging, only to get home and discover most of what's inside the box is air.

● **Check yourself out.** Yes, they have those creepy mechanical voices and half the time you need to signal someone for help anyway, but self-checkout aisles offer one massive advantage, especially when you're shopping with kids: no checkout-line items for sale. Impulse purchases drop by 16.7 percent for men—and by 32.1 percent for women—when they use the self-checkout aisle, according to a study by the IHL Group research firm. (And you'll eat healthier too— 80 percent of candy and 61 percent of salty snacks are bought on impulse.)

● **Stay local.** A 2004 Tulane University study found that easy access to supermarket shopping was associated with increased household use of fruits (an extra 84 grams per adult daily).

● **Eat before you shop.** This is critical! A 2008 study in the *Journal of Consumer Research* found that consumers, even on a tight budget, are more likely to spend more if their appetite is stimulated before making a purchase. The study tested the reaction of women shoppers by placing hidden chocolate chip–scented candles in the room. Nearly 70 percent who got a whiff of the cookie scent said they would buy a new sweater even though they were on a tight budget, compared with only 17 percent of those who weren't exposed to the cookie smell. You just know the guys who run the bake shop at the supermarket have read this study too!

● **Stop the retail therapy.** Sadness increases the amount of money that shoppers are willing to spend, according to a 2008 study in *Psychological Science*. Study participants who watched a sad film were willing to pay four times as much for a product as those who watched a neutral film about nature.

● **Make Wednesday grocery night.**
One impetus to extra spending is being stuck on the checkout line for 15 minutes. But according to *Progressive Grocer,* only 11 percent of shoppers go to the store on Wednesdays, and only 4 percent of customers shop on any day after 9 p.m. If your store's open late, it might be the best way to avoid the crowds.

For more simple ways to save cash while maximizing nutrition, check out **eatthis.com**

The Growing Cost of *Not* Having a Shopping Strategy

Knowing which foods pack the most nutrition for the money is more important today than at any time in the last 35 years!

Food Price Inflation (average annual percent change by decade) FPI		Consumer Price Index for Food at Home 2002–2007 CPI	
1970s	8.1%	2002	1.3%
1980s	4.6%	2003	2.2%
1990s	2.8%	2004	3.8%
2000s	2.7%	2005	1.9%
2007	4.2%	2006	1.7%
April '08	5.1%	2007	4.2%

Source: Trends and Economic Research Service, through Anne-Marie Roerink, director of research at Food Marketing Institute

287

Cook This, Not That!

10 American Classics, Redefined

Even in these lean times, Americans will still spend half of their food dollars—nearly $500 billion—eating out this year. That's a staggering number, especially when you consider the type of slop they're serving us: 1,500-calorie salads at IHOP, a pancake at Bob Evans with more sugar than 2 pints of Ben & Jerry's Butter Pecan ice cream, a plate of Aussie Cheese Fries at Outback with more calories than 10 Krispy Kreme Original Glazed Doughnuts! To add insult to injury, they expect us to shell out three to four times what it would cost us to make the same lousy dish at home. Enough.

The best way to take control of your diet at the same time as taking control of your food finances is to grab a chef's knife and a sauté pan and start cooking. According to studies, people consume 50 percent more calories, fat, and sodium when they eat out than when they cook at home. Add to that the fact that you're likely to save some serious coin with a bit of savvy shopping and you have a potent case for the power of a little down-home cooking.

In hopes of inspiring you to turn up the heat in your kitchen, we've taken 10 of America's most popular dishes and remade them, with quality nutrition, prudent spending, and maximum gustatory pleasure all considered in equal measure. As you'll see with the calorie comparisons we provide, these also happen to be 10 dishes the restaurant industry has egregiously hijacked and corrupted. To help you take back the food you love most, we built each recipe around some of the finest products in the supermarket which, when combined together, make for some top-notch eating on a shoestring.

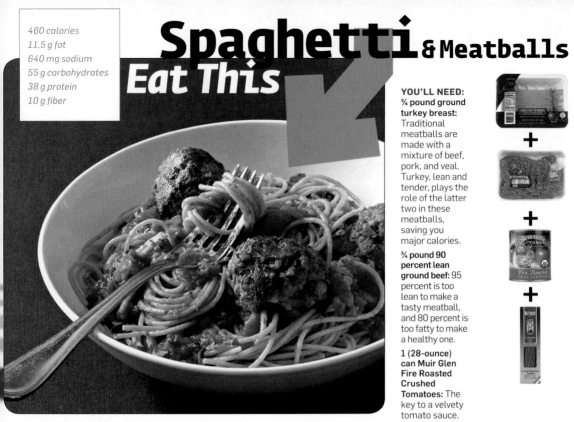

460 calories
11.5 g fat
640 mg sodium
55 g carbohydrates
38 g protein
10 g fiber

Spaghetti &Meatballs
Eat This

YOU'LL NEED:

¾ pound ground turkey breast: Traditional meatballs are made with a mixture of beef, pork, and veal. Turkey, lean and tender, plays the role of the latter two in these meatballs, saving you major calories.

¾ pound 90 percent lean ground beef: 95 percent is too lean to make a tasty meatball, and 80 percent is too fatty to make a healthy one.

1 (28-ounce) can Muir Glen Fire Roasted Crushed Tomatoes: The key to a velvety tomato sauce. And the fire-roasting makes it taste like it cooked all day.

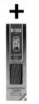

12 ounces DeCecco Whole Wheat Spaghetti: 7 grams of fiber and 8 grams of protein a serving make a strong case for wheat over white pasta.

How to make it

Mix the meat, egg, bread crumbs, parsley, half of the onion and garlic, and the salt and pepper. Form into golf balls.

Heat half the olive oil in a large nonstick skillet and cook the meatballs over medium heat until well browned. Reserve.

Heat the remaining olive oil in a saucepan and cook the remaining onion and garlic over medium heat until translucent. Add the tomatoes and bring to a simmer. Add the meatballs into the sauce and cook for 15 to 20 minutes.

Cook the pasta according to the package instructions. Divide it among plates, top with a few meatballs and sauce, and garnish with parsley.

Makes 6 servings / Price per serving: $2.28

YOU'LL ALSO NEED:

1	egg
½	cup bread crumbs
½	cup chopped parsley
1	onion, minced
3	garlic cloves, minced
¾	tsp salt
½	tsp black pepper
1	Tbsp olive oil

Not That!

Romano's Macaroni Grill Spaghetti & Meatballs

1,430 calories
81 g fat (41 g saturated)
4,540 mg sodium

ChickenWings

260 calories
10 g fat
(5 g saturated)
740 mg sodium
5 g carbohydrates
34 g protein
1 g fiber

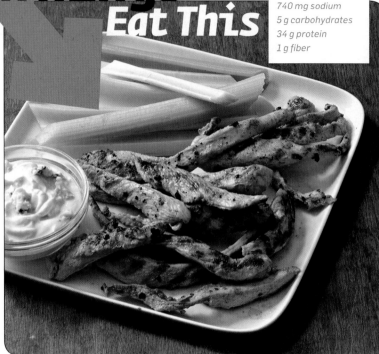

+

+

+

YOU'LL NEED:
1 pound boneless, skinless chicken breast, cut into ½-inch-thick strips: At just 31 calories an ounce, each strip will cut nearly 40 calories from a traditional fried wing. Save extra cash by buying a bag of frozen chicken breasts, then cutting each breast into ½-inch-thick strips.

½ cup Frank's Red Hot Wing Sauce: Most restaurants make their wing sauce with half butter, half hot sauce. Frank's comes without a lick of fat—just vinegar and chili pepper.

⅛ teaspoon cayenne pepper: Capsaicin, found prominently in both the cayenne and the hot sauce, has been shown to boost metabolism.

½ cup Fage 2% Yogurt: It's not just the wings that cost calories—it's the ubiquitous vat of blue cheese that accompanies them. This yogurt-based version gives you the same cooling effect without all of the unnecessary fat.

Not That!

Uno Chicago Buffalo Wings (6 wings)

450 calories
35 g fat
(7 g saturated)
700 mg sodium
24 g protein

YOU'LL ALSO NEED:

½ tsp garlic powder

½ tsp black pepper

¼ cup blue cheese

Worcestershire sauce

1 Tbsp white wine vinegar

16 celery sticks

How to make it

Mix the tenders, hot sauce, cayenne, garlic powder, and black pepper in a large sealable bag and let marinate in the refrigerator for at least 30 minutes and up to 4 hours.

Preheat a grill or a broiler. Remove tenders from the bag and cook for 3 to 4 minutes a side until lightly browned all over.

Combine the yogurt, blue cheese, a few shakes of Worcestershire, and vinegar. Serve the wings with the blue cheese dressing and the celery sticks on the side.

Makes 4 servings / Cost per serving: $2.69

Hearty Lasagna
Eat This

430 calories
13 g fat
(4.5 g saturated)
810 mg sodium
47 g carbohydrates
28 g protein
2 g fiber

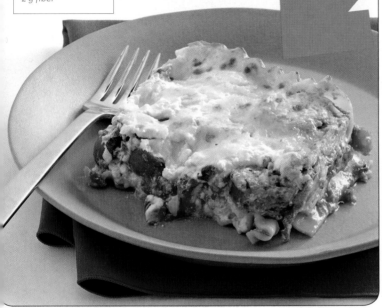

How to make it

Mix the ricotta, basil, sausage, milk, garlic, chili flakes, and salt.

Spread ½ cup of the tomato sauce on the bottom of an 8 × 8-inch baking dish. Lay two noodles over the sauce; cover with ⅓ of the ricotta mixture and another ½ cup of the tomato sauce. Repeat with noodles, ⅓ cheese mixture, and ½ cup sauce twice more. Top with last layer of pasta, remaining ricotta mixture and sauce, and Parmesan.

Cover with foil and bake at 425°F for 20 minutes. Remove the foil and bake another 15 minutes, until the top is golden.

Makes 4 servings / Cost per serving: $3.50

YOU'LL ALSO NEED:
¼ cup milk

2¼ cups Muir Glen Tomato Basil Pasta Sauce

2 garlic cloves, minced

½ tsp red chili flakes

⅛ tsp salt

¼ cup grated Parmesan cheese

YOU'LL NEED:
1 (15-ounce) container part-skim ricotta: Real Italian lasagna isn't made with mozzarella, and neither is this one. Instead, ricotta is thinned out with a touch of fat-free milk, which cuts calories and cash and gives this lasagna a more authentic taste.

½ bunch fresh basil, chopped: Tons of flavor and antioxidants and calorie free: why not use it? Use the other half to make fresh pesto or fold it into your next scramble.

2 links Al Fresco Sundried Tomato and Basil Chicken Sausage, diced: One of the best sausages in the supermarket. Low on ingredients and calories, heavy on flavor and protein.

8 Barilla Oven Ready Lasagne noodles: Most lasagna noodles need to be fully cooked before baking, but these sheets are ready for building right out of the box. Just make sure they're fully covered with sauce.

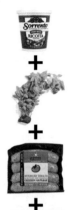

Not That!

Sbarro's Meat Lasagna
650 calories
37 g fat
1,170 mg sodium

Eggs Benedict

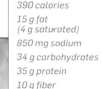

390 calories
15 g fat
(4 g saturated)
850 mg sodium
34 g carbohydrates
35 g protein
10 g fiber

YOU'LL NEED:

1 cup Fage 2% Yogurt: Traditional hollandaise—made from egg yolks and melted butter—is a disaster. Thinned out with a bit of fresh lemon juice and hot sauce, this low-fat yogurt makes a perfect substitute.

1 package Hormel Canadian Bacon, sliced into thin pieces: Considerably leaner than standard bacon, the Canadian kind is the best of all breakfast meats.

1 box frozen spinach, thawed and squeezed dry: Fresh spinach is 90 percent water, which is why that $3 bunch is reduced to a tiny pile as soon as it hits the pan. Frozen spinach is pre-cooked, so it maintains its mass.

8 large Eggland's Best Eggs: Eggs are one of the planet's great sources of low-cost protein. This brand comes infused with healthy omega-3s.

4 Thomas' Light Multi-Grain English Muffins, toasted: 8 grams of fiber per muffin turn these muffins into potent hunger killers.

Not That!

Bob Evans Spinach, Bacon & Tomato Country Benedict

729 calories
48 g fat (16 g saturated, 5 g trans)
1,885 mg sodium

YOU'LL ALSO NEED:

8–10 dashes of your hot sauce

Juice of 1 lemon

Salt and pepper

½ tsp extra-virgin olive oil

¼ tsp white distilled vinegar

How to make it

Mix the yogurt, hot sauce, and lemon juice. Season to taste with salt and pepper. Heat a skillet, add the oil, and cook the bacon until firm. Add the spinach and cook until warm.

Bring 2 inches of water to a simmer in a large skillet; stir in the vinegar and bring to a boil. Crack an egg into a small cup and carefully slip into the water. Repeat. Cook each egg until the white is firmly set, about 3 to 4 minutes, and remove.

Top each English muffin half with the spinach, a poached egg, and the yogurt sauce.

Makes 4 servings / Cost per serving: $3.94

350 calories
10 g fat
(3 g saturated)
670 mg sodium
31 g carbohydrates
40 g protein
6 g fiber

Turkey-Swiss-Guac Burger

Eat This

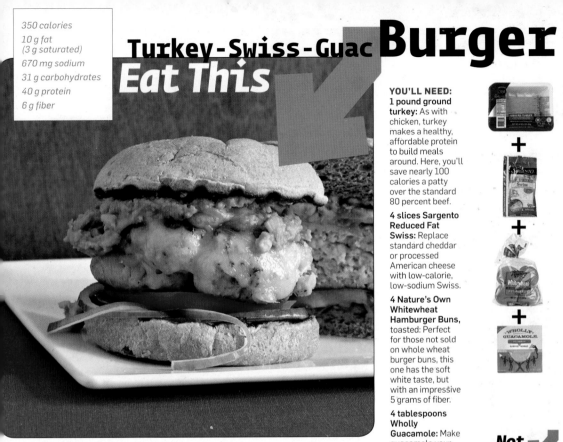

YOU'LL NEED:
1 pound ground turkey: As with chicken, turkey makes a healthy, affordable protein to build meals around. Here, you'll save nearly 100 calories a patty over the standard 80 percent beef.

4 slices Sargento Reduced Fat Swiss: Replace standard cheddar or processed American cheese with low-calorie, low-sodium Swiss.

4 Nature's Own Whitewheat Hamburger Buns, toasted: Perfect for those not sold on whole wheat burger buns, this one has the soft white taste, but with an impressive 5 grams of fiber.

4 tablespoons Wholly Guacamole: Make guacamole your go-to secret sauce: It has more than half of the calories of mayo and three times the nutrition.

How to make it

Mix the turkey, salt, and pepper and shape into 4 patties.

Preheat a grill, grill pan, or cast-iron skillet. Cook the patties over medium-high heat until lightly charred on the outside, about 4 minutes, then flip. Place a tablespoon of the chiles on top of each patty, then cover with a slice of Swiss. Cook until the patty is firm, about 8 to 10 minutes total.

Dress buns with tomato and onion slices, top with the burgers, and slather with the guacamole.

Makes 4 servings / Cost per serving: $3.76

YOU'LL ALSO NEED:
½ tsp salt
½ tsp black pepper
4 Tbsp Ortega chopped green chiles
2 tomatoes, sliced
1 red onion, sliced

Not That!

Ruby Tuesday Avocado Turkey Burger

1,026 calories
62 g fat
(0 g saturated)
49 g carbohydrates
7 g fiber

293

Steak Tacos

YOU'LL NEED:

2 chipotle peppers in adobo: A super-versatile secret weapon. These smoked jalapeños, canned in a spicy vinegar and tomato sauce, make great instant marinades, salsa bases, and soup enhancers. A $2 can will provide enough flavor for dozens of meals.

1 pound flank steak: Flank is a perfect lean cut for tacos. Plus it's much cheaper than nutritionally inferior steaks like strip and rib eye.

8 (6") Mission White Corn Tortillas: Tacos in Mexico are made with corn tortillas, which have 50 percent more fiber and less than half the calories of the flour tortillas American restaurants favor.

¼ cup Wholly Guacamole: Skip the sour cream and shredded cheese—neither is traditional or particularly nutritious. Guac, however, is both. Making it at home is simple, but if you buy it, make sure avocado is the first ingredient.

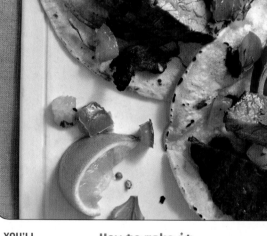

Eat This

250 calories
7 g fat
(1.5 g saturated)
310 mg sodium
31 g carbohydrates
16 g protein
5 g fiber

Not That!

Chevy's Grilled Steak Tacos

1,090 calories
43 g fat
(13 g saturated)
2,600 mg sodium

YOU'LL ALSO NEED:

1 cup OJ
1 tsp cumin
2 garlic cloves
2 cups cilantro
½ tsp salt
½ tsp black pepper
Your favorite salsa
1 red onion, minced
2 limes, quartered

How to make it

Combine the chipotle, OJ, cumin, garlic, and cilantro in a blender and puree. Place the steak and marinade in a sealable plastic bag and refrigerate for 30 minutes or more.

Remove the steak from the marinade. Season with salt and pepper. Heat a grill or cast-iron skillet over high heat. Cook the beef for 3 to 4 minutes per side (for medium-rare).

Heat the tortillas until warm and pliable. Slice the steak into thin pieces and divide it among the tortillas. Top with guacamole, salsa, onions, extra cilantro, and a squirt of fresh lime juice.

Makes 4 2-taco servings / Cost per serving: $3.69

Fish and Chips

Eat This

320 calories
3.5 g fat
(0 g saturated)
770 mg sodium
23 g carbohydrates
46 g protein
3 g fiber

How to make it

Toss the sweet potatoes with the oil, half of the salt and pepper, and the paprika. Arrange on a baking tray and place in a 425°F oven.

While the fries cook, whisk the egg whites, Dijon, cayenne, and remaining salt and pepper. Combine the bread crumbs and thyme in a shallow dish. Dip the fish in the egg whites, then carefully roll in the crumb mixture.

After the fries have cooked for 15 minutes, add the fish and return to the oven. Cook for another 12 to 15 minutes, until the fish flakes easily with a fork. Serve with lemon or vinegar.

Makes 4 servings / Cost per serving: $4.92

YOU'LL ALSO NEED:

½ Tbsp olive oil
1   tsp salt
1   tsp black pepper
2   egg whites
1   Tbsp Dijon mustard
⅛   tsp cayenne pepper
½   tsp dried thyme
Lemon slices or malt vinegar

YOU'LL NEED:

2 medium sweet potatoes, peeled and cut into large wedges: Russet potatoes are long on antioxidants, but sweet potatoes bring to the table extra fiber and beta-carotene.

+

½ teaspoon smoked paprika (called pimentón): If you try one new spice this year, make this it. Made from slow-smoked Spanish red peppers, it adds big flavor to any meat or vegetable it touches.

+

1 cup panko bread crumbs: These flat, delicate Japanese-style bread crumbs produce a lighter, less dense but no less crispy crust on whatever they cover.

+

4 (6-ounce) halibut fillets, skin removed: Halibut ranks number 3 in "The Eat This, Not That! Fish Finder" on page 53, which takes into account omega-3 levels, contaminants, and environmental friendliness. Want to save a little bit more cash? Pick up catfish fillets instead (they rank number 4).

Not That!

Denny's Fish and Chips

1,080 calories

*49 g fat
(9 g saturated)*

1,650 mg sodium

117 g carbohydrates

40 g protein

8 g fiber

Blueberry **Pancakes**
Eat This

310 calories
8 g fat
(3.5 g saturated)
500 mg sodium
47 g carbohydrates
20 g protein
6 g fiber

YOU'LL NEED:

2 cups frozen wild blueberries: Cheap syrup is made from pure high-fructose corn syrup, and real maple syrup can run up to $12 per bottle. Instead, top your pancakes with this super-simple blueberry compote. It takes 10 minutes to make and brings the fruit's potent cache of phytonutrients to the breakfast table.

1 cup cottage cheese: A great, inexpensive way to force out some of the troublesome carbs in pancakes and replace them with protein.

1 cup Fage 0% Yogurt: Yogurt adds another shot of lean protein, plus a host of stomach-friendly bacteria. More important, it helps make these unique pancakes creamy and super tender.

1 cup King Arthur Whole Wheat Flour: Cut back on the refined flour by replacing regular all-purpose flour with a bag of whole wheat flour. King Arthur's brings 33 percent more protein and three times the fiber to baked goods.

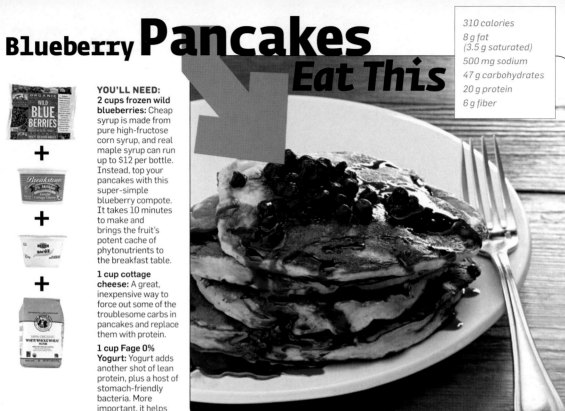

Not That!

IHOP Blueberry pancakes

710 calories

(IHOP does not provide anything other than calorie counts for its menu items.)

YOU'LL ALSO NEED:

½ cup water
¼ cup sugar
3 eggs
Juice of 1 lemon
½ tsp baking soda
Pinch of salt

How to make it

Combine the blueberries, water, and sugar in a saucepan and cook over low heat for 10 minutes, stirring often, until the blueberries begin to break apart.

Beat together the cottage cheese, yogurt, eggs, and lemon juice. Mix the baking soda, flour, and salt. Stir the flour mixture into the dairy and mix just enough to blend.

Heat a skillet over medium-low heat. Coat with nonstick spray and add batter in large spoonfuls (about ¼ cup). Flip when the tops begin to bubble, 3 to 5 minutes, and cook the second side until browned. Serve with the warm compote.

Makes 4 servings / Cost per serving: $2.23

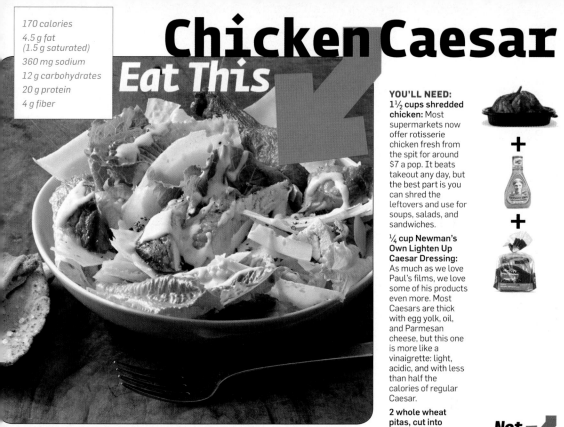

170 calories
4.5 g fat
(1.5 g saturated)
360 mg sodium
12 g carbohydrates
20 g protein
4 g fiber

Chicken Caesar

Eat This

YOU'LL NEED:
1½ cups shredded chicken: Most supermarkets now offer rotisserie chicken fresh from the spit for around $7 a pop. It beats takeout any day, but the best part is you can shred the leftovers and use for soups, salads, and sandwiches.

¼ cup Newman's Own Lighten Up Caesar Dressing: As much as we love Paul's films, we love some of his products even more. Most Caesars are thick with egg yolk, oil, and Parmesan cheese, but this one is more like a vinaigrette: light, acidic, and less than half the calories of regular Caesar.

2 whole wheat pitas, cut into wedges, tossed with olive oil, and toasted: Don't trust food companies with croutons—they'll just drop bread in the fryer and call it quits. By starting with a low-carb, fiber-rich pita, you get the crunch you want with the salad for a tiny fraction of the calories.

How to make it

Combine the chicken, romaine, dressing, and Parmesan cheese. Mix thoroughly until all leaves are evenly coated. Serve the salad with the pita croutons and lots of fresh cracked pepper.

Makes 4 servings / Cost per serving: $2.13

YOU'LL ALSO NEED:
1 head romaine lettuce, roughly chopped
¼ cup grated Parmesan cheese
Cracked black pepper

Not That!

Chili's Caesar Salad with Grilled Chicken and Caesar Dressing

1,010 calories
76 g fat
(13 g saturated)
1,910 mg sodium

Pizza

YOU'LL NEED:

12" Boboli 100% Whole Wheat Thin Crust: Swapping Boboli's standard dough for their new whole wheat crust will save you 370 calories per pie, plus add an extra 17 grams of fiber. Or make personal pizzas on Thomas' Light Multi-Grain English Muffins.

1 cup Muir Glen Tomato Basil Pasta Sauce: One of our favorite products from one of our favorite companies. Can't find this? Try Classico.

2 cups Kraft Natural Low-Moisture Part-Skim Mozzarella Shreds: Real Italian pizza is made with fresh buffalo mozzarella, but at $12 a pound, it's not cheap. These part-skim shreds do the trick for a fraction of the coin and calories.

Hormel Turkey Pepperoni: The most popular topping in America is also the most fattening, at least when it's made with pork. This turkey version cuts the calories in half and the fat in third.

Not That!

Pizza Hut Supreme Pan Pizza (2 slices)

620 calories
32 g fat (12 g saturated)
1,440 mg sodium

298

YOU'LL ALSO NEED:

- ½ onion, sliced
- ½ cup roasted red peppers
- ½ cup chopped green olives
- 2 garlic cloves, minced
- ½ tsp chili flakes
- 1 (6-oz) jar artichoke hearts
- 1 cup fresh basil

Eat This

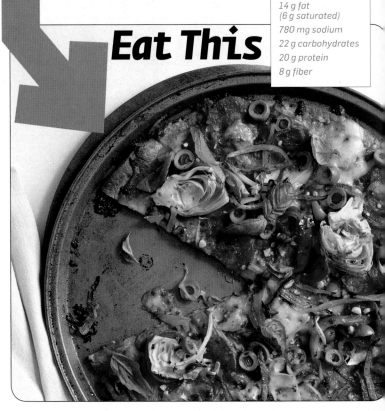

300 calories
14 g fat (6 g saturated)
780 mg sodium
22 g carbohydrates
20 g protein
8 g fiber

How to make it

Preheat the oven to 400°F. Cover the crust with sauce and then cheese. Sprinkle the remaining ingredients (minus the basil) over the pizza. Bake for 12 to 15 minutes, until the cheese is melted and bubbling. Top with the basil and serve immediately.

Makes 4 servings / Cost per serving: $4.07

Shop Once, Eat for a Week

10 simple-to-make meals that fight fat, build muscle, and save you time—all for less than 50 bucks

You might not use the terms "pizza box" and "serving dish" interchangeably, but if you're like most people, you probably could. That's because 64 percent of people spend little or no time preparing their meals. Their excuse? Time and money constraints. Unfortunately—and perhaps not coincidentally—that number parallels the 66 percent who are overweight or obese. It's no wonder: The inexpensive, time-saving foods that people choose most often are also the ones that are the highest in sugar, fat, and calories, according to a recent study from the University of Washington.

Thankfully, we have a culinary solution that'll perfectly fit your budget, schedule, and diet. The plan: Set aside 20 minutes on Sunday to fulfill our 16-item shopping list, then forget about your wallet—and collection of takeout menus—for the rest of the work week. By following our 5-day menu, you'll have the precise number of ingredients to create 10 fast, flavorful meals, all of which are designed to help melt fat while saving you money. (The average price of 10 meals eaten out: about $120; the total price of our meals: $47.96.) Each night, you'll simply prepare a quick and easy dinner and then creatively use the leftovers to assemble the next day's lunch. Call it the mixologist's guide to eating. The best part? While others are stuck on hold in drive-thrus, you'll be rolling through the express line with your next 10 meals in tow.

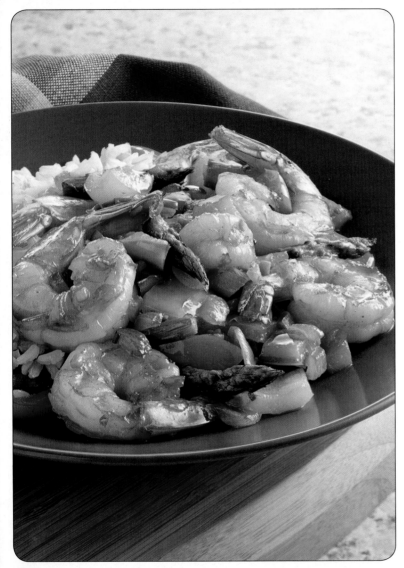

Rotisserie Chicken
with Vegetables

YOU'LL NEED:

¾ bunch asparagus (about 8
    spears)

3 portobello mushroom caps,
   sliced ¼" thick

2 onions, cut in ¼"-thick rings

½ Tbsp extra-virgin olive oil

Salt and pepper

1 rotisserie chicken breast or leg

1 cup mixed greens, dressed with
   olive oil and balsamic vinegar

HOW TO MAKE IT

Preheat the oven to 400°F.
Remove the woody ends of the
asparagus by gently bending
each stalk until it breaks—it'll
naturally snap off at the right
spot. In a baking dish, toss the
vegetables with the oil and
season with salt and pepper.
Roast for 15 to 20 minutes, until
the vegetables have developed
a light brown crust. Serve half
of the vegetables with the
chicken and the salad.

Makes 1 serving

Reserve the other half of the
vegetables and the remaining
chicken for other meals this
week. To chop the chicken,
remove the skin and use a fork
to pull the meat from the bones.
Then place the meat on your
cutting board and cut it into
bite-size pieces—it should yield
about 3 cups' worth for later in
the week.

*Per serving: 430 calories, 25 g fat
(7 g saturated), 36 g protein,
18 g carbohydrates, 5 g fiber*

Chicken Portobello Wrap with Balsamic Aioli

YOU'LL NEED:

1 cup chopped rotisserie chicken (left over from Sunday's dinner)

3 bell peppers

1 clove garlic, minced

1 Tbsp reduced-fat mayonnaise

1 tsp balsamic vinegar

1 whole-wheat tortilla

2 Tbsp shredded mozzarella

1 small handful mixed greens

1 cup leftover asparagus, mushrooms, and onions

HOW TO MAKE IT

Measure out the chicken and put the rest away for later in the week. Chop the peppers into ½" pieces: They should yield about 4 cups; use ½ cup today and save the rest in a plastic bag for tonight's dinner, Wednesday's dinner, and Thursday's lunch and dinner.

Mix the garlic, mayonnaise, and vinegar to make the aioli. Brush the tortilla with the aioli, then put the cheese down the middle, followed by the greens, chicken, and vegetables. To make a tight wrap, fold the bottom of the tortilla up first, then roll it from the side.

Makes 1 serving

Per serving: 400 calories, 15 g fat (4.5 g saturated), 43 g protein, 29 g carbohydrates, 5 g fiber

Shrimp Fajitas

YOU'LL NEED:

¼ cup instant brown rice (measured dry)

½ can black beans, drained and heated

½ Tbsp canola or other cooking oil

1 onion, sliced

1 cup chopped bell pepper (left over from Monday's lunch)

2 garlic cloves, chopped

8 oz frozen shrimp, defrosted

Cayenne pepper, crushed red pepper, or Tabasco to taste

½ tsp cumin

Salt and black pepper

½ avocado, pitted, peeled, and thinly sliced

1 whole-wheat tortilla, warmed

HOW TO MAKE IT

Cook the rice according to the package directions, then add the beans. Heat the oil in a large skillet or wok over high heat. Add the onion, the bell pepper, and garlic; cook for 5 to 7 minutes, until the vegetables begin to brown. Mix in the shrimp and spices; cook for another 3 minutes, until the shrimp are pink and firm. Serve half of the shrimp fajita mix with a small scoop of the rice and beans, the avocado slices, and the tortilla.

Makes 1 serving

Reserve the rest of the rice and beans in a microwavable bowl or plastic container along with the leftover fajita mix and use them for tomorrow's lunch.

Wrap the leftover avocado well and refrigerate to minimize browning.

Per serving: 602 calories, 22.5 g fat (3 g saturated), 42 g protein, 71 g carbohydrates, 15 g fiber

Classic Kitchen Skill #178: Mincing Garlic

You can buy the jarred stuff, but precut garlic lacks many of the essential oils that give this classic vegetable its intense (and addictive) flavor. For the full garlicky effect, you need to mince it yourself—preferably just before using it. Here's how: Lay a clove, still in its papery skin, on a cutting board. Place a heavy knife flat on top and whack it with a tight fist to flatten the clove. Peel off the skin and use the knife to slice the clove lengthwise into thin planks. Rotate the slices 90 degrees and repeat for a fine mince.

Fiesta Rice Bowl

YOU'LL NEED:

Rice, beans, and fajita mix
(left over from Monday's dinner)

½ avocado, peeled and thinly sliced

Salsa (optional)

HOW TO MAKE IT

Heat the leftovers in a plastic
container or a microwavable
bowl for 60 seconds. Top with
the avocado and salsa to taste,
if desired.

Makes 1 serving

*Per serving: 650 calories,
20 g fat (3 g saturated),
37 g protein, 85 g carbohydrates,
20 g fat (3 g saturated), 16 g fiber*

Fettuccine with Chicken, Roasted Vegetables, and Sun-Dried Tomato Pesto

YOU'LL NEED:

6 oz 100% whole-wheat fettuccine

½ Tbsp canola oil

1 cup chopped rotisserie chicken
(left over from Sunday's dinner)

1 cup roasted vegetables
(left over from Sunday's dinner)

1½ Tbsps sun-dried-tomato pesto

Salt and black pepper

Parmesan cheese

1 cup mixed greens, dressed with
olive oil and balsamic vinegar

HOW TO MAKE IT

Cook the fettuccine according to
the package directions. Drain.
Toss half of the pasta with the
oil and reserve in a container for
Thursday's lunch. Mix the chicken,
vegetables, and pesto with the
remaining pasta. Season with salt
and pepper. Grate some Parmesan
and sprinkle on top. Serve with the
greens.

Makes 1 serving

*Per serving: 490 calories, 20 g fat
(5 g saturated), 46 g protein,
34 g carbohydrates, 6 g fiber*

Italian Quesadilla

YOU'LL NEED:

1 Tbsp sun-dried-tomato pesto

1 whole-wheat tortilla

½ cup shredded mozzarella cheese

½ cup chopped rotisserie chicken
(left over from Sunday's dinner)

1 cup roasted vegetables
(left over from Sunday's dinner)

HOW TO MAKE IT

Spread the pesto on the tortilla.
Top with the cheese, chicken,
and vegetables. Microwave
open-faced for 1 minute, until
the cheese has fully melted.
Fold over and slice into
quarters. If you have time, try
cooking it over low heat in a
skillet for a crispier result.

Makes 1 serving

*Per serving: 440 calories, 19 g fat
(8 g saturated), 38 g protein,
32 g carbohydrates, 4 g fiber*

Spicy Shrimp-and-Asparagus Stir-Fry

YOU'LL NEED:

½ cup instant brown rice
(measured dry)

1 tsp canola or other cooking oil

½ onion, chopped

1 cup chopped bell peppers
(left over from Monday's lunch)

2 garlic cloves, chopped

1 cup chopped raw asparagus
spears (the remainder of the
bunch from Sunday's dinner)

8 oz frozen shrimp, defrosted

1 Tbsp low-sodium soy sauce

Hot sauce (we like Thai sriracha)

Salt and black pepper

HOW TO MAKE IT

Cook the rice according to the
package directions. Add the oil
to a large skillet or wok and
place over high heat. When the
oil is smoking, add the onion,
bell peppers, garlic, and
asparagus, then stir-fry for 5
minutes, until the vegetables
have browned slightly. Stir in
the shrimp, soy sauce, and hot
sauce to taste; cook for an
additional 3 minutes. Season
with salt and pepper and serve
half of it over the brown rice.

Makes 1 serving

Reserve the remaining stir-fry
for lunch tomorrow.

*Per serving: 592 calories, 11 g fat
(2 g saturated), 36 g protein,
88 g carbohydrates, 9 g fiber*

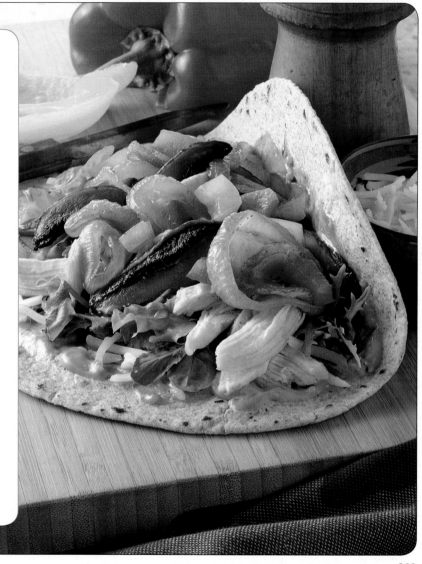

The Pantry List

Buy these crucial building blocks every couple of months and you'll always have them on hand to construct meals around the clock.

- Balsamic vinegar
- Mayonnaise, reduced fat
- Dijon mustard
- Olive oil, extra virgin
- Parmesan cheese
- Peanut butter
- Salsa
- Soy sauce, low sodium
- Tabasco or other hot sauce

Thai Peanut Noodles

YOU'LL NEED:
- 1 cup shrimp stir-fry (left over from Wednesday's dinner)
- 3 oz cooked whole-wheat fettuccine (left over from Tuesday's dinner)
- 1 Tbsp peanut butter
- ½ Tbsp low-sodium soy sauce
- 1 Tbsp water
- Splash of vinegar or orange juice
- ½ tsp black pepper
- Hot sauce
- 1 Tbsp chopped peanuts (optional)

HOW TO MAKE IT
Toss the shrimp stir-fry with the leftover pasta. In a separate bowl, whisk together the peanut butter, soy sauce, water, vinegar, and pepper. Add the peanut-butter mixture and hot sauce to taste to the pasta mixture and mix thoroughly. Top with peanuts, if desired. Eat cold or at room temperature.

Makes 1 serving

Per serving: 530 calories, 12 g fat (2 g saturated), 43 g protein, 63 g carbohydrates, 7 g fiber

The Grocery List

A balance of protein-packed meats, fresh produce, and a few versatile extras is all you need to feed yourself well week after week.

- **Frozen shrimp** 1 pound uncooked, medium size
- **Rotisserie chicken** 1 cooked
- **Pork tenderloin** 1 herb-flavored or lemon-garlic marinated (about ¾ pound)
- **Bell peppers** 1 tray tricolor (or pick out 1 red, 1 yellow, and 1 orange)
- **Yellow onions** 2½ pounds, medium size
- **Baby mixed greens** 4-ounce bag, washed
- **Portobello mushrooms** 3 large caps
- **Asparagus** 1 bunch
- **Garlic** 1 head
- **Sun-dried-tomato pesto** 8-ounce jar
- **Avocado** 1 ripe
- **Mozzarella** 8-ounce bag of shredded
- **Instant brown rice** 1-pound box
- **Black beans** 12-ounce can
- **100% whole wheat fettuccine** 16-ounce box
- **100% whole wheat tortillas** 1 package, 10" size

Roasted Pork Loin
With Peppers And Balsamic Onions

YOU'LL NEED:
- 1 pork tenderloin, about ¾ pound (herb or lemon-garlic marinated, if available; check the meat section)
- 1 onion, quartered
- 1½ cups chopped peppers (left over from Monday's lunch)
- 2 garlic cloves, crushed
- 1 Tbsp extra-virgin olive oil
- 1 Tbsp balsamic vinegar
- Salt and pepper

HOW TO MAKE IT
Preheat the oven to 450°F. In a baking dish, toss together the pork, onion, peppers, garlic, oil, and vinegar. Season with salt and pepper. Bake for 20 to 25 minutes, depending on the thickness of the tenderloin (to an internal temperature of 150°F, if using a meat thermometer). Enjoy half of the pork and vegetables tonight. (If

you want a bigger meal, prepare ¼ cup of instant brown rice, measured dry. It'll add 170 calories, 4 g protein, 36 g carbohydrates, 1 g fat, and 2 g fiber to the nutrition information below.)

Makes 1 serving

Save the remainder of the pork and vegetables—storing both together in a sealed container—for lunch tomorrow.

Per serving: 350 calories, 17 g fat (3.5 g saturated), 37 g protein, 12 g carbohydrates, 2 g fiber

FRIDAY LUNCH

Roasted Pork Wrap

YOU'LL NEED:
- ½ Tbsp sun-dried-tomato pesto
- ½ Tbsp reduced-fat mayonnaise
- 1 whole-wheat tortilla
- 2 Tbsps shredded mozzarella cheese

Vegetables and pork tenderloin, thinly sliced (left over from Thursday's dinner)

HOW TO MAKE IT
Mix the pesto and mayonnaise and spread over the tortilla. Layer the cheese, pork slices, and leftover vegetables on top and wrap it up.

Makes 1 serving

Per serving: 480 calories, 16 g fat (5 g saturated), 48 g protein, 37 g carbohydrates, 3 g fiber

Five Cheap Eats You Can't Beat
Stretch your dollar and maximize nutrition with these prudent picks

Frozen chicken breasts: A tremendous source of lean protein for about half the price of fresh chicken. In our taste tests, where we seasoned and grilled chicken breasts, we found it impossible to tell the difference between fresh and frozen.

Canola oil: Save the pricey olive oil for dressing salads or drizzling lightly over grilled vegetables. Canola's neutral flavor is great for cooking, and it happens to have an even better ratio of monounsaturated to saturated fat than the vaunted extra virgin. Olive can cost as much as a dollar per ounce, while high-end canola oil costs about $.25.

Dry lentils: For about the price of a bottle of water you can boil up a massive pot of soup- and salad-ready lentils. A pound-size bag has 11 grams of fiber and 10 grams of protein in each of its 13 servings. It's also one of the world's richest sources of folate, a B vitamin that helps form oxygen-carrying red blood cells and promotes communication between nerve cells.

Salsa: Not only is salsa more nutritious than ketchup, it's twice as versatile. Look to the bottom shelf for store-brand bulk containers and you'll find a half-gallon for less than 6 bucks, a month's supply for about the price of a Chipotle Burrito.

Popcorn: Paper-bag popcorns run about $3.50 for nine ounces, versus $1.25 a pound for straight kernels. Why pay a premium for grease? Instead, make popcorn the old fashioned way: straight from the jar. Just fill the bottom of a large saucepan with kernels and a touch of oil and cover. You'll have fresh popcorn ready in a few minutes for a third of the price. Flavor it with fresh herbs, citrus, or chili powder.

Food Additive Glossary

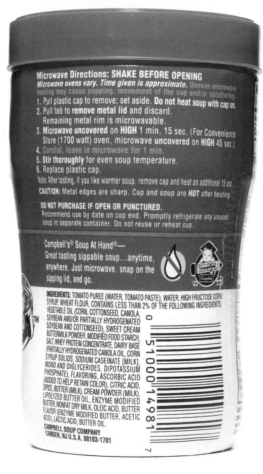

Microwave Directions: **SHAKE BEFORE OPENING**
Microwave ovens vary. Time given is approximate. Uneven microwave heating may cause popping, movement of the cup and/or splattering.

1. Pull plastic cap to remove; set aside. **Do not heat soup with cap on.**
2. Pull tab to **remove metal lid** and discard.
   Remaining metal rim is microwavable.
3. Microwave uncovered on **HIGH** 1 min. 15 sec. (For Convenience Store (1700 watt) oven, microwave uncovered on **HIGH** 45 sec.)
4. Careful, leave in microwave for 1 min.
5. Stir thoroughly for even soup temperature.
6. Replace plastic cap.

Note: After tasting, if you like warmer soup, remove cap and heat an additional 15 sec.

CAUTION: Metal edges are sharp. Cup and soup are **HOT** after heating.

DO NOT PURCHASE IF OPEN OR PUNCTURED.
Recommend use by date on cup end. Promptly refrigerate any unused soup in separate container. Do not reuse or reheat cup.

Campbell's® Soup At Hand®—
Great tasting sippable soup...anytime, anywhere. Just microwave, snap on the sipping lid, and go.

INGREDIENTS: TOMATO PUREE (WATER, TOMATO PASTE), WATER, HIGH FRUCTOSE CORN SYRUP, WHEAT FLOUR, CONTAINS LESS THAN 2% OF THE FOLLOWING INGREDIENTS: VEGETABLE OIL (CORN, COTTONSEED, CANOLA, SOYBEAN AND/OR PARTIALLY HYDROGENATED SOYBEAN AND COTTONSEED), SWEET CREAM BUTTERMILK POWDER, MODIFIED FOOD STARCH, SALT, WHEY PROTEIN CONCENTRATE, DAIRY BASE (PARTIALLY HYDROGENATED CANOLA OIL, CORN SYRUP SOLIDS, SODIUM CASEINATE [MILK], MONO AND DIGLYCERIDES, DIPOTASSIUM PHOSPHATE), FLAVORING, ASCORBIC ACID (ADDED TO HELP RETAIN COLOR), CITRIC ACID, SPICE, BUTTER (MILK), CREAM POWDER (MILK), LIPOLYZED BUTTER OIL, ENZYME MODIFIED BUTTER, NONFAT DRY MILK, OLEIC ACID, BUTTER FLAVOR (ENZYME MODIFIED BUTTER, ACETIC ACID), LACTIC ACID, BUTTER OIL.

CAMPBELL SOUP COMPANY
CAMDEN, NJ U.S.A. 08103-1701

One glance at the back of a label and you'll see the food industry has kidnapped real ingredients and replaced them with science experiments. And lots of them. Milkshakes with 78 ingredients? Bread with 27?

This glossary describes and analyzes the most common food additives in the aisles, from the nutritious (inulin) to the downright frightening (interesterified fat). Consider it your Ph.D. in food chemistry.

Acesulfame Potassium (Acesulfame-K)

A calorie-free artificial sweetener 200 times sweeter than sugar. It is often used with other artificial sweeteners to mask a bitter aftertaste.

FOUND IN: More than 5,000 food products worldwide, including diet soft drinks and no-sugar-added ice cream.

WHAT YOU NEED TO KNOW: Although the FDA has approved it for use in most foods, many health and industry insiders claim that the decision was based on flawed tests. Animal studies have linked the chemical to lung and breast tumors and thyroid problems.

Alpha-Tocopherol

The form of vitamin E most commonly added to foods and most readily absorbed and stored in the body. It is an essential nutrient that helps prevent oxidative damage to the cells and plays a crucial role in cell communication, skin health, and disease prevention.
FOUND IN: Meats, foods with added fats, and foods that boast vitamin E health claims. Also occurs naturally in seeds, nuts, leafy vegetables, and vegetable oils.
WHAT YOU NEED TO KNOW: In the amount added to foods, tocopherols pose no apparent health risks, but highly concentrated supplements might bring on toxicity symptoms such as cramps, weakness, and double vision.

Artificial Flavoring

Denotes any of hundreds of allowable chemicals such as butyl alcohol, isobutyric acid, and phenylacetaldehyde dimethyl acetal. The exact chemicals used in flavoring are the proprietary information of food processors, used to imitate specific fruits, butter, spices, and so on.
FOUND IN: Thousands of highly processed foods such as cereals, fruit snacks, beverages, and cookies.

WHAT YOU NEED TO KNOW: The FDA has approved every item on the list of allowable chemicals, but because they are permitted to hide behind a blanket term, there is no way for consumers to pinpoint the cause of a reaction they might have had.

Ascorbic Acid

The chemical name for the water-soluble vitamin C.
FOUND IN: Juices and fruit products, meat, cereals, and other foods with vitamin C health claims.
WHAT YOU NEED TO KNOW: Although vitamin C is associated with no known risks, it is often added to junk foods to make them appear healthy.

Aspartame

A near-zero-calorie artificial sweetener made by combining two amino acids with methanol. Most commonly used in diet soda, aspartame is 180 times sweeter than sugar.
FOUND IN: More than 6,000 grocery items including diet sodas, yogurts, and the tabletop sweeteners NutraSweet and Equal.
WHAT YOU NEED TO KNOW: Over the past 30 years, the FDA has received thousands of consumer complaints due mostly to neurological symptoms such as headaches, dizziness, memory loss, and, in rare cases, epileptic seizures. Many studies have shown aspartame to be com-

pletely harmless, while others indicate that the additive might be responsible for a range of cancers.

BHA and BHT (Butylated HydroxyAnisole and Butylated Hydroxytoluene)

Petroleum-derived antioxidants used to preserve fats and oils.

FOUND IN: Beer, crackers, cereals, butter, and foods with added fats.

WHAT YOU NEED TO KNOW: Of the two, BHA is considered the most dangerous. Studies have shown it to cause cancer in the forestomachs of rats, mice, and hamsters. The Department of Health and Human Services classifies the preservative as "reasonably anticipated to be a human carcinogen."

Blue #1 (Brilliant Blue) and Blue #2 (Indigotine)

Synthetic dyes that can be used alone or combined with other dyes to make different colors.

FOUND IN: Blue, purple, and green foods such as beverages, cereals, candy, and icing.

WHAT YOU NEED TO KNOW: Both dyes have been loosely linked to cancers in animal studies, and the Center for Science in the Public Interest recommends that they be avoided.

Brown Rice Syrup

A natural sweetener about half as sweet as sugar. It is obtained by using enzymes to break down the starches in cooked rice.

FOUND IN: Protein bars and organic and natural foods.

WHAT YOU NEED TO KNOW: Brown rice sugar has a lower glycemic index than table sugar, which means it provides an easier ride for your blood sugar.

Carrageenan

A thickener, stabilizer, and emulsifier extracted from red seaweed.

FOUND IN: Jellies and jams, ice cream, yogurt, and whipped topping.

WHAT YOU NEED TO KNOW: In animal studies, carrageenan has been shown to cause ulcers, colon inflammation, and digestive cancers. While these results seem limited to degraded carrageenan—a class that has been treated with heat and chemicals—a University of Iowa study concluded that even undegraded carrageenan could become degraded in the human digestive system.

Casein

A milk protein used to thicken and whiten foods and appearing often by the names sodium caseinate or calcium caseinate. It is a good source of amino acids.

FOUND IN: Protein bars and shakes, sher-

bet, ice cream, and other frozen desserts.
WHAT YOU NEED TO KNOW: Although casein is a byproduct of milk, the FDA allows it and its derivatives—sodium calcium caseinates—to be used in "non-dairy" and "dairy-free" creamers. Most lactose intolerants can handle casein, but those with broader milk allergies might experience reactions.

Cochineal Extract or Carmine

A pigment extracted from the dried eggs and bodies of the female *Dactylopius coccus*, a beetlelike insect that preys on cactus plants. It is added to food for its dark-crimson color.
FOUND IN: Artificial crabmeat, fruit juices, frozen-fruit snacks, candy, and yogurt.
WHAT YOU NEED TO KNOW: Carmine is the refined coloring, while cochineal extract is comprised of about 90 percent insect-body fragments. Although the FDA receives fewer than one adverse-reaction report per year, some organizations are asking for a mandatory warning label to accompany cochineal-colored foods. Vegetarians, they say, should be forewarned about the insect juices.

Corn Syrup

A liquid sweetener and food thickener made by allowing enzymes to break corn starches into smaller sugars. USDA subsidies to the corn industry make it cheap and abundant, placing it among the most ubiquitous ingredients in grocery food products.
FOUND IN: Every imaginable food category including bread, soup, sauces, frozen dinners, and frozen treats.
WHAT YOU NEED TO KNOW: Corn syrup provides no nutritional value other than calories. In moderation, it poses no specific threat, that is, other than an expanded waistline.

Dextrose

A corn-derived caloric sweetener. Like corn syrup, dextrose contributes to the American habit of more than 200 calories of corn sweeteners per day.
FOUND IN: Bread, cookies, and crackers.
WHAT YOU NEED TO KNOW: As with other sugars, dextrose is safe in moderate amounts.

Erythorbic Acid

A compound similar to ascorbic acid but with no apparent nutritional value of its own. It is added to nitrite-containing meats to disrupt the formation of cancer-causing nitrosamines.
FOUND IN: Deli meats, hot dogs, and sausages.
WHAT YOU NEED TO KNOW: Erythorbic acid poses no risks, and like ascorbic acid,

might actually improve the body's ability to absorb iron.

Evaporated Cane Juice

A sweetener derived from sugarcane, the same plant used to make refined table sugar. It's also known as crystallized cane juice, cane juice, or cane sugar. Because it's subject to less processing than table sugar, evaporated cane juice retains slightly more nutrients from the grassy cane sugar.

FOUND IN: Yogurt, soy milk, protein bars, granola, cereal, chicken sausages, and other natural or organic foods.

WHAT YOU NEED TO KNOW: Although pristine sugars are often used to replace ordinary sugars in "healthier" foods, the actual nutritional difference between the sugars is miniscule. Both should be consumed in moderation.

Fully Hydrogenated Vegetable Oil

Extremely hard, waxlike fat made by forcing as much hydrogen as possible onto the carbon backbone of fat molecules. To obtain a manageable consistency, food manufacturers will often blend the hard fat with unhydrogenated liquid fats, the result of which is called interesterified fat.

FOUND IN: Baked goods, doughnuts, frozen meals, and tub margarine.

WHAT YOU NEED TO KNOW: In theory, fully hydrogenated oils, as opposed to partially hydrogenated oils, should contain zero trans fat. In practice, however, the process of hydrogenation isn't completely perfect, which means that some trans fat will inevitably occur in small amounts, as will an increased concentration of saturated fat.

Guar Gum

A thickening, emulsifying, and stabilizing agent made from ground guar beans. The legume, also known as a cluster bean, is of Indian origin but small amounts are grown domestically.

FOUND IN: Pastry fillings, ice cream, and sauces.

WHAT YOU NEED TO KNOW: Guar gum is a good source of soluble fiber and might even improve insulin sensitivity. One Italian study suggested that partially hydrolyzed guar gum might have probiotic properties that make it useful in treating patients with irritable bowel syndrome.

High-Fructose Corn Syrup (HFCS)

A corn-derived sweetener representing more than 40 percent of all caloric sweeteners in the supermarket. In 2005, there were 59 pounds produced per capita. The liquid sweetener is created by a complex process that involves breaking down cornstarch with enzymes, and the result is a roughly 50/50 mix of fructose and glucose.

FOUND IN: Although about two-thirds of the HFCS consumed in the United States is in beverages, it can be found in every grocery aisle in products such as ice cream, chips, cookies, cereal, bread, ketchup, jam, canned fruits, yogurt, barbecue sauce, frozen dinners, and so on.

WHAT YOU NEED TO KNOW: Since around 1980, the US obesity rate has risen proportionately to the increase in HFCS, and Americans are now consuming at least 200 calories of the sweetener each day. Some researchers argue that the body metabolizes HFCS differently, making it easier to store as fat, but this theory has not been proven.

Hydrogenated Vegetable Oil: See Fully Hydrogenated Vegetable Oil.

Hydrolyzed Vegetable Protein
A flavor enhancer created when heat and chemicals are used to break down vegetables—most often soy—into its component amino acids. It allows food processors to achieve stronger flavors from fewer ingredients.

FOUND IN: Canned soups and chili, frozen dinners, beef and chicken flavored products.

WHAT YOU NEED TO KNOW: One effect of hydrolyzing proteins is the creation of MSG, or monosodium glutamate. When MSG in food is the result of hydrolyzed protein, the FDA does not require it to be listed on the packaging.

Interesterified Fat
A semi-soft fat created by chemically blending fully hydrogenated and non-hydrogenated oils. It was developed in response to the public demand for an alternative to trans fats.

FOUND IN: Pastries, pies, margarine, frozen dinners, and canned soups.

WHAT YOU NEED TO KNOW: Testing on these fats has not been extensive, but the early evidence doesn't look promising. A study by Malaysian researchers showed a 4-week diet of 12 percent interesterified fats increased the ratio of LDL to HDL cholesterol. Furthermore, this study showed an increase in blood glucose levels and a decrease in insulin response.

Inulin
Naturally occurring plant fiber in fruits and vegetables that is added to foods to boost the fiber or replace the fatlike mouthfeel in low-fat foods. Most of the inulin in the food supply is extracted from chicory root or synthesized from sucrose.

FOUND IN: Smoothies, meal-replacement

bars, and processed foods trying to gain legitimacy among healthy eaters.

WHAT YOU NEED TO KNOW: Like other fibers, inulin can help stabilize blood sugar, improve bowel functions, and help the body absorb nutrients such as calcium and iron.

Lecithin

A naturally occurring emulsifier and anti-oxidant that retards the rancidity of fats. The two major sources for lecithin as an additive are egg yolks and soybeans.

FOUND IN: Pastries, ice cream, and margarine.

WHAT YOU NEED TO KNOW: Lecithin is an excellent source of choline and inositol, compounds that help cells and nerves communicate and play a role in breaking down fats and cholesterol.

Maltodextrin

A caloric sweetener and flavor enhancer made from rice, potatoes, or, more commonly, cornstarch. Through treatment with enzymes and acids, it can be converted into a fiber and thickening agent.

FOUND IN: Canned fruit, instant pudding, sauces, dressings, and chocolates.

WHAT YOU NEED TO KNOW: Like other sugars, maltodextrin has the potential to raise blood glucose and insulin levels.

Maltose (Malt Sugar)

A caloric sweetener about a third as sweet as honey. It occurs naturally in some grains, but as an additive it is usually derived from corn. Food processors like it because it prolongs shelf life and inhibits bacterial growth.

FOUND IN: Cereal grains, nuts and seeds, sports beverages, deli meats, and poultry products.

WHAT YOU NEED TO KNOW: Maltose poses no threats other than those associated with other sugars.

Mannitol

A sugar alcohol that's 70 percent as sweet as sugar. It provides fewer calories and has a less drastic effect on blood sugar.

FOUND IN: Sugar-free candy, low-calorie and diet foods, and chewing gum.

WHAT YOU NEED TO KNOW: Because sugar alcohols are not fully digested, they can cause intestinal discomfort, gas, bloating, flatulence, and diarrhea.

Modified Food Starch

An indefinite term describing a starch that has been manipulated in a nonspecific way. The starches can be derived from corn, wheat, potato, or rice, and they are modified to change their response to heat or cold, improve their texture, and create efficient emulsifiers, among other reasons.

FOUND IN: Most highly processed foods, low-calorie and diet foods, pastries, cookies, and frozen meals.
WHAT YOU NEED TO KNOW: The starches themselves appear safe, but the nondisclosure of the chemicals used in processing causes some nutritionists to question their effects on health, especially of infants.

Mono- and Diglycerides

Fats added to foods to bind liquids with fats. They occur naturally in foods and constitute about 1 percent of normal food fats.
FOUND IN: Peanut butter, ice cream, margarine, baked goods, and whipped topping.
WHAT YOU NEED TO KNOW: Aside from being a source of fat, the glycerides themselves pose no serious health threats.

Monosodium Glutamate (MSG)

The salt of the amino acid glutamic acid, used to enhance the savory quality of foods. MSG alone has little flavor, and exactly how it enhances other foods is unknown.
FOUND IN: Chili, soup, and foods with chicken or beef flavoring.
WHAT YOU NEED TO KNOW: Studies have shown that MSG injected into mice causes brain-cell damage, but the FDA believes these results are not typical for humans. The FDA receives dozens of reaction complaints each year for nausea, headaches, chest pains, and weakness.

Neotame

The newest addition to the FDA-approved artificial sweeteners. It's chemically similar to aspartame and at least 8,000 times sweeter than sugar. It was approved in 2002, and its use is not yet widespread.
FOUND IN: Clabber Girl Sugar Replacer, Domino Pure D'Lite, and Hostess 100-Calorie Packs.
WHAT YOU NEED TO KNOW: Neotame is the second artificial sweetener to be deemed safe by the Center for Science in the Public Interest (the first was sucralose). It's considered more stable than aspartame, and because it's 40 times sweeter, it can be used in much smaller concentrations.

Olestra

A synthetic fat created by pharmaceutical company Procter & Gamble and sold under the name Olean. It has zero-calorie impact and is not absorbed as it passes though the digestive system.
FOUND IN: Light chips and crackers.
WHAT YOU NEED TO KNOW: Olestra can cause diarrhea, intestinal cramps, and flatulence. Studies show that it impairs the body's ability to absorb fat-soluble vitamins and vital carotenoids such as beta-carotene, lycopene, lutein, and zeaxanthin.

Oligofructose: See Inulin.

Partially Hydrogenated Vegetable Oil

A manufactured fat created by forcing hydrogen gas into vegetable fats under extremely high pressure, an unintended effect of which is the creation of trans fatty acids. Food processors like this fat because of its low cost and long shelf life.
FOUND IN: Margarine, pastries, frozen foods, cakes, cookies, crackers, soups, and nondairy creamers.
WHAT YOU NEED TO KNOW: Trans fat has been shown to contribute to heart disease more so than saturated fats. While most health organizations recommend keeping trans-fat consumption as low as possible, a loophole in the FDA's labeling requirements allows processors to add as much as 0.49 grams per serving and still claim zero in their nutrition facts. Progressive jurisdictions such as New York City, California, and Boston have approved legislation to phase trans fat out of restaurants, and pressure from watchdog groups might eventually lead to a full ban on the dangerous oil.

Pectin

A carbohydrate that occurs naturally in many fruits and vegetables and is used to thicken and stabilize foods.
FOUND IN: Jellies and jams, sauces, pie filling, smoothies, and shakes.
WHAT YOU NEED TO KNOW: Pectin is a source of dietary fiber and might help to lower cholesterol.

Polysorbates

A class of chemicals usually derived from animal fats and used primarily as emulsifiers, much like mono- and diglycerides.
FOUND IN: Cakes, icing, bread mixes, condiments, ice cream, and pickles.
WHAT YOU NEED TO KNOW: Polysorbates allow otherwise fat-soluble vitamins to be dissolved in water, an odd trait that seems to have a benign effect. Watchdog groups have deemed the additive safe for consumption.

Propyl Gallate

An antioxidant used often in conjunction with BHA and BHT to retard the rancidity of fats.
FOUND IN: Mayonnaise, margarine, oils, dried meats, pork sausage, and other fatty foods.
WHAT YOU NEED TO KNOW: Rat studies in the early '80s linked propyl gallate to brain cancer. Although these studies don't provide sound evidence, it is advisable to avoid this chemical when possible.

Red #3 (Erythrosine) and Red #40 (Allura Red)

Food dyes that are orange-red and cherry red, respectively. Red #40 is the most widely used food dye in America.

FOUND IN: Fruit cocktail, candy, chocolate cake, cereal, beverages, pastries, maraschino cherries, and fruit snacks.

WHAT YOU NEED TO KNOW: The FDA has proposed a ban on Red #3 in the past, but so far the agency has been unsuccessful in implementing it. After the dye was inextricably linked to thyroid tumors in rat studies, the FDA managed to have the lake (or liquid) form of the dye removed from external drugs and cosmetics.

Saccharin

An artificial sweetener 300 to 500 times sweeter than sugar. Discovered in 1879, it's the oldest of the five FDA-approved artificial sweeteners.

FOUND IN: Diet foods, chewing gum, toothpaste, beverages, sugar-free candy, and Sweet 'N Low.

WHAT YOU NEED TO KNOW: Rat studies in the early '70s showed saccharin to cause bladder cancer, and the FDA, reacting to these studies, enacted a mandatory warning label to be printed on every saccharin-containing product. The label was removed after 20 years, but the question over saccharin's safety was never resolved. More recent studies show that rats on saccharin-rich diets gain more weight than those on high-sugar diets.

Sodium Ascorbate: See Ascorbic Acid.

Sodium Caseinate: See Casein.

Sodium Nitrite and Sodium Nitrate

Preservatives used to prevent bacterial growth and maintain the pinkish color of meats and fish.

FOUND IN: Bacon, sausage, hot dogs, and cured, canned, and packaged meats.

WHAT YOU NEED TO KNOW: Under certain conditions, sodium nitrite and nitrate react with amino acids to form cancer-causing chemicals called nitrosamines. This reaction can be hindered by the addition of ascorbic acid, erythorbic acids, or alpha-tocopherol.

Sorbitol

A sugar alcohol that occurs naturally in some fruits. It's about 60 percent as sweet as sugar and used to both sweeten and thicken.

FOUND IN: Dried fruit, chewing gum, and reduced-sugar candy.

WHAT YOU NEED TO KNOW: Sorbitol digests slower than sugars, which makes it a better choice for diabetics. But like other sugar alcohols, it can cause intestinal discomfort, gas, bloating, flatulence, and diarrhea.

Soy Lecithin: See Lecithin.

Sucralose

A zero-calorie artificial sweetener made by joining chlorine particles and sugar molecules. It's 600 times sweeter than sugar and largely celebrated as the least damaging of the artificial sweeteners.

FOUND IN: Sugar-free foods, pudding, beverages, some diet sodas, and Splenda.

WHAT YOU NEED TO KNOW: After reviewing more than 110 human and animal studies, the FDA concluded that use of sucralose does not cause cancer. The sweetener is one of only three artificial sweeteners deemed safe by the Center for Science in the Public Interest.

Tartrazine: See Yellow #5.

Vegetable Shortening: See Partially Hydrogenated Vegetable Oil.

Yellow #5 (Tartrazine) and Yellow #6 (Sunset Yellow)

The second and third most common food colorings, respectively.

FOUND IN: Cereal, pudding, bread mix, beverages, chips, cookies, and condiments.

WHAT YOU NEED TO KNOW: Several studies have linked both dyes to learning and concentration disorders in children, and there are piles of animal studies demonstrating potential risks such as kidney and intestinal tumors. One study found that mice fed high doses of sunset yellow had trouble swimming straight and righting themselves in water. The FDA does not view these as serious risks to humans.

Xanthan Gum

An extremely common emulsifier and thickener made from glucose in a reaction requiring a slimy bacteria called *Xanthomonas campestris*—the same bacterial strain that appears as black rot on cruciferous vegetables like broccoli.

FOUND IN: Whipped topping, dressings, marinades, custard, and pie filling.

WHAT YOU NEED TO KNOW: Xanthan gum is associated with no adverse effects.

Xylitol

A sugar alcohol that occurs naturally in strawberries, mushrooms, and other fruits and vegetables. It is most commonly extracted from the pulp of the birch tree.

FOUND IN: Sugar-free candy, yogurt, and beverages.

WHAT YOU NEED TO KNOW: Unlike real sugar, sugar alcohols don't encourage cavity-causing bacteria. They do have a laxative effect, though, so heavy ingestion might cause intestinal discomfort or gas.

Learn more about the science of the supermarket and how to fill your shopping cart with the simplest, healthiest choices in the aisles at **eatthis.com**

Index

Boldface page references indicate photographs.
Underscored references indicate boxed text.

319

Get the most up-to-date nutrition secrets and breaking research science from

EAT THIS, NOT THAT!

Sign up for the free weekly newsletter at

eatthis.com

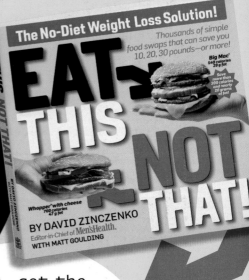

The No-Diet Weight Loss Solution!
Thousands of simple food swaps that can save you 10, 20, 30 pounds—or more!

Big Mac®
540 calories
29 g fat

EAT THIS NOT THAT!

Save more than 200 calories and nearly 20 grams of fat

Whopper® with cheese
760 calories
47 g fat

BY DAVID ZINCZENKO
Editor-in-Chief of Men'sHealth.
WITH MATT GOULDING

Plus, get the exclusive, healthy eating info you need at any market, restaurant, or roadside stand—instantly! with

EAT THIS, NOT THAT! Mobile!

Sign up at
eatthis.com

And look out for

EAT THIS, NOT THAT! FOR KIDS!

Wherever books are sold!